# Lifespan Development: Biopsychosocial Perspectives

Bassim Hamadeh, CEO and Publisher
Laura Pasquale, Specialist Acquisitions Editor
Gem Rabanera, Project Editor
Alia Bales, Production Editor
Jess Estrella, Senior Graphic Designer
Trey Soto, Licensing Coordinator
Natalie Piccotti, Director of Marketing
Kassie Graves, Vice President of Editorial
Jamie Giganti, Director of Academic Publishing



Printed in the United States of America.

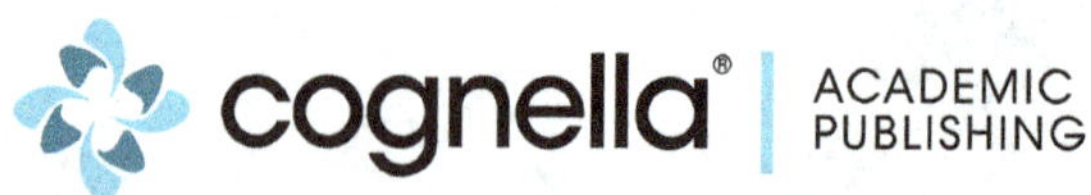

# Lifespan Development: Biopsychosocial Perspectives

**Susan Krauss Whitbourne and Cynthia R. Davis**

*University of Massachusetts Amherst*

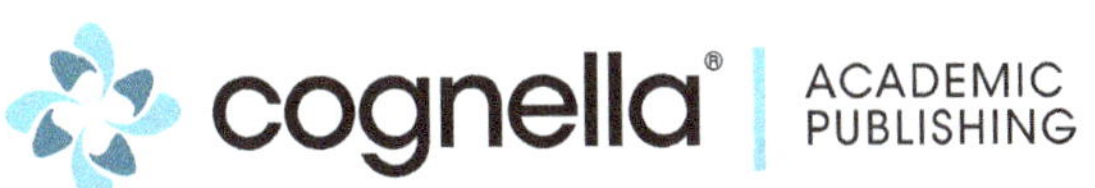

# CONTENTS

# ACTIVE LEARNING

Throughout the text, when you see this Active Learning icon

an interactive activity is available to complement your reading.

Your instructor may have customized the selection of activities available for your unique course. Please check with your professor to verify whether your class will access this content through the Cognella Active Learning portal (http://active.cognella.com) or through your home learning management system.

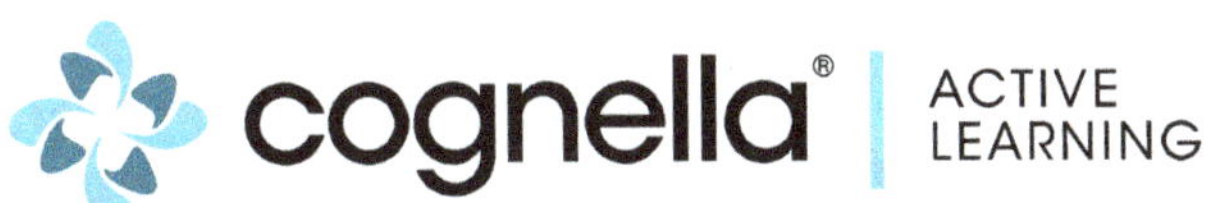


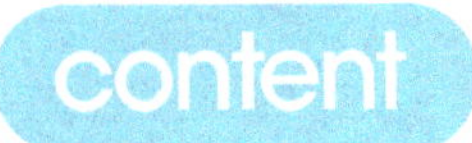

We would like to thank Kate Rusillo for her efforts toward earlier drafts of the manuscript.

-C.D and S.W.

# CHAPTER 1

# An Introduction to Development

Both development and the aging process begin the moment you are born and unfold until the day you die. We grow and age simultaneously. Perhaps growth is something you think about more often if you are a traditional-aged college student. On the other hand, if this is your first time back in the classroom after a number of years away from an educational institution, you may be thinking more about aging. Even still, neither of these assumptions may necessarily be valid. Regardless of which is true for you, we hope you use this book to understand better development across the lifespan and to understand the complex processes that underlie how we make our way through life. In the process, we'll ask you to consider your own and others' developmental experiences—some of which you have already experienced, those you will experience, and those experiences you may never come to know.

Let's start with a few questions. How old are you? What comes to mind when you think of your current age? Are you very similar to others this age? Is it an important part of who you are or do you not think about your current age much? Do you consider yourself an adult? What do the words "young" and "old" mean to you? Do you consider those younger than you young and those older than you old? What are your thoughts on development and aging? Does development happen when we are young, but aging happens when we're old? Now we'll give you some examples of ways that people think about individuals of different ages. When you think of infants, do you think of them as sponges? What about older adults? Do you immediately regard them as unable to care for themselves? What is the "typical" child or "typical" adult like, in your eyes? What about all those age groups in between?

Just by thinking about these questions, you've already started to focus on what age means in terms of your overall sense of self. These are the types of questions we'll explore throughout the book. Even as we discuss in-depth the effects of development and the aging process across the life span, we will often come back and question how much we really know about a person based on age alone. We'll also show you that some age distinctions are almost arbitrary. Someone decided that a certain age means you're in a certain stage of life; from that point forward, people attribute a great deal of meaning to that particular number. In reality, however, the developmental process isn't completely linked to the passage of time alone.

**LO 1-1** **Compare biological age and chronological age**

**LO 1-2** **Define functional age, psychological age, and social age**

# The Meaning of Age and Aging

The study of development and aging implies that age is the major variable of interest. However, the scientific study of aging faces a challenge in that age carries with it many problems as the major variable of interest (for example, a variable such as personality or metabolism rate). To be sure, there is some value in categorizing individuals based on their age for convenience if nothing else. At the same time, attaching a numerical value to people on the basis of their date of birth carries with it a certain amount of randomness. Chronological age is a number based on measures of Earth's movement around the sun. However, we don't know how much the changes in the physical universe relate to what goes on inside the body in any kind of precise fashion.

Consider what happens when people's ages change on a major birthday such as reaching the age of 40. The crossing from an age that ends in 9 to an age that ends in 0 may lead people to engage in self-scrutiny simply because many of us have been socialized to believe that 40 means something important. This belief is reinforced by birthday cards that invoke the "over the hill" metaphor as we've concluded the first half of our life (going up the hill) and are now in the second half of our life (over the hill and going down). In truth, your body does not change in discrete fits nor starts when you pass a particular birthday. Nevertheless, birthdays are important social markers, and the numbers associated with certain birthdays, such as your 1st, 16th, 18th, 21st, and so on, carry with them certain meanings and even certain social permissions. Chronological age does have some value in describing a person, but like other descriptive features of a person, such as gender or eye color, it is the social meaning attached to chronological age that often outweighs any intrinsic usefulness.

The body does keep time in a cycle that approximates a 24-hour period, as shown in Figure 1-1, but there is no clear evidence at the moment to suggest how time's pacemaker is related to aging. Based on current evidence, it is questionable to say chronological age (or time) "means" anything with regard to the status of the body's functioning. The popularity of such phrases as "30 being the new 20" and "60 the new 50" capture the difficulty of defining people's aging processes based solely on a number. People of the same age can vary substantially from one another, and people of different ages can be more similar to each other than their differing age might lead you to expect.

**FIGURE 1-1** A typical 24-hour circadian clock.

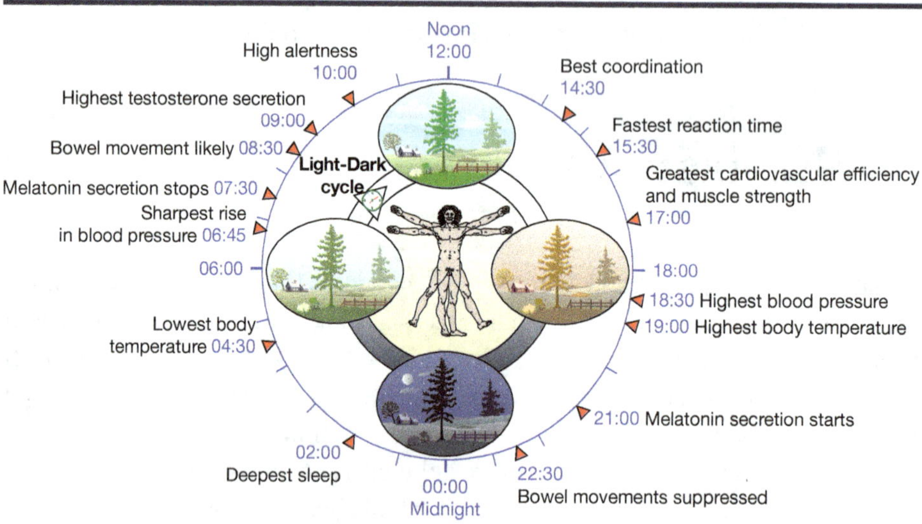


*Source*: Copyright © YassineMrabet (CC BY-SA 3.0) at https://commons.wikimedia.org/wiki/File:Biological_clock_human.PNG.

## Using Age to Define Developmental Periods

Now that we have you thinking about the meaning of age, we will move on to the next challenge—the meanings of various terms that describe different periods along the life span: newborn, infant, toddler, child, preteen, adolescent, young adult, middle aged, older adult. Think about each of these terms and what you associate with each one. Now think about the shift from one developmental period to the next. When does a newborn stop being a newborn? Is it at 1 week or 1 month? What about the infant born premature who is finally allowed home at 4 months? When does the preteen become an adolescent? Some define adolescence as the period between the ages of 12 and 18, whereas others define it using different age ranges. When do you become an adult?

Now think about the word "maturity." You may conjure up images of a person reaching a certain level of accomplishment or growth. Consider, for example, the term "mature" in reference to a banana. A mature banana is ready to be eaten, and you can judge that by examining its yellow color and firm texture. A piece of fruit's maturity level is relatively easy to measure compared with judging the maturity of humans. The complexity of the biopsychosocial processes that occur within us are far more difficult to quantify.

You might think that the most logical definition of maturity should be based on physical development. Yet, you also know that a 14-year-old female who may appear outwardly to have reached her full physical development would, in contemporary Western society, be regarded as anything but an adult. Although her physical attributes define her as an adult, her own psychological development and social standards likely would not. However, when is it exactly that we become adults? Perhaps standards of development and their associated labels based on ability rather than age are better options. Consider 16 years, the age when most people can legally drive. Or, alternatively, consider age 18, when U.S. society ordains the person with the right to vote.

Using the age of 21 presents another possible point of entry into adulthood. Because it is the age when American adults can legally drink alcohol, for many, the turning of 21 represents a defining mark of the beginning of adulthood. However, the United States is in a small minority of nations that set the drinking age at 21. Some Canadian provinces set the drinking age at 19 (though it is 18 in most); countries such as Germany, Barbados, and Portugal set it at 16. These conflicting age demarcations for even such a seemingly concrete behavior as drinking alcohol show that deciding when a person is an adult on this basis has limited utility. The variations in the legal drinking age shown from country to country (and even within a country) illustrate the interaction of biological and sociocultural factors in setting age-based limits around human behavior. People in Canada who are 18 years old are, on average, not all that physiologically distinct from 18-year-olds who live in France. For that matter, they are probably not even psychologically different. It's culture that distinguishes whether they're able to drink alcohol without getting arrested. The physiological effects and risks remain the same.

If you're like many students, the age of 25 may hold special importance for you. This is the age where, in the United States, you can rent a car (without having to pay a tremendous surcharge). This age has no inherent meaning, but it is used by car rental companies because the chances of having an auto accident are lower after the age of 25. It's possible that a switch is flicked on a person's 25th birthday so that the unsafe driver now has become a model of good behavior on the road. However, it's more rational to argue the odds are statistically higher that people under age 25 are more likely to engage in the risky combination of drinking and driving. It is this behavioral index, supported by actuarial evidence, that leads to the higher insurance premiums. Another social convention that highlights the randomness of how we associate chronological age with development pertains to when people can marry without the consent of their parents. Within the United States alone, the age of consent varies from state to state (in South Carolina it is 14, whereas other states deem 16 or 18 the appropriate age). The age when people actually marry, as opposed to when they're allowed to marry, reflects factors such as the health of the economy. In bad economic times, the median age of marriage goes well above the age of consent. During these times, a person in her 20s (or older) may also find she's forced to move back in with her parents because she isn't earning sufficient income to rent or buy her own place. Does this person become an adult only when she moves out of her parents' house? What if that never happens? Is that person never truly an adult, even if she's 60? Does this mean people become less "adult" when the economy lags?

We've highlighted the contradictory definitions of developmental periods and milestones and their associated age ranges. Therefore, we will differentiate between developmental periods based on two factors. First, we will bear in mind the chronological age range associated with a set of abilities typical for those of that age range. For example, the characteristics, abilities, and experiences that are typical for most children between the ages of 3 and 5 will be considered toddlerhood. Second, we will take into account the expectations and privileges of a given society or subculture. For example, in the United States, individuals may be considered to have reached adulthood at the age when they are eligible to vote, drink, drive, and get married. For the majority of U.S. states, the age of 21 is therefore considered the threshold to adulthood. In other countries, these criteria may be reached at the age of 18.

## Defining Age

**Chronological age** refers to the amount of time, typically in number of years, that has elapsed since the day you were born. **Biological age** is the age of an individual's bodily systems. Using biological age instead of chronological age would tell us exactly how well people's minds and bodies are able to perform mental and physical functions such as the heart's pumping blood through the arteries and getting oxygen to the lungs. It is important to consider not only with regard to vital functions such as these, but in other domains as well, for example, in childhood when it comes to school readiness at the age of 5, or placement on a sports team at the age of 15. With biological age, you could also help people learn how best to improve things such as muscle and bone strength.

To be able to use biological age as an index as we do chronological age, we would need a large repository of data showing what's to be expected for each major biological function at each age. For example, we'd need to know the population values for blood pressure readings in people with different chronological ages. Then, we would assign people a "blood pressure age" according to which chronological age of healthy people most closely match their numbers. A 50-year-old whose blood pressure was in the range of normal 25- to 30-year-olds would then have a biological age that was 20 or 25 years younger than their chronological age. Similarly, we could assign a child a "mathematics age" that could potentially be a number of years ahead of her peers.

Popular culture has certainly caught on to the notion of biological rather than chronological age. In terms of longevity, there are a multitude of online calculators in which you answer various questions to estimate how long you will live. In addition, there are slightly more sophisticated "biological age tests" that let you calculate your "lung age," for example.

On the other end of the spectrum, when we think about development earlier in the life span, there are certainly established standards in educational settings regarding reading, mathematics and social skills. Some are more objective than others, such as mathematical abilities expected by "the average" 7-year-old, whereas others are based on more subjective ratings, such as emotional maturity.

Discontented with the entire concept of chronological age, a number of developmental scientists are devising a new classification system that is based not on what the calendar says but on **functional age**, which is how people actually perform. With functional instead of chronological age as the basis for a system of studying aging, we could gain a better grasp of a person's true characteristics and abilities. **Psychological age** refers to the performance an individual achieves on measures of certain cognitive abilities such as reaction time, memory, learning ability, and intelligence (all of which are known to change with age). Like biological age, a person's performance on these tasks would be compared with those of others and then scaled accordingly.

**FIGURE 1-2** Defining age.

**Functional** age offers advantages over chronological age

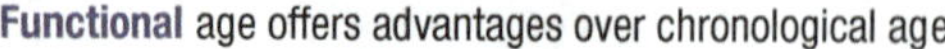

**a**

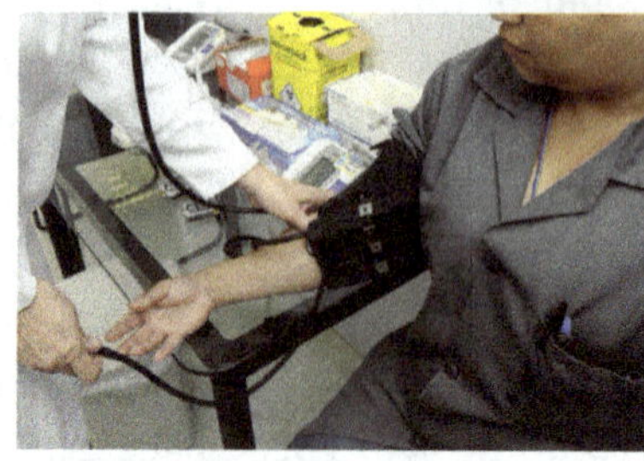

**Biological age**
Heart rate
Blood pressure
Glucose levels
Muscle and bone strength

**b**

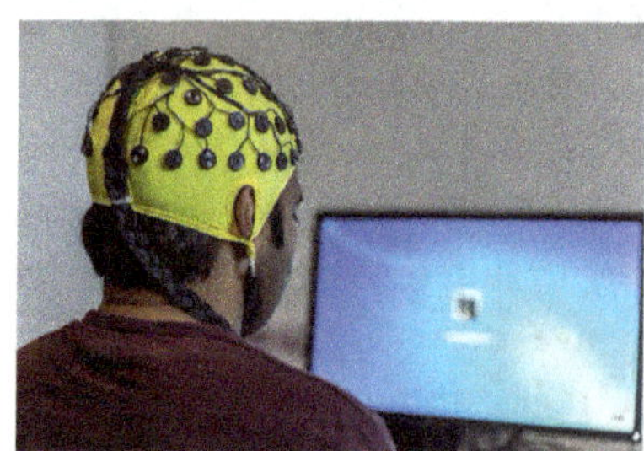

**Psychological age**
Reaction time
Learning ability
Memory
Intelligence

**c**

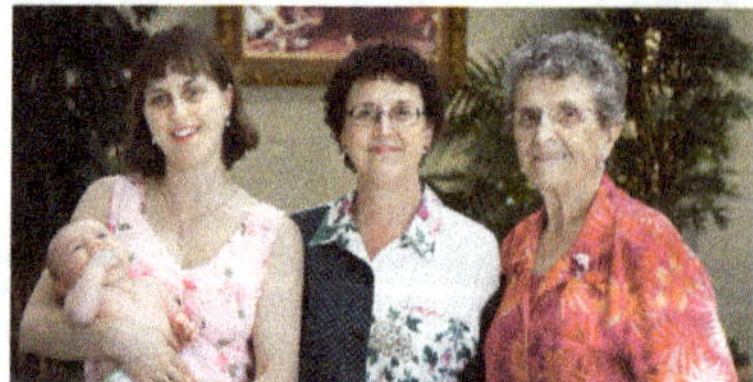

**Social age**
Parental, grandparental status
Work role
Retirement status

*Sources*:
Fig. 1.2a: https://pixabay.com/en/heart-control-treatment-evaluation-1698840/.
Fig. 1.2b: https://pixabay.com/en/eeg-integration-2680957/.
Fig. 1.2c: Copyright © Azoreg (CC BY-SA 3.0) at https://commons.wikimedia.org/wiki/Category:Generations#/media/File:Baby_Mother_Grandmother_and_Great_Grandmother.jpg.

**Social age** is calculated by evaluating where people are compared with the "typical" ages expected of people when they reach certain milestones in life. For children, these milestones may include entry to school and for adults they tend to center on family and work roles. For example, you may be in your early 20s and in your 3rd year of college, while your classmate may be in his late 40s and also in his 3rd year of college. Another example may be a 20-year-old's biological grandparent at 87 who has older social and biological ages than the 20-year-old's biological parent who's 65. This person could have a friend who is 21 years old, but he has a biological grandparent who's 64, who's socially older but biologically younger than the 20-year-old's biological parent.

Social age can have some interesting twists. For example, it's entirely possible for someone to become a grandparent in their late 20s (with a social age of 60 or older). Conversely, people can become parents in their late 60s. Perhaps you have a friend whose grandmother is 93 and another whose grandmother is 57. We see the same issue with regard to work roles. A 70-year-old who is still working has a younger social age than a 66-year-old who has retired. Athletes and politicians present a similar contrast. A figure skater may be forced to give up her sport at 18 years of age and thus have an older social age than a still-employed legislator in her 60s.

As we stated earlier, an advantage of using functional indices of aging is that they can be more accurate than chronological age. However, it's much easier to use chronological age than these sophisticated calculations. Adding to the problem is the need for functional ages to be constantly calibrated and recalibrated to ensure they continue to be accurate. For example, a biological index based in part on blood pressure may require adjustments as health practitioners change the definition of what is considered "normal." Changes in both medical knowledge and population norms for particular age groups may mean that the definition of normal blood pressure for an average 60-year-old shifts to be more typical of a person in the 70s. Psychological age and social age indices are also likely to change over time. In terms of educational standards, years ago children were not expected to develop the basics of reading until first grade, but in many cases this expectation has now shifted earlier to kindergarten. Despite its faults, chronological age may be the best index for many areas of functioning. Just keep in mind it does not tell us everything.

## Personal Versus Social Development and Aging

The development and aging process occurs within the individual, but as you have learned already, it is shaped by events occurring in the individual's social context. When developmental scientists study the development and aging process, it is difficult to disentangle those internal changes from those that reflect a changing world, though we try to do so by applying the appropriate controls in our research.

**Personal development** is considered those aspects of the individual related to the self, such as certain abilities or one's identity. **Social development** has to do with how we develop skills related to social relationships, such as emotion regulation and perspective-taking. **Personal aging** refers to changes that occur within the individual and reflect the influence of time's passage on the body's structures and functions. This is how people ordinarily think of the aging process. **Social aging** refers to the effects of a person's exposure to a changing environment. Over time, the changes we see within the individual represent the unique blend of personal and social development and aging as these play out in that individual's life.

Within the category of social aging, the changes that take place in an individual's life are seen as reflecting a multitude of interacting factors. At any one time, the individual's life reflects one or more of three basic categories of three social influences. These influences, identified by psychologist Paul Baltes (1979) and still seen as relevant today, include normative age-graded influences, normative history-graded influences, and nonnormative influences. We'll look at each of these in turn.

**Normative age-graded influences** lead people to choose experiences that their culture and historical period attach to certain ages or points in the life span. The term "normative" stems from the term "**norm**," which is a social expectation for behavior. In Western society, age norms traditionally dictate that individuals enter educational institutions roughly around the age of 5, graduate from high school in their teenage years, graduate from college in their early 20s, get married and begin a family in their 20s or 30s, retire in their 60s, and become grandparents in their middle to later years, usually in the decades of the 50s, 60s, and beyond. These are influences on behavior to the extent that people believe they should structure their lives according to these age demarcations.

Events that occur in response to normative age-graded influences occur in part because a given society has developed expectations about what is assumed appropriate for people of certain ages. Graduation from high school generally occurs at the age of 18 for most because in most industrialized societies children start school at the age of 5 or 6 and the educational system is based on 12 or 13 grades. Becoming independent of one's family of origin typical occurs during the 3rd decade of life in many Western countries, but norms may vary from culture to culture and be dependent on a variety of family and environmental circumstances. The decision to retire at the age of 65 years can be seen as a response to the norm, "*65 is the correct age to leave the labor market*" was truer in the past than today. Normative age-graded influences exert their impact beyond what the norms themselves imply because people are socialized into believing that they *should* structure their lives so they conform to these influences. When people don't adhere to these norms, for whatever reasons, they may feel there is something wrong with them. Puberty is a particularly relevant normative age-graded influence. Reaching puberty early or being a late bloomer may be a source of self-consciousness for many teenagers. Parents may also feel pressures due to these influences, for example if their child is held back a grade in kindergarten. In adulthood, a 35-year-old may prefer not to marry or to have children but feel pressured into doing so by other family members, friends, or the society at large by virtue of having reached their mid-30s. A 40-year-old office worker may consider retiring but feel reluctant to do so because it is not what is expected for a person of that age in that field of employment, whereas a 75-year-old may feel frustrated that he must remain at his job because he cannot afford to retire.

The normative age-graded influences are partly linked to the biological aging process. Parenthood in most cultures in Western societies traditionally occurs between the ages of 20 and 40, coinciding with a woman's reproductive cycle. This age range sets the normative age period for biologically becoming a parent. Once this age is set, then a lower limit is set on the age at which the adult can become a grandparent. If the child also follows certain normative age-graded influences, the parent will likely become a grandparent for the first time between the ages of 55 and 65 years. This, of course, varies from culture to culture. Similarly, manual laborers or athletes may be at peak physical capacity up to their 40s, when they may experience loss of strength and speed.

Now let's turn to the second set of influences on development, those that relate to the impact of events in the outside world on the individual. **Normative history-graded influences** are events that occur to everyone within a certain culture or geopolitical unit (regardless of age) and include large-scale occurrences, such as world wars, economic trends, or sociocultural changes in attitudes and values. The impact of these events on people's lives may be felt immediately. They can continue to have a lasting impact for many years on the subsequent patterns of work, family, and quality of life of the people affected by those events. A study of World War II veterans showed that those who entered the military after their families were already established were more likely upon their return to get divorced or separated, to suffer career setbacks, and to experience poorer physical health after they turned 50 (Elder et al., 1994). Had they not gone off to war, their lives may have taken a more stable course.

An individual does not have to experience a historical event directly to be affected by a normative history-graded influence. For example, in 2015, several large terrorist attacks took place in Paris, France. The impact of these events reverberated throughout Europe and North America, in particular. Anytime there is a significant enough event or set of events affecting a large number of people, the event's aftermath may continue to affect aspects of each person's life for years to come.

If the life course was influenced only by normative age- and history-graded influences, predicting the course of development of people of the same age living in the same culture would not be easy, but it would be manageable. Plug in a person's age and the year of the person's birth, and you'd be able to figure out which combination of age-graded and history-graded influences set the course of that person's life. However, people's lives are also affected by **nonnormative influences**, the random idiosyncratic events that occur throughout life. They are "nonnormative" because they occur with no regular predictability.

There are almost an infinite number of examples of nonnormative influences. Some are due to good luck, such as winning the lottery or making a smart investment. Nonnormative influences can also be negative, such as a child experiencing the death of a parent, a car accident, or an earthquake. These types of events reflect acute adversities that happen in a singular moment but whose effects can be long-lasting. One moment your life is routine and predictable, and in the next a single event irrevocably alters it. Other nonnormative influences may unfold over a longer period, such as neighborhood violence, experiencing divorce, or developing a chronic illness not related to the aging process. Both acute and gradual adversities can have long-lasting impacts on a person psychologically and physically, as we will discuss.

We're sure it has occurred to you while reading about these influences that the social environment is an important contributor toward development. Consider the example of divorce. Although society's norms have changed considerably regarding this life event, many would still consider this a nonnormative occurrence because the norm or expectation (and certainly the hope) of married couples is to remain married. And although a divorce is a personal occurrence, it may be seen in part as a response to larger social forces. For example, a couple who is exposed to financial hardship because one or both partners lost a job because of living in harsh economic times (normative historical influence) is now faced with severe emotional stress. If they are in their middle years, when couples are expected to have reached a degree of financial comfort (age-graded normative influence), their problems may be exacerbated. Yet, some couples may feel closer to each other when exposed to such adversity, and this is where the idiosyncratic nonnormative factors come into play.

This example illustrates the dilemmas faced by researchers in human development who attempt to separate not only personal from social aging but also the impact of particular influences that fall into the category of social aging. Though challenging, the very complexity of the equation fascinates those of us who try to understand what makes humans "tick" and what causes that ticking to change over the decades of the human lifespan.

**LO 1-3 Define the four principles of human development**

# Four Principles of Human Development

We begin our study of human development with four principles that form the foundation of our biopsychosocial approach. As you read the book, you'll find we return to these principles. If you begin to understand them now, you will find the course material much easier to master.

## First Principle: The Continuity Principle

Many changes over the life span happen in a continuous fashion. According to the **continuity principle**, the changes people experience build on previous experiences. This means we can never isolate a later period of life without considering what preceded it. Given that time moves in a forward direction, the changes throughout life build on themselves in a cumulative fashion. If a child develops good reading habits early on, these will contribute to his abilities across the school years. If you were hard on your body as a young adult, chances are the changes you'll undergo when you're older will be more negative than if you took good care of yourself.

When others look at you, however, they don't necessarily consider this perspective. People don't meet you for the first time and think about what you were like when you were younger—they see you as you are now. Unless they are close relatives or friends, they have no way of knowing what you were like when you were in your childhood or teenage years. Anyone meeting you now judges you on the basis of your current characteristics because they have no other data from which to draw.

Similarly, when interacting with a child or looking at an adult, it's unlikely you judge that person on based on how they may have been in the past. You may see a third grader struggle with reading, but do you consider the reading habits his parents instilled in him (or not) when he was 2 years old? You may see an older woman, walking with a little difficulty, and don't stop to think that she might have been a marathon runner in her youth. However, that older woman knows that she is the "same" person she's always been. True, she can no longer compete for a marathon, but this accomplishment is part of her identity. She knows her physical abilities have changed, but to herself she's still the Sophia, Sherry, or Ann she has been her entire life. The continuity principle also applies to the way that people think about their own identities. You know you're the same person you always were. Birthdays don't transform you into a different person. You don't look the same as you did when you were 7, but you feel essentially the "same" on the inside.

There's an important implication of the continuity principle for anyone working with older adults. You need to remember they would prefer to be treated as the people they always were, rather than as "old people." As we'll see later, older adults are often stereotyped as weak and infirm, when in reality they want to be viewed as individuals who possess strengths and experiences they have built over their entire lives. They don't want to be stereotyped on the basis of the way they look to the world right now. Some nursing home administrators, eager to remind their employees of this fact, display pictures of the residents from their younger years on the nameplates outside their doors. The residents and their visitors think of them in this way, and it's helpful if those who work with them are reminded of this fact.

Even though we often think of development as continuous and that experiences build on each gradually, there can be examples of discontinuous growth when big leaps, rather than small progressions, are made, for example the infant who never crawls but all of a sudden begins to walk. Similarly, there can be regressions, when development seems to go backward. This may be the 6-year-old who has been potty trained for 2 years but starts first grade 1 week after his baby sister is born and begins to have accidents.

## Second Principle: Only the Survivors Grow Old

The **survivor principle** states that the people who live to old age are the ones who managed to outlive the many threats that could have caused their deaths at earlier ages. Perhaps this is obvious because clearly, to grow old, you have to not die. However, the survivor principle is a bit more complex than that. Some of the factors that can lead to death prior to old age are random, to be sure, such as being killed by someone else in an accident, by an act of war, or in a natural disaster. However, many other factors that lead some to survive into old age are nonrandom. Survivors not only manage to avoid random causes of their own fatalities but also are more likely to take care of their health, not engage in risky behaviors (such as driving too fast or getting involved in crime, or use drugs and alcohol excessively.

The survivor principle has important theoretical implications. Survivors are not like the people born during the same time period they were. They may have been born with greater resilience, but they likely took care to maintain their health and preserve their longevity. There are so many ways to lose one's life, especially in adulthood, from causes such as terminal illness or accidents, that to become an older adult you have to possess some incredibly special characteristics. The survivor principle also affects the way we understand research on aging. Clearly, all older adults who participate in research are survivors of genetic conditions and predispositions that may have affected their longevity, have managed to maintain their physical abilities (biological factors), are cognitively and emotionally healthy (psychological factors), and have surrounded themselves with a good support system (social factors). Furthermore, these factors build on and interact with each other. People with stronger cognitive skills are more likely to attend college that, in turn, provides them with greater economic resources that can sustain their health and well-being. A combination of mental and physical health and adequate resources, plus a dose of good luck, allow them to be with us today. Others do not endure. As time goes by, more and more of the older population will die. Those who reach age 90 or 100 most likely represent a different population than their now-deceased age mates. The older they get, the more select they become in key characteristics such as physical functioning, health, intelligence, and even personality (Baird et al., 2010).

Consequently, when we examine differences between younger and older people, we must keep in mind that younger adults have not yet been subjected to the same conditions that could threaten their lives, and some of them will die before they reach old age. Because of this, the younger group is really not equivalent to the older group on all things with the exception of age. Knowing who will be the survivors is almost impossible to predict, of course, meaning we may be comparing highly select older adults with a wider range of younger adults. We cannot conclude that age "causes" certain characteristics or behaviors of older adults because they may always have been different from their own age group when they were younger.

To help illustrate this principle, consider data on the psychological characteristic of conscientiousness. Personality research shows that older adults are more conscientious than young adults. It's possible that aging has nothing to do with this, but that it's only the more conscientious people who live a long time. The less conscientious people who made poor health decisions would be less likely to have survived into old age. As a result of the survivor principle, you need to remind yourself that the older adults we study may have become more attentive to details, schedules, and obligations. On the other hand, they may not have changed at all—only survived long enough for us to study them.

## Third Principle: Individuality Matters

A long-held myth or misconception regarding development is that as people age they all become alike. This view is refuted by the principle of **individuality**, which asserts that as people develop they become more different from each other. This divergence occurs in people's physical functioning, psychological performance, relationships, interest in work, economic security, and personality. In fact, we know that from very early on, individual differences in human beings are vast. As we make our way through this book, we will highlight common myths and misconceptions like this one related to biopsychosocial aspects of various developmental stages and related to development itself.

Studies on infant and child behaviors and characteristics, such as cognitive capabilities and temperament, demonstrate that we are all different from the moment we are born (Colombo & Fagen, 2014). Likewise, research in adult developmental and aging continues to underscore the notion that individuals continue to become less alike from each other with age. Such findings suggest that diversity becomes an increasingly prominent theme during the adult years (Nelson & Dannefer, 1992).

The idea of increasing divergence among older adult populations does not mean everyone starts out at exactly the same point when they're young, or even when they're born. There are always going to be differences within any sample of people in almost any characteristic you can name. Even if you have a sample of older adults who were exactly the same age, it's likely they will differ more among themselves as a group, despite sharing certain characteristics such as age, than they would have when they were younger because they've lived through more experiences affecting everything from their health to their psychological well-being. Those experiences have cumulative effects, causing them to change at different rates and to differing degrees.

Consider what's happened to you and the people you grew up with by this point in your life. You have made the decision to go to college, whereas others in your age group may have enlisted in military service. You may meet your future spouse in college, while your best friend remains on the dating scene for years. After graduation, some may choose to pursue graduate studies as others enter the workforce. You may or may not choose to start a family, or perhaps have already begun the process. With the passage of time, your differing experiences build on each other to help mold the person you become. The many possibilities that can stem from the choices you make help illustrate that the permutations of events in people's lives are virtually endless. Personal histories move in increasingly idiosyncratic directions with each passing day, year, and decade of life.

Two types of differences come into play when we talk about individuality. **Intraindividual differences** refer to the variations within the same individual, for example, how fast you can count backward from 100 now, compared with when you were 6. Chances are good you're a lot faster now. Also, not all aspects of the individual develop at the same rate. Some aspects may develop quickly, whereas others develop more gradually; some may increase over time, others decrease, and others stay the same. Even within a construct such as intelligence, an individual may show gains in one area, losses in another, and stability in yet another domain. Intraindividual differences illustrate the fact that development can proceed in multiple directions within the same person (Baltes, 1996), a concept known as **multidirectionality**.

**Interindividual differences** are differences between people. We see interindividual differences between people over the course of the life span in numerous areas. Think about characteristics such as personality traits, like extroversion. You may be a less extroverted person who prefers staying in on a Friday night and talking with one or two close friends, while your roommate may be out and about with his fellow fraternity members at a bar or club. Chances are good, but not necessarily true, you would have made similarly different choices about how you spent your time when you were younger. You may have preferred to be listening to music in your room, while he was involved in Boy Scouts, soccer, and student council. Chances are good, but not guaranteed, that in 20 years' time, you'll again make these same sorts of differing decisions and how to spend your time. This is an example of how interindividual differences remain stable across the life span. If we think about something like reading, or athletic abilities, these types of interindividual differences may be less stable across one's life. Another example of interindividual differences is shown in hippocampal size, a part of the brain involved in memory thought to grow smaller as people get older. People of the same age can vary so dramatically from one another that they may more closely resemble people from different age groups. A hippocampus of a 70-year-old may actually equal that of a one 20-year-old. Many 70-year-olds have hippocampal sizes that are equal to those of people in their 40s. These interindividual differences clearly show that not all 70-year-olds are alike.

This example supports the idea that some older adults can outperform younger adults on tasks typically shown to decline with age. This sort of occurrence happens in many areas of study. Although traditionally younger adults have faster reaction times than older adults, exceptions to the norm are common. Although you may think of average-age college students as being able to run faster, lift heavier weights, or solve crossword puzzles in a shorter time than people three times their age, consider the differences between a sedentary 21-year-old and a 72-year-old triathlete. Chances are the triathlete will outperform the sedentary adult in all categories.

Looking at the other end of the life span, we often see in childhood intraindividual as well as interindividual examples. For example, a 7-year-old may be still need training wheels to ride her bike, while her 4-year-old neighbor hasn't used training wheels for months. This is an example of an interindividual difference that contradicts simpler ideas about aging and ability. At the same time, that very same 7-year-old is able to ride a horse at a trotting speed independently with great ease. This is an example of an intraindividual difference in the 7-year-old's physical abilities.

## Fourth Principle: "Normal" Aging Occurs Across the Life Span

**Primary aging** (or **normal aging**) refers to the normal changes over time that occur due to universal, intrinsic, and progressive alterations in the body's systems. What are some universals of aging that you can think of? Do they all occur roughly around the same age? What about that kid you know whose hair started thinning in high school? Presbycusis, or age-related hearing loss, is something we'll discuss in our chapter on later life, but did you know that presbycusis begins at about age 20? It's just that we tend not to notice its effects until we're in our 60s and beyond.

Changes over time leading to impairment due to disease rather than normal aging are referred to as **secondary** or **impaired aging**. These changes are not due to universal, intrinsic processes but are a function of an abnormal set of changes afflicting a segment rather than the entirety of the population (Aldwin & Gilmer, 1999). Skin wrinkling and discoloration are examples of the development of skin cancer and secondary aging, and they don't only occur when we've reached much older ages.

The third type of aging process sets in toward the very end of life, when individuals experience a rapid loss of functions across multiple areas of functioning. This precipitous decline is called **tertiary aging** (Gerstorf et al., 2013). Representing the impact of disease on already compromised areas of functioning, tertiary aging deserves mention in its own right as distinct from primary or even secondary aging.

Primary, secondary, and tertiary aging refer to processes that, over time, accumulate, and perhaps occur sooner than you may think. In the absence of accident or injury, the accumulation of these types of aging can lead to an individual's death. More gradual changes due to optimal aging may reflect the preventative or compensatory measures we take across the life span, from your dad putting sunscreen on you during your summer vacations when you were 5 to the water aerobics class you'll take when you're 85. These efforts can counter the toll that aging would normally take on a person's physical, psychological, or social functioning. There are also factors early on in life that seem to contribute to our health and may play a role in secondary and tertiary aging. For example, childhood adversity is associated metabolic system impairments in midlife. Similarly, post-traumatic stress disorder (PTSD) is associated with earlier onset and increased occurrence of disease for veterans from the wars in Iraq and Afghanistan. We will discuss several potential reasons for these links throughout this book {Davis, 2014 #2505;Joung, 2014 #2506}. On the other hand, some individuals don't make any special efforts to alter certain aging processes but, for reasons not always entirely clear, seem to age at a slower rate than their peers. They may be the ones who never seem to get sick right until the very end of their lives, when a sudden illness leads to their death (i.e., tertiary aging).

Throughout life, age-related losses due to primary, secondary, and tertiary aging can occur simultaneously. Thus, even while optimal aging can slow the deleterious changes of primary and secondary aging, eventually tertiary aging takes over and the individual's life comes to an end. Remember though, according to the principles of intraindividual and interindividual variability, the rates of each type of aging vary within individuals and from person to person. Gerontologists believe that despite changes in the body that lead to loss, aging also involves gains.

Primary, secondary, and tertiary aging all tie into the principle that **normal aging is different from disease**. This means growing older doesn't necessarily mean growing sicker. It is important for both practical and scientific reasons to distinguish between normal aging in adulthood and disease. Health care specialists who work with middle-age and older adults need to recognize and treat the onset of a disease rather than dismiss it simply as "getting older."

## Key Social Factors in Studying Human Development

As we've just seen, social factors play an important role in shaping the course of our lives. Here we make explicit exactly how we define and use the key social factors that we will refer to in this book.

## Sex and Gender

As you will see, there are important male-female differences related to biology, as well as differences related to the socialization experiences of men and women. We will use the term **gender** to refer to the individual's identification as being a man or a woman. Gender is distinct from biological **sex**, which refers to the individual's inherited predisposition to develop the physiological characteristics typically associated with maleness or femaleness. Both sex and gender are important in the study of development and aging. Physiological factors relevant to sex influence the timing and nature of physical development and aging processes, primarily through the operation of sex hormones (Whitbourne & Bookwala, 2015). For example, during puberty the activation of sex hormones and adrenal hormones affect the physical appearance of the body, the brain, and behavior. Later across the life span, the sex hormone estrogen is thought to play at least some role in affecting a woman's risks of heart disease, bone loss, and possibly cognitive changes (Whitbourne & Bookwala, 2015).

Social and cultural factors relevant to gender are important to the extent that the individual assumes a certain role in society based on being viewed as a man or a woman. Opportunities in education and employment are two main areas in which gender influences the course of development and becomes a limiting factor for women. Although progress has certainly occurred in both domains over the past several decades, women continue to face a more restricted range of choices and the prospects of lower earnings than do men. Furthermore, these differences are important to consider when studying the current generation of older adults, as they were raised in an era with more traditional gender expectations (Whitbourne & Whitbourne, 2012).

In recent years, mainstream Western society has become more exposed to the experiences of transgendered individuals (i.e., those whose sense of their own personal gender is different from the sex they were born with), as well as other noncisgender individuals (i.e., those whose sex and gender do not correspond, but who do not necessarily identify as transgender). It is too soon for researchers to have produced enough information related to development and aging for us to include these individuals as distinct groups. We might expect this will become an area of study, particularly because it also highlights the role of social influences on development. Prior to the 2010s, there was relatively little social awareness of the experience of transgendered and other noncisgender individuals and development, but this is rapidly changing (Orel & Fruhauf, 2015).

## Race

A person's **race** is defined in biological terms as the classification within the species based on physical and structural characteristics. However, the concept of race as commonly used is broader than these biological features. Race is used in a more widespread fashion to refer to the cultural background associated with being born in a particular biologically defined segment of the population. The "race" people use to identify themselves is more likely to be socially than biologically determined. Also, because few people are only one race in the biological sense, social and cultural background factors have even greater prominence.

The U.S. Census, a count of those living in the United States conducted every 10 years, attempts to provide an accurate depiction of the size and make-up of the country. The 2010 U.S. Census defined race on the basis of a person's self-identification. The categories provided by the U.S. Census include White; Black or African American; American Indian or Alaska Native; Asian (including Asian Indian, Chinese, Filipino, Japanese, Korean, Vietnamese, or Other Asian); Native Hawaiian or other Pacific Islander (including Guamanian or Chamorro, and Samoan); and some other race.

To the extent that race is biologically determined, racial differences in functioning along developmental lines may reflect differences in genetic inheritance. For example, people who have inherited a risk factor that has been found to be higher within a certain race are more likely to be at risk for developing that illness during their adult years (Whitbourne & Whitbourne, 2012). Racial variations in risk factors may also interact with different cultural backgrounds and practices associated with a particular race. For example, people at risk for a disease with a metabolic basis (such as inability to metabolize fats) will be more likely to develop that disease if cooking foods high in fat content are a part of their culture (Whitbourne & Whitbourne, 2012).

Social and cultural aspects of race may alter an individual's development through the structure of a society and systematic biases against people who identify with that race. We will demonstrate throughout this book how social and cultural factors associated with race, such as an exposure to certain environments and access to opportunities related to biopsychosocial development, are well documented and remain important from birth to death, such as living in low- versus high-crime neighborhoods and having access to health care. Illnesses have higher prevalence rates among certain races as well, such as the Black population in comparison with the White population in the United States, which has led to significant disparities in the health of the two groups. Part of the differences in health may be attributed to lack of opportunities for education and well-paying jobs, but systematic discrimination is also believed to take a toll on health by increasing the levels of stress experienced by African Americans (Green & Darity, 2010).

## Ethnicity

The concept of **ethnicity** captures the cultural background of an individual, reflecting the predominant values, attitudes, and expectations in which the individual has been raised. Along with race, ethnicity is often studied in development as an influence on a person's familial attitudes and experiences. For example, people of certain ethnic backgrounds are thought to show greater respect for older adults and feel a stronger sense of obligation to care for their aging parents. Ethnicity also may play a role in influencing the development and aging of various physiological functions, in part through genetic inheritance, and in part through exposure to cultural habits and traditions. Finally, discrimination against people of certain ethnic backgrounds may serve the same function as race in limiting the opportunities for educational and occupational achievements.

The term "ethnicity" is gradually replacing the term "race" as a way of categorizing individuals into groups in social research. We will follow that tradition in this book unless there is a clear-cut reason to refer specifically to race (i.e., if we are describing research that also uses this term). However, there are occasional points of confusion in that the U.S. Census occasionally combines race (White or Black) and ethnicity (Hispanic or non-Hispanic). Many Census statistics break down the distributions they report into White non-Hispanic, White Hispanic, Black non-Hispanic, and Black Hispanic.

## Socioeconomic Status

**Socioeconomic status (SES)** reflects a person's position in the educational and occupational ranks of a society. Technically, SES is calculated through a weighted formula that takes into account a person's highest level of education and the prestige level of their occupation. There is no one set way to calculate SES, however. Various researchers have developed scales of socioeconomic status that give differing weights to these values in coming up with a total score. People with higher levels of education tend to have occupations that are higher in prestige, and so some researchers use level of education alone as the index of SES (Whitbourne & Whitbourne, 2012).

**TABLE 1-1**

| Social Class Reflects |
| --- |
| Occupational Prestige + Educational Level but Not Income |

Income levels are not necessarily associated with socioeconomic status. High-prestige jobs (such as teachers) can have mid- or low-level salaries. However, as a substitute for or in addition to SES, some researchers use income as the basis for analyzing social class differences in health and opportunities (Whitbourne & Whitbourne, 2012). When we study children and are concerned with features of their SES, we measure this using the characteristics described but as they relate to their parents. However, if we're examining adults and are concerned with how childhood factors are associated with current functioning in adulthood, there can be issues with recall and errors in accurately reporting these characteristics of their parents from years ago.

## Religion

**Religion**, or an individual's identification with an organized belief system, is surprisingly one of the least well-understood but presumably important influences on aging. Organized religions form a set of social structures that transcend nationality and that, additionally, are partly connected with race and ethnicity. More important, religion provides many people with a source of coping strategies, social support in times of crisis, and a systematic basis for interpreting life experiences (Klemmack et al., 2007).

Religion is distinct from spirituality, or the set of beliefs that an individual holds about such areas as the afterlife, a sense of meaning in life, and feelings of connections to others. Spirituality and its relation to psychological well-being is becoming an increasing focus of researchers in the field and will undoubtedly grow in importance over the coming years (Tomás et al., 2016).

# Development Around the World

Trends in development certainly vary across each of the social factors we described, from variations in certain biological predispositions to differing social norms. These factors also interact with one another to form an even more complex picture. When possible, we will present information from both developed and developing countries and within unique subcultures. World population statistics are often reported in terms of "developed" and "developing" countries. Developed countries include all those in Europe, North America, Japan, Australia, and New Zealand, plus some nations formerly in the Soviet Union. All other nations of the world are classified as developing. The developing countries are those that have an agrarian-based economy, typically with lower levels of health care, education, and income (Whitbourne & Whitbourne, 2012).

Our goal is to present a complete picture of development across the life span that goes beyond what you may see inside and out of the classroom. We hope you will understand there are diverse pathways through life that impact our health and well-being and are impacted by and impact the world around us.

**LO 1-4 Explain the biopsychosocial perspective.**

# The Biopsychosocial Perspective

We organize the book around the **biopsychosocial perspective**, a view of development as a complex interaction of biological, psychological, and social processes. Development is not a simple, straightforward progression through time. Your body undergoes biological changes largely influenced by your genetics or physiology. At the same time, you change psychologically in ways that reflect what's happening to your body that, in turn, affect your body's changes. All of this takes place in a social context. Holding biology and psychology constant, people age differently depending on the environment, where and when they live, with whom they interact, and the resources available to them.

Biological processes refer to how the body's functions and structures change throughout the life span. Psychological processes include the individual's identity, behaviors, personality characteristics, motivations, thoughts, and feelings. The social processes of development reflect the cultural, historical, interpersonal, and environmental influences on the individual. You'll find that there's a great deal more to human development than you may have initially thought.

As you can see from the biopsychosocial model, we intend to go beyond "psychology" in teaching you about the processes involved in development. People who devote their professional lives to the study of human development come from many different academic and applied areas—psychology, biology, medicine, nursing, sociology, history, and even the arts and literature. Knowledge, theories, and perspectives from all disciplines contribute importantly to the study of the individual over time.

Our goal is to encourage you to make personal explorations and connections as you gain factual information about biopsychosocial processes. Not only will this material help you in your career regardless of what field you go into, but it will also help you understand yourself, how you develop and change over time, and what may be at the root of certain changes you experience. You'll also learn, perhaps surprisingly, that development and aging are ongoing and that both processes are not simply things you passively experience. There are active steps you have took and will take that impact your functioning and that can help ensure you continue functioning as well as possible for as long as possible throughout your entire life.

If you're a traditional college-age student heading into your 20s, we hope to help you appreciate that it is never too early to start incorporating changes into your lifestyle that impact your aging. For our readers of nontraditional college ages, we hope you see development is a lifelong process. A key goal we have in writing this book is to involve you in an understanding of the processes related to your development during earlier stages of life and the progression of your aging processes and show you ways to be an active part of your development.

# CHAPTER 2

# Conception and Prenatal Development

If you ask a cross section of individuals to define pregnancy, you will likely get a variety of responses. Pregnancy is "a choice," "time to prepare," "like nothing else you will ever experience," "the longest, most uncomfortable 8 months you'll ever endure," "a wonderfully scary and glorious experience," and "a miracle, exciting, all encompassing, worrying, amazing, the point of life."

The pregnancy experience depends on who you ask—a single woman, a pregnant woman, an expectant father, an adoptive parent, or a surrogate. It depends on many psychological factors—is it planned, are there infertility issues, is the health of the fetus at risk? There are also the physiological factors, or side effects of the biological processes, going on in the woman's body.

**TABLE 2-1** Stages of Prenatal Development

| Name | Process | Approximate Time During Pregnancy |
|---|---|---|
| 1st day of menstrual period | A dominant follicle begins to grow that will eventually become an ovum | 0 weeks |
| Ovum | An unfertilized female gamete is now present | 2 weeks, 0 days |
| Zygote | A fertilized ovum with 23 chromosomes merges with a sperm (male gamete) with 23 chromosomes to create one cell with 46 chromosomes | 2 weeks, 0 days to 2 weeks, 4 days |
| Embryo | A developing set of cells, beginning with the first cell division into two cells, gradually becomes an organism with a developing circulatory system, organs, facial features, arms, legs, fingers, and toes | 2 weeks, 4 days to 11 weeks, 0 days |
| Fetus | Progressive growth from a nonviable embryo to a completely developed infant | 11 weeks, 0 days to birth |

# Fertilization

**LO 2-1** **What happens at the cellular and molecular levels during fertilization?**

**LO 2-2** **What role do chromosomes have in determining the sex of a child?**

What makes us different from one another begins with **fertilization**. Fertilization happens when a sperm and an ovum come together to form a new cell. Currently there are many different ways in which fertilization can occur with the advent of assisted reproductive technologies (ART). However, in the more traditional sense, when mobile sperm are introduced into the female body, it can take anywhere from 30 minutes to 5 days for the sperm to reach the ovum, or egg, inside a female's fallopian tube.

## What Would You Do? Edwina's Story

I am the youngest of my parents' four children. The first, a son, was born in 1965. They took him home from the hospital where it quickly became apparent that he was very unwell and, after just 1 night, he needed to go back to the hospital. Initially my mother's concerns were dismissed as that of an overanxious first-time mother, but unfortunately her instincts were proven correct and her baby was diagnosed with cystic fibrosis (CF), a disease of which they had never heard. The diagnosis came as a shock; although CF is a genetic disorder, there was no family history that they were aware of and no other family members or any of their siblings' children were affected. The baby remained in the hospital where my parents kept vigil for the remainder of his short life and he died, unexpectedly, within 3 months. My parents were informed that they were both carriers of the CF gene and that if they were going to have more children they would quite possibly have another with the same disorder. Knowing this risk they took a chance and 2 years later my sister Mary was born. She too was diagnosed with CF. Four years later and after much agonizing over whether to take the risk again, my parents had another daughter.

This time the news was good and she was healthy. Another 4 years passed before I was born, also free of the disorder.

My sister Mary was relatively healthy throughout childhood and her teenage years, thanks in part to a rigorous regime of physical therapy, administered by my mother, alongside numerous pills. My parents made the decision to keep her condition secret from her schools and friends. They were concerned that knowledge of the condition would change the way her teachers interacted with her and that perhaps ignorance of the condition might prevent parents from allowing their children to be her friend, and they wanted her to have as normal a life as possible. The secret extended to me. I knew that she had regular check-ups at the hospital and I saw the prescriptions and nightly physiotherapy sessions, but whenever I questioned it I was either disregarded or told simply that she was sick. I understand now that they were doing their best to allow the three of us to have as normal a childhood as possible.

At the age of 12, while watching television, an advertisement for a CF fundraising event aired. It was just the two of us in the room and Mary said, "that's what I've got." I was a bit confused. I didn't know anything about it or what it meant. She explained that it was why she always had a cough and followed that with "I will probably die young." In my mind, at that time, I had heard people talking about an aunt who had died in her 40s and how young that had been, so the thought of my sister dying at about 40 seemed sufficiently far away for me not to worry and, apart from a persistent cough, she was fine as far as I knew.

Five years later she asked me to accompany her to an information session at her hospital, primarily for new parents of children with CF. We took our seats and the CF consultant began the presentation by showing a chart detailing the average life expectancy of CF patients over the decades since its discovery. The outlook in the 1960s had been particularly grim, with most patients not living beyond childhood. The 1970s showed a gradual improvement but were not much better. This was the early 1990s, and at this point I was 17 and my sister was 26. The life expectancy on the chart in front of us read approximately 18 years of age. For me, this was a major, sickening shock. Her health had begun to deteriorate at this point, and she had been hospitalized a couple of times for intravenous antibiotics to help her fight infections. The reality of the disease hit home and I felt that she had already defied the odds and was likely living on borrowed time. However, it was not all bleak, and scientific advancements were, and continue to be, made all the time. It was around this time that she was started on what was then a pioneering new "gene therapy" treatment that she breathed in every night through a

The sperm, created in the testes of the male, and the ovum, created in the female's ovaries, are called gametes. A gamete is a single cell that fuses with another gamete during sexual reproduction to produce a new, single-celled **zygote**. Although females are born with all the gametes (ova or eggs) they will ever possess, males continually make new gametes (sperm) throughout the life span. Amazingly it is typical for only one sperm, out of approximately 250,000,000 that are created in any single male ejaculation, to reach the ovum and penetrate its outer layer to achieve fertilization. Fertilization triggers a release of calcium from inside the ovum to form around the egg, preventing other sperm from entering. Before we learn what happens to this newly formed zygote after the fertilization process, let's take a moment to talk about what is happening inside the new cell that has been created.

## Chromosomes

When the sperm and the ovum join, they interact on the chromosomal level. **Chromosomes** are structures found in the nucleus of cells that store the genetic material passed on from the male and female gametes. Almost all cells in the human body contain 46 chromosomes total that are linked in 23 pairs. These cells are known as **diploid cells**. However, sperm and ova contain only 23 chromosomes. Sperm and ova are referred to as **haploid cells**. When the ovum is fertilized by the sperm, these haploid cells, each with 23 chromosomes, join to produce a new diploid cell, a zygote, with 46 chromosomes total. This diploid cell then reproduces, passing on the genetic material contained in the chromosomes. Table 2-2 presents a comparison of diploid and haploid cells.

**TABLE 2-2** A Comparison of Diploid and Haploid Cells

| | Diploid Cells | Haploid Cells |
|---|---|---|
| Examples | Hair, blood, skin, muscle, and many more | Sperm, ova |
| Number of chromosomes | 46 | 23 |
| How they are made | **Mitosis**<br>They are produced from identical diploid cells | **Meiosis**<br>They are produced from diploid sex cells that divide to produce gametes |
| How they reproduce | They produce identical diploid cells | They merge with another haploid cell during fertilization to produce a diploid cell |

## DNA

Chromosomes are made of protein and an organized molecule of deoxyribonucleic acid (DNA). **DNA** is a long, informational molecule in the shape of a spiral ladder, or double helix. Like a blueprint used to build a house, DNA is the blueprint for the development and functioning of all living things. The double helix in a diploid cell contains approximately six billion base pairs that make up the rungs of the ladder, while the sides of the ladder are comprised of sugars and phosphates. The base pairs are pairs of nucleotide molecules (adenine, thymine, cytosine, and guanine) held together by a hydrogen bond. A natural set of rules pertains to pairing the nucleotides contained in each rung. For example, because the size of each nucleotide differs, adenine is always paired with thymine, and cytosine is always paired with guanine to create the right size rung to fit the ladder. An adenine molecule will only form a hydrogen bond with thymine. Likewise, cytosine will only form a hydrogen bond with guanine. Therefore, the amount of adenine in a DNA molecule will always equal the amount of thymine, and the amount of cytosine will always equal the amount of guanine.

nebulizer machine. A year later she was married. Unfortunately, her health deteriorated greatly from this point forward. Her doctors discussed with her the possibility of a heart and lung transplant, but after much consideration she decided that was not for her. She died on July 20, 1996, at the age of 29.

The loss of my sister was hugely traumatic and witnessing the rapid deterioration in her condition was immensely difficult for me and the rest of my family. At the time of her death and the years that immediately followed, I felt adamant that I did not want to take any risks when it came to having children and potentially passing the condition to another generation. I just did not feel strong enough to go through this illness again with someone I loved and vowed I would not have children without knowing for certain if I carried the CF gene.

The passage of time, the birth of my other sister's three healthy children, and a greater understanding regarding genetic conditions as a whole have made me review this decision. Having spoken to a genetic counselor I have chosen not to undergo screening at this time. There are so many genetic conditions, and although I could be tested for CF and find that I am not a carrier, I could well be a carrier for another disorder. In addition, if I became pregnant, I would not want to have my unborn child tested for CF. To me, the only good it would serve would be to enable me to prepare mentally if the test came back positive. And I would never terminate the pregnancy. Had these tests been available in the 1960s and 1970s and my parents had undertaken them my sister would not have been born. If my child was born with CF would it really be such bad news? It is certainly not the death sentence it once was; today the prognosis for CF patients has improved, with the average life expectancy now estimated to be 37 years. Although certainly this is still very young, I am hopeful there is a cure within sight.

Think about what you would do in this situation after reading the chapter, and then decide the following:

- If you were Edwina, would you be screened for cystic fibrosis? If you were a carrier, would this knowledge affect your decision on having children? If you were pregnant, would you have prenatal screening?
- If you were a doctor or genetic counselor, how would you advise Edwina on screening and pregnancy?
- If you were the doctor or family counselor for a family of a child diagnosed with CF, what recommendations would you have for coping with the diagnosis?

The long DNA molecule is made up of sections, referred to as sequences, which contain either genes (coding DNA that is the basis of our characteristics, behaviors, etc.) or noncoding DNA (DNA sequences that, at this stage of genetics research, seem to have no biological function). Scientists believe that only 1% of human DNA serves a purpose in making us human; the rest of what is found on the double helix is junk.

**FIGURE 2-1** The location and structure of a chromosome.

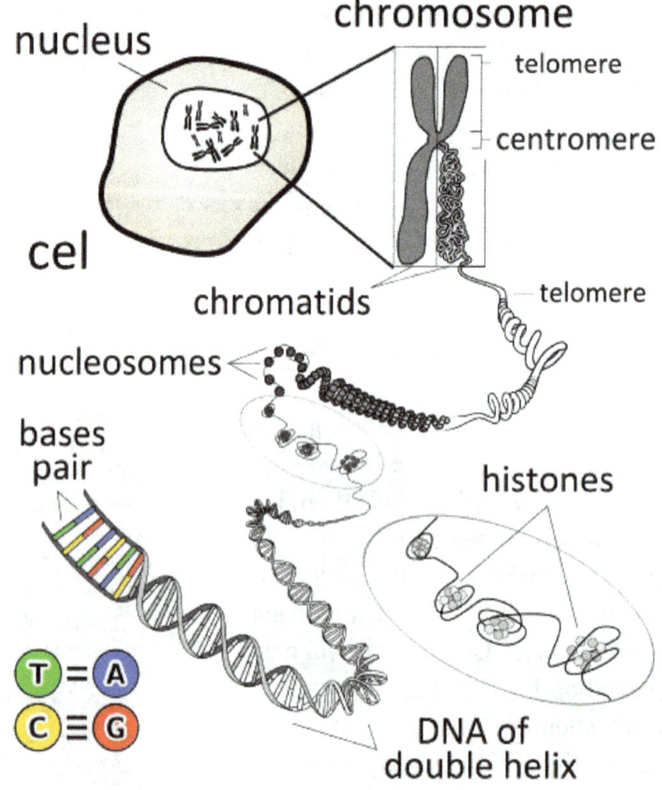


*Source*: Copyright © Kes47 (CC BY 3.0) at https://commons.wikimedia.org/wiki/File:Chromosome_en.svg.

## Male or Female?

Sex organs do not develop until roughly the 8th week of pregnancy (6 weeks after fertilization). The sex is determined by the sperm that penetrates the ovum, because the sperm contains the chromosome that determines the sex. In any given ejaculate, there are roughly an equal number of sperm with either a male chromosome or a female chromosome. Typically, "female" sperm are more hardy swimmers, but "male" sperm are faster swimmers.

Male and female gametes have specific sex chromosomes that when combined at fertilization determine whether the embryo will be male or female. Females are called homogametic because they have a pair of chromosomes in their diploid cells responsible for sex that are two "X" chromosomes or XX. Males also have a pair of chromosomes in their diploid cells, but one is X and one is Y. They are XY or heterogametic. When you split the XX chromosome in females, each haploid cell or ova will get an X chromosome. When you split the XY chromosome in males, one sperm will get an X chromosome and the other sperm will get a Y chromosome. When the male sperm (X or a Y) joins with the female ovum (X) this new diploid cell will have either an XX or an XY sex chromosome, as you can see in Table 2-3.

**TABLE 2-3** The Division of Diploid Sex Chromosomes XX and XY Into Haploid Cells and the Possible Outcomes

| | | **Females** | |
|---|---|---|---|
| | | **X** | **X** |
| **Males** | **X** | XX | XX |
| | **Y** | XY | XY |

**Sex and gender.** There can often be confusion between the terms "sex" and "gender." Typically, when we refer to someone's sex, we are referring to the biological anatomy of that individual. Do they have male reproductive organs or do they have female reproductive organs? The terms "male" and "female" describe an individual's sex. Gender relates to someone's self-identification as a "man" or "woman" regardless of their sex, and these are the terms we may use to describe a person's gender.

**FIGURE 2-2** A woman whose sex is male.

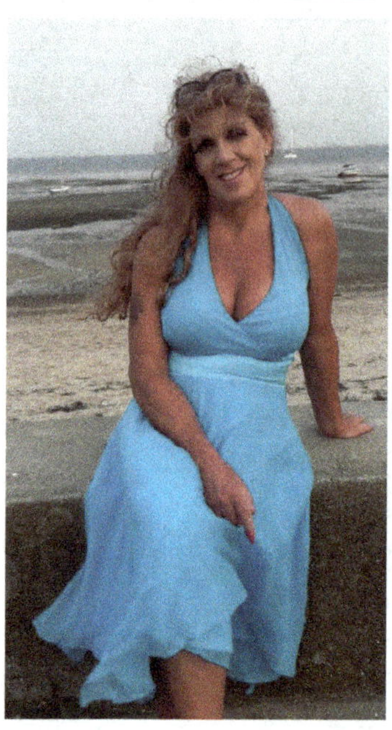

Photo Credit: Cynthia R. Davis

# Assisted Reproductive Technologies (ARTs)

ARTs have become very prevalent as ways to help individuals and couples who may have difficulty becoming pregnant. These technologies are also helpful to those without a partner of the opposite sex who want to achieve pregnancy. Common ART methods include medication, intrauterine insemination (IUI), and in vitro fertilization (IVF), as well as variations on these methods that utilize egg donors, sperm donors, and surrogate carriers. In each of the methods, the chances of having fraternal twins increases because of the types of hormones and methods that are used.

**Medication.** There are several medications, taken orally and injected, that help the ovaries develop **follicles**. Follicles contain cells and an immature ovum that may eventually grow to become a mature ovum. Medication increases the likelihood of pregnancy for those who may have difficulties with egg production.

**Intrauterine insemination (IUI).** Intrauterine insemination occurs when sperm is injected directly into a woman's uterus. The woman will often inject medications prior to insemination to facilitate the growth and development of follicles that become ova.

**In vitro fertilization (IVF).** In vitro fertilization is a process in which follicles are retrieved from the ovaries. In most cases, shortly thereafter these follicles become ova and are introduced to sperm, outside of a woman's body in a laboratory culture dish (or Petri dish) that is then place into an incubator, to create a zygote. After the zygote has developed into a multicellular embryo it is inserted into the uterus. Prior to the retrieval of the follicles, women typically inject medications to increase the number of follicles that are produced, and therefore the potential number of ova that can be fertilized. Although many follicles can be retrieved, there may be a limited number of embryos that survive outside the body that are suitable to be transferred to the uterus. Doctors typically transfer one to three embryos into a woman based on the number of cells in the embryo and the quality of those cells. Women often have the choice to freeze any remaining high-quality embryos. However, not all embryos can withstand the freezing and unfreezing process.

Some research shows an association between in vitro fertilization and a greater likelihood of birth defects, including genetic disorders, low birth weight, and preterm birth. However, researchers emphasize that there are other factors potentially related to the health of the biological parents and/or donors that may contribute to this (Kelley-Quon et al., 2012). There may also be some risks for women who undergo ART. Researchers point to a link between starting IVF treatments at a young age and an increased risk for breast cancer (Stewart et al., 2012). However,

ART and, in particular, IVF are relatively new sciences. In general, there is a lack of consensus on the risks of IVF because research on risks is at an early stage.

The Centers for Disease Control and Prevention recently reported that more than 1% of births in the United States were a result of ART methods. In 2010 there were 147,260 ART procedures, resulting in 47,090 live births and 14,474 twin births, giving ART an overall success rate of 32% (Centers for Disease Control and Prevention, 2011a).

The cost of ART varies from place to place and depends largely on the method used. In the United States, the cost of one attempt at in vitro fertilization can be anywhere between $10,000 and $30,000. In some states, this cost is covered by health insurance or even employers. However, in many states it is the parents who pay directly out of pocket. Coupled with the chance that more than one attempt may be needed, ART methods can be very costly for those with fertility issues looking to have a child, keeping in mind, too, the psychological challenges that may go along with the need for ART.

# Genes

**LO 2-3** **How do genes influence the development of human characteristics?**

**LO 2-4** **What role does the environment play in the link between genes and human characteristics?**

There are roughly 20,000 to 25,000 **genes** or "gene sequences" contained in the DNA of our 46 chromosomes, with anywhere from 100 genes on the shorter chromosomes to thousands of genes on the longer chromosomes. The sum total of our genes in called the human **genome**, which contains all the genetic material for any one human being. Much of our recent knowledge of genes comes from the Human Genome Project, a 13-year project funded by the U.S. Department of Energy's Office of Health and Environmental Research and National Institutes of Health National Human Genome Research Institute. The project was conducted at several research institutes across the United States and one in the United Kingdom. It finished in 2003 and aimed at determining the sequences of all the base pairs and identifying every gene found in human DNA (U.S. Department of Energy Genome Programs, 2019). The Human Genome Project found that humans have roughly the same number of genes as mice and roundworms, but the expression of those genes into physical characteristics and behaviors are what make us humans and not small and furry or long and slimy. The hope of those involved with the Human Genome Project was that these types of discoveries would provide information on how certain diseases develop and how to potentially treat those diseases.

Researchers on the Human Genome Project collected blood and sperm samples from many donors across the United States. However, relatively few samples were used in the project. Given that so many donors were available but so few were used, this allowed for better anonymity among the participants who provided their samples. Both the donors and the scientists never knew whose samples were being examined. In fact, more than 70% of what was discovered about the human genome came from one donor, a man from Buffalo, New York.

A person's genome is certainly unique to them (except in the case of identical twins). Mapping the genome involves understanding the sequences that occur in certain genes. Think of these sequences as place holders for the specific genes a person can have. Scientists now know how the sequences are organized, but what goes into each place holder is unique to every individual. The Human Genome Project made great strides in understanding the structure of our DNA and the sequences of genes. However, we only know how a small number of genes translate into specific human characteristics.

## Alleles

Genes tell us the basis for an individual's characteristics, and each gene that we possess in our diploid cells contains two **alleles**. When diploid cells and their 46 chromosomes divide to create reproductive cells or gametes, those cells are now haploid cells and contain 23 chromosomes. Because of this, haploid cells contain only one of the two alleles for a particular gene. When male and female reproductive cells combine during fertilization to create a new diploid cell, there is now a pair of alleles, one from the male and one from the female, that constitutes a gene, or genotype. The **genotype** is the combination of alleles at the genetic level, but the **phenotype** is the expression of that gene that we can observe in everyday life. For example, someone may have a genotype combination of two alleles for being tall contained somewhere on one of their chromosomes, but the outward expression of that genotype, their height, is the phenotype for that allele combination. Genotypes can make one person look very different from another, for example, having blonde hair versus brown hair is a noticeable difference. However, even though we possess a great number of genes, the various combinations of alleles result in relatively few striking differences in human characteristics.

**Heredity and dominant and recessive alleles.** Alleles can be dominant or recessive. In most cases, if an allele is dominant it will override the other allele and the phenotypic expression will be whatever is dictated by the **dominant allele**. Some examples of dominant physiological traits are brown eyes, farsightedness, dark hair, thick hair, detached earlobes, double jointedness, and the ability to roll your tongue into a U shape. In the study of heritability, dominant alleles are represented by English upper-case letters (A) and **recessive alleles** are represented by English lower case letters (a). We use Punnett squares to understand the potential for variations in alleles for any trait and to determine the probability of a particular phenotype, as shown in Table 2-4.

**TABLE 2-4** All Possible Combinations of Punnett Squares

| Two homozygous dominant pairs | A | A |
|---|---|---|
| A | AA | AA |
| A | AA | AA |

| Two heterozygous pairs | A | a |
|---|---|---|
| A | AA | Aa |
| a | Aa | aa |

| One homozygous dominant, one heterozygous pair | A | a |
|---|---|---|
| A | AA | Aa |
| A | AA | Aa |

| One homozygous recessive, one heterozygous pair | A | a |
|---|---|---|
| a | Aa | aa |
| a | Aa | aa |

| One homozygous dominant, one homozygous recessive pair | a | a |
|---|---|---|
| A | Aa | Aa |
| A | Aa | Aa |

| Two homozygous recessive pairs | a | a |
|---|---|---|
| a | aa | aa |
| a | aa | aa |

If you have the same alleles for a gene, whether it be dominant (AA) or recessive (aa), you are considered **homozygous**. If you have two different alleles for a gene (Aa), you are considered **heterozygous** for that gene. If both the male and female have dominant, homozygous genotypes for a particular trait (AA), then the offspring can have nothing but a dominant, homozygous genotype for that trait. If both partners have recessive, homozygous genotypes for a trait (aa), then the offspring can have nothing but a recessive, homozygous genotype for that trait. If both partners are heterozygous, that is, one dominant allele and one recessive allele (Aa genotype), then a variety of outcomes are possible, ranging from dominant homozygous (AA) to recessive homozygous (aa) or heterozygous (Aa). These are all the possible outcomes for two alleles coming together to create one new genotype.

If one of those two alleles for any genotype is dominant, then most often the dominant trait will prevail, regardless of whether the other allele is dominant or recessive. Generally, the recessive trait will prevail only when both alleles in a genotype are recessive. And when a person has the Aa genotype, they are often referred to as a "carrier" for the recessive gene. In this case, the recessive gene is not typically expressed as a phenotype. In other words, you wouldn't know by just looking at them whether the person was AA or Aa because the dominant phenotype would be expressed.

**FIGURE 2-3** The possible distribution of two heterozygous genotypes. Two heterozygous individuals have a 25% chance of having a child with a dominant homozygous genotype, a 50% chance of having a child with a heterozygous genotype, and a 25% chance of having a recessive homozygous genotype.

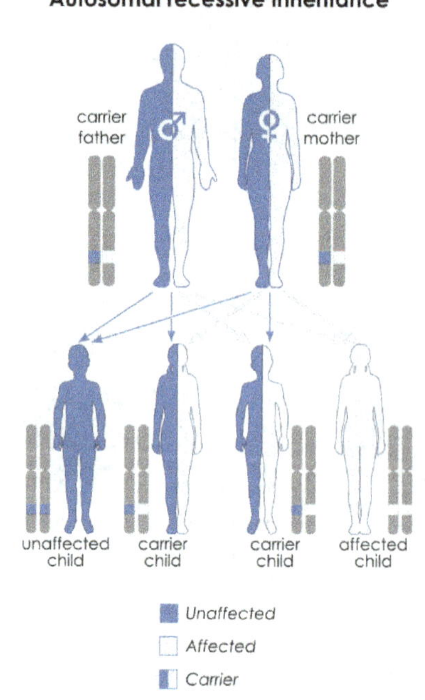


*Source*: Copyright © Kashmiri (CC BY-SA 3.0) at https://commons.wikimedia.org/wiki/File:Autosomal_recessive_-_en.svg.

## Gene-Environment Interaction

Our genes predispose us to many of the characteristics we possess in terms of our traits and our behaviors. Our phenotypes are not only a result of underlying genes, but they are also influenced by our environment. For example, a child may have the genotype to be tall (TT). However, if this child is raised in an environment in which malnutrition is a problem, that child may never reach his full height potential because the environment failed to support it. Therefore, phenotypically this child will be short, even though he possesses the genotype for tall stature. If we think back to the blueprint metaphor, our DNA provides the blueprint, but the environment provides the type and quality of building materials we have to work with. The field of **epigenetics** concerns how environmental factors such as diet, certain behaviors, stress, and exposure to toxins can alter the phenotypic expression of an underlying genotype. As in this example, the expression of certain genes can be silenced or turned off. Much like genetic material itself, a silenced gene can also be passed on to future generations. This means, if your grandparents experienced malnutrition, this may have silenced the expression of certain genes for them, which could mean silenced genes were passed on to your parents and eventually to you. There is a question about whether these epigenetic changes can be reversed. In other words, can a silenced gene be turned back on? Some studies have shown this may be the case, but more research is needed.

In terms of psychological disorders, gene and environment interaction is often referred to alongside the **diathesis-stress model**. The diathesis-stress model states that certain characteristics that an individual possesses (for example, certain genes we have) set the stage for a predisposition or vulnerability (diathesis) to a particular outcome later on in life. This predisposition, coupled with an environmental stressor, like low socioeconomic status or parental neglect, can contribute to some of the psychological disorders we see today. This theory argues, for example, that a person may inherit a genetic predisposition for schizophrenia. However, if there is not a significant environmental stressor, then the gene may never be activated for that person and schizophrenic symptoms may never manifest.

What other psychological traits are heritable? It is widely held the certain psychological disorders, such as schizophrenia, are heritable, given that those with a sibling or parent with schizophrenia have roughly a 6% chance of developing the disorder themselves. The risk is 40% for those with an identical twin with schizophrenia (Picchioni, 2007). Researchers are now trying to determine whether personality traits such as attitudes and emotional expression are also heritable (Kato et al., 2012). The jury is still out, but researchers believe that some of the more broad personality traits, such as extroversion and neuroticism, are more heritable than others (Loehlin, 2012).

## Genetic Disorders and Genetic Testing

Genetic testing examines the enzymes and proteins of chromosomes and DNA sequences to determine whether specific genetic disorders exist. Common genetic tests involve determining whether individuals are carriers of particular diseases and disorders that have a genetic basis such as cystic fibrosis. Gene disorders may be due to a missing chromosome, an extra chromosome, or both, or a mutation

**TABLE 2-5** Genetic Disorders That Are Screened Prenatally: Their Causes, Prevalence, and Symptoms

| Genetic Disorder | Genetic Cause | Prevalence | Predominant Symptoms |
|---|---|---|---|
| Down Syndrome or Trisomy 21 | An extra 21st chromosome resulting in 47 chromosomes total | 1 in 800 | Causes head and eye shape abnormalities, impulsive behavior, poor judgment, short attention span, and slow learning. |
| Edwards Syndrome or Trisomy 18 | An extra 18th chromosome resulting in 47 chromosomes total | 1 in 6,000 | Heart and kidney abnormalities. Most fetuses do not survive until birth. Only 8% of those who do live beyond one year. |
| Neural Tube Defects | Undetermined | 1 in 1,000 | An opening in the spinal cord or brain. Most infants do not survive birth. |
| Abdominal Wall Defect/ Omphalocele | Likely due to an extra 13th or 18th chromosome | 1 in 4,000 | Liver and intestines protrude from the abdomen. Can be treated with surgery. 25% of cases are fatal and most cases have other genetic disorders such as trisomy 18 or neural tube defects. |

within a gene sequence, the absence of a gene sequence, or a gene sequence that is too long. According to the American Medical Association, there are more than 1,200 genetic tests currently available to help diagnose more than 1,000 different genetic disorders. However, science has identified more than 10,000 diseases caused by single genetic mutations, so there is no one test or set of tests that can detect all possible genetic disorders (World Health Organization, 2013a). An additional challenge of genetic testing is that they are not entirely straightforward; some results are vague and cannot prove or disprove whether a person is a carrier of a genetic disorder. Nor are genetic tests 100% accurate. A false-positive result (saying that a genetic disorder is present, when, in fact, one is not) on a prenatal screening can have significant consequences for those involved. Because of this, genetic testing often goes hand in hand with genetic counseling, given the psychological and ethical implications of the outcomes.

There are various methods of genetic testing depending on the type of test and the type of information that is sought. Prenatal genetic testing typically involves an initial blood test to determine the likelihood of the fetus having a genetic disorder and the need for additional testing, most often via an amniocentesis. An amniocentesis takes a sample of the amniotic fluid that surrounds the fetus. This procedure also involves weighing the risk of having a fetus with a genetic disorder alongside the risk of losing the fetus as a result of the test procedure itself. It is estimated that approximately 1 to 2 pregnancies out of every 100 amniocentesis procedures results in miscarriage (Tabor et al., 2009). Table 2-5 shows causes, prevalence, and symptoms of some well-known genetic disorders.

**Newborn genetic testing.** Widely used, it tests for genetic disorders that can sometimes be successfully treated early on, such as phenylketonuria (PKU). PKU is the inability to breakdown certain amino acids that can lead to mental decline in young children. However, if diagnosed, PKU can be treated with a special diet.

**Diagnostic genetic testing.** Used for people of all ages, these tests typically analyze blood samples to determine whether a person has a certain genetic disorder. They can be done if a person has an identified risk for a disorder (such as having a diagnosed relative) and shows symptoms of the disorder, is presymptomatic, or is nonsymptomatic. These tests can also determine whether someone is a carrier for certain diseases, such as cystic fibrosis, and the likelihood that they may pass this risk onto a biological child.

**FIGURE 2-4** Possibilities for passing on cystic fibrosis for two "carrier" individuals. There is a genetic test that can determine whether a male and a female are carriers for cystic fibrosis. If both are carriers, they have a 25% chance of having a child with the disorder. Cystic fibrosis affects the lungs and the pancreas and has a median survival age of 37.4 (American Lung Association, 2010).

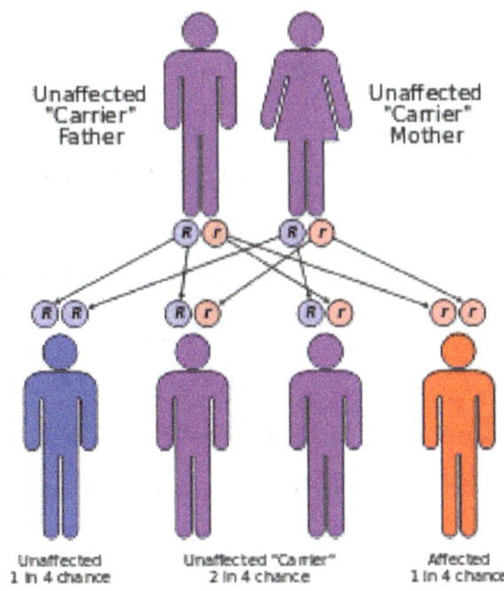


*Source*: Copyright © Cburnett (CC BY-SA 3.0) at https://commons.wikimedia.org/wiki/File:Autorecessive.svg.

There are also diagnostic genetic tests for certain types of cancer. For example, the results can tell a person about their genetic predisposition and the potential need for frequent routine cancer screenings. Lastly, there are many forensic genetic tests used within the justice system that identify genetic sequences unique to individuals, such as victims or perpetrators of crimes, through saliva, hair, and skin, among others. Genetic blood tests can also be used to determine paternity and ancestry.

**The Embryo**

As soon as the first cell division occurs, the zygote becomes an embryo and will be an embryo until it becomes a fetus at approximately 9 weeks after fertilization in the 11th week of pregnancy.

FIGURE 2-5 A six-celled embryo.

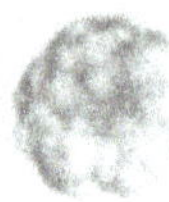

*Source*: Cynthia R. Davis

# Fetal Development

**LO 2-5 Which senses begin to develop during the fetal stage?**

**LO 2-6 What are some psychological characteristics that may be influenced by the fetal environment?**

Now that we know what's happening on the chromosomal level and how this can influence the health and development of the fetus, let's return to the single-celled zygote. The zygote begins to divide, from one cell to two cells.

It continues to divide, from two cells to four cells, four cells to eight cells, and so on. During this process, cell division occurs approximately once every 12 to 20 hours. Approximately 5 days postfertilization, the embryo has 70 to 100 cells and becomes a **blastocyst** with an inner cell mass that will eventually form the fetus and an outer layer of cells that will form the placenta, the membranes that nourish and protect the fetus. In the first few days postfertilization, from fertilization to blastocyst stage in typical pregnancies, the embryo slowly travels down the fallopian tubes toward the uterus. However, in some ART pregnancies, this embryo, created outside the body, is transferred into the uterus 3 to 4 days postfertilization.

## Implantation

Anywhere from 6 to 12 days after fertilization, as cells continue to divide and structures continue to develop, the blastocyst is also working to implant in the uterus. Upon entering the uterus it typically takes 72 hours for the blastocyst to implant. Throughout this process the blastocyst receives its nourishment from chemical processes inside the uterus that are triggered by the menstrual cycle and the presence of the blastocyst itself (Boron & Boulpaep, 2004). Chemical changes also draw the blastocyst to the uterine wall, or **endometrium**, and work to immobilize it. The blastocyst starts the process of implantation by connecting to the endometrium and decreasing its movement to a slow roll on the endometrial surface. There it typically connects to the uterus within a small crypt so that there is greater contact between the blastocyst and the endometrium. The volume of the uterus also decreases so that it is brought closer to the blastocyst. The purpose of this connection is to obtain oxygen and nutrients from the woman's bloodstream, and as time passes it grows from a loose connection to becoming deeply embedded within the endometrium. During this process, the blastocyst secretes substances to communicate with the endometrium cells so that they change on a molecular level to support and not reject the "invading" blastocyst. Because the blastocycst's cells are different from the woman's cells, her immune system secretes immunosuppressive chemicals to tell the body there is a pregnancy and to not reject the blastocyst. Regardless of whether a blastocyst is present at this stage of the menstrual cycle, endometrium cells change and the uterine wall increases in thickness to facilitate implantation and support an embryo. These thicker cells remain throughout the first trimester and are largely replaced by the placenta as the pregnancy progresses. If there's no fertilization, the cells that are produced to form the thicker layer of the endometrium prepared for implantation are shed during menstruation.

The blastocyst is fully attached to the uterine wall approximately 9 days after fertilization, and it will stay attached for the remainder of the pregnancy. Some women experience light bleeding during the implantation process, which can often be mistaken for a light period. At the same time, the blastocyst can be spontaneously flushed from the woman's uterus through natural processes at any time during these

**FIGURE 2-6** From fertilization to implantation.

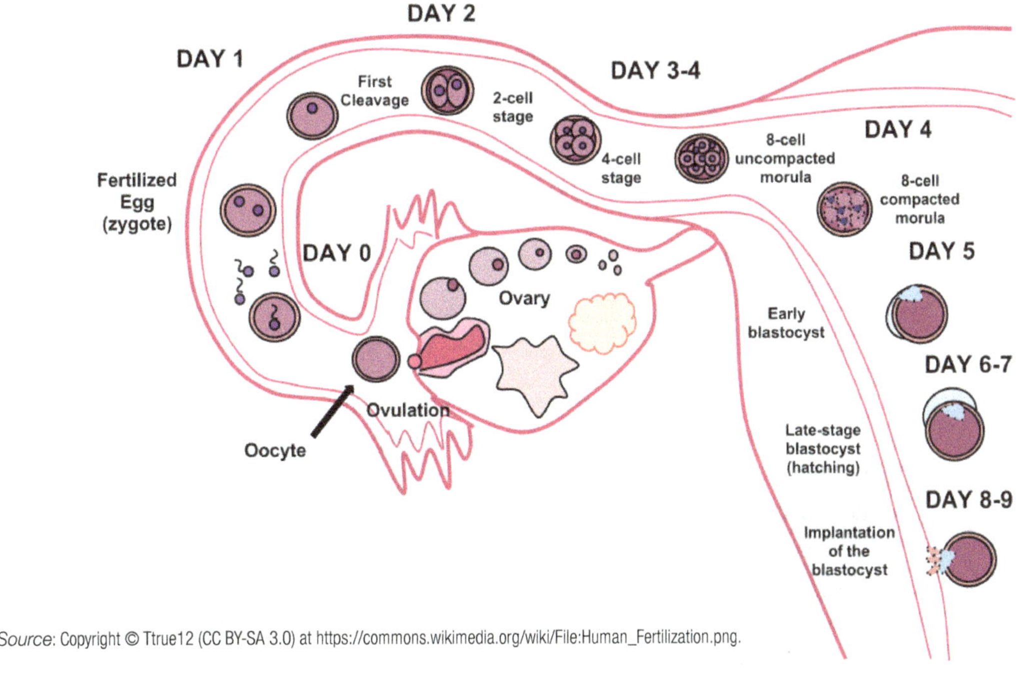


*Source*: Copyright © Ttrue12 (CC BY-SA 3.0) at https://commons.wikimedia.org/wiki/File:Human_Fertilization.png.

**Myths and Misconceptions**

A mother carries a gene for identical twins. **Misconception**

Science has yet to determine why identical twins occur. However, hyperovulation, and thus the likelihood of having fraternal twins, may be passed on genetically to females. **Fact**

early stages. In fact, around 22% of all fertilizations do not make it through the implantation stage and the majority of women cannot detect that fertilization ever occurred (Wilcox et al., 1988).

**Gastrulation** occurs approximately 10 days postfertilization when the implanted blastocyst develops endoderm, mesoderm, and ectoderm layers. The development of a twin fetus can occur at any time until gastrulation occurs. Once gastrulation occurs, these new layers create specific organs and tissues. The **endoderm** is the foundation for the digestive system and organs such as the liver and the stomach, as well as the respiratory system and organs such as the heart and lungs. The **mesoderm** is the basis for muscles, cartilage, blood vessels, bones, and connective tissues. The **ectoderm** will become the nervous system and skin.

The embryo now begins the complex process of developing the fundamental systems of the body and their supporting organs, glands, vessels, muscles, bones, cartilage, ligaments, tendons, tissues, and hormones. Once it has reached the 11th week, it is now in the fetal period of prenatal development and will remain a fetus until birth.

## The Placenta, Umbilical Cord, and Amniotic Sac

The **placenta** is a flat, disc-shaped organ connected to the woman's blood supply that provides nutrients and allows waste elimination in the developing fetus via the **umbilical cord**. The placenta is fully developed by the 13th week of pregnancy. Part of the placenta contains the outer wall of the **amniotic sac**, a fluid-filled structure that cushions the fetus and allows it to move freely to promote musculoskeletal development. The fetus breathes the amniotic fluid, which promotes lung development, and it swallows the fluid and eliminates it as urine or **meconium** (digestive waste).

## Duration of Pregnancy

Pregnancy consists of three trimesters, from 0 to 12 weeks, 13 to 27 weeks, and 28 weeks to birth. **Gestational age** is the age of a fetus that begins at the start of a woman's last menstrual cycle. Fetuses are generally not viable until 24 weeks of pregnancy, with survival rates and the health of the newborn increasing with each progressive week of pregnancy. In the United States, a fetus has a 50% survival rate if born at 24 weeks, but will likely experience developmental complications, whereas those born at 32 weeks have excellent survival rates (Breborowicz, 2001). A woman is considered "early term" for the 2 weeks during her 37th and 38th weeks of pregnancy, and "full term" after she has completed her 39th week of pregnancy until her 41st week of pregnancy (American College of Obstetricians and Gynecologists, 2013). After that, she is considered "late term." The typical pregnancy lasts 40 weeks, but a woman is considered "term" through 42 weeks. Many believe that that once a woman reaches term there are relatively few effects on fetal health. However, new research shows that there is considerable variation in infants born across the 5 weeks from the 37th to the 42nd week (Fleischman et al., 2010). Developmental milestones on a week-by-week basis throughout pregnancy are presented in Table 2-6 (MedlinePlus, 2020).

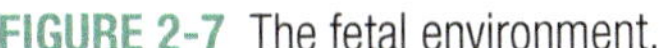

**FIGURE 2-7** The fetal environment.

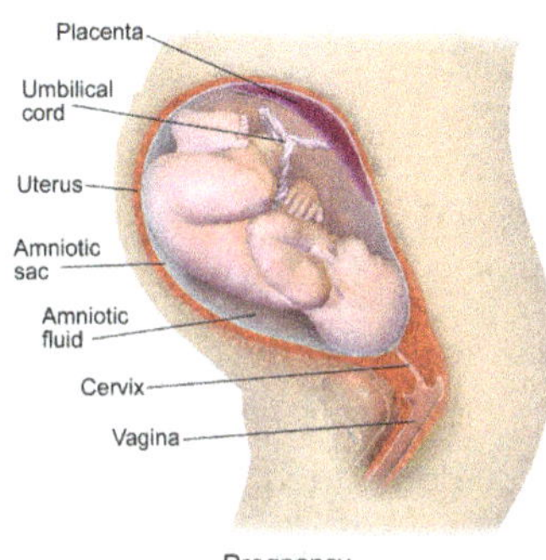


*Source*: Copyright © BruceBlaus (CC BY-SA 3.0) at https://commons.wikimedia.org/wiki/File:Blausen_0747_Pregnancy.png.

**TABLE 2-6** Gestational Age and Corresponding Developmental Milestones (Cunningham et al., 2010; Ross et al., 2007)

| Gestational Age in Weeks | Milestone |
|---|---|
| 5 | • Brain, spinal cord, heart, gastrointestinal tract develop |
| 6–7 | • Eyes, ears, arm and leg buds form, heart beats at regular rhythm |
| 8 | • Fingers and toes develop, lungs form |
| 9 | • All essential organs start to form |
| 10 | • Intestines rotate, facial features develop |
| 11–14 | • Face well formed, eyelids close (don't reopen until ~28th week), genitals well differentiated, red blood cells produced, first can be made, tooth buds appear |
| 15–18 | • Skin transparent, fine hair (lanugo) on head develops, meconium produced in intestinal tract, muscle tissue develops, fetus makes active movements (sucking) |
| 9–21 | • Women may feel fluttering |
| 22 | • Lanugo covers entire body; eyebrows, lashes, nails appear; fetal heartbeat detectable with stethoscope; women can feel fetus moving |
| 23–25 | • Bone marrow makes blood cells, lower airways of lungs develop, fetus stores fat |
| 26 | • Air sacs form in lungs, all eye parts developed, foot and fingerprints forming, hand and startle reflex present |

| Gestational Age in Weeks | Milestone |
|---|---|
| 27–30 | • Rapid brain development, nervous system can control some body functions, respiratory systems allow for gas exchange |
| 31–34 | • Rapid increase in body fat, rhythmic breathing movements (lungs not mature), bones fully developed (soft and pliable) |
| 38 | • Lanugo begins to disappear |
| 39–42 | • Small breast buds present, head hair course and thicker |

Adapted from F. Gary Cunningham, et al., Fetal Growth and Development, Williams Obstetrics. McGraw-Hill Education, 2010 and M. G. Ross, M. G. Ervin, and D. Novak, ?Fetal Physiology,? Obstetrics: Normal and Problem Pregnancies, ed. Steven G. Gabbe, Joe Leigh Simpson, and Jennifer R. Niebyl. Churchill Livingstone, 2007.

## Sensory Development and the Fetal Environment

Touch may be one of the first senses to develop. Studies have shown that a twin will react to the touch of the other twin as early as 8 weeks (Arabin et al., 1996). However, researchers have also concluded that fetuses likely do not perceive pain until the third trimester of pregnancy (Lee et al., 2005).

The ear drum develops during approximately the 10th week of pregnancy, and around 20 weeks hearing develops. At this stage, the fetus can respond to sounds, and hearing continues to develop over the course of the pregnancy. Research suggests that in the later weeks of pregnancy a fetus can show physiological responses (measured by heart rate) to the woman's voice, and newborns show a preference for her voice compared with others, likely because of repeated exposure during the pregnancy (Kisilevsky et al., 2009; Querleu et al., 1988). Prenatal hearing also seems to help establish our ability to learn a native language. Infants only a few hours old prefer the phonics of the woman's native language to the sounds of a foreign language (Moon et al., 2013). All these things not only support the notion that fetuses hear, but that they have the capacity for attention and learning and the ability to develop short-term auditory memories toward the end of pregnancy.

At roughly 14 weeks, taste buds begin to develop in the mouth, and the ability to taste develops at 27 weeks. Between 34 and 38 weeks, the fetus begins to develop food preferences based on the woman's diet (Endowment for Human Development, 2013). For example, one experimental study had women drink carrot juice for a period of time during pregnancy, and those infants later showed a preference for carrot-flavored cereal (Mennella et al., 2001).

The nerves necessary for smell are developed by the 13th week of pregnancy. However, the ability to smell doesn't come until later because the nasal cavity is plugged with other tissues until roughly the 30th week of pregnancy. The prenatal environment has particular smells—for example, one experimental study showed that women who ate garlic capsules had amniotic fluid with a distinct smell compared with those who did not (Mennella et al., 1995). Research has also shown that newborns prefer and are soothed by the smell of their own amniotic fluid (Varendi et al., 1998).

Vision is the last of the senses to develop, with the pupils able to react to light at 29 weeks. However, we still do not know how the fetus processes this information (Arabin, 2009). Much of what we do know about prenatal visual development is based on studies of infants born preterm. These studies show that infants have the ability to focus and track vertically and horizontally by 32 weeks (Chamberlain, 2013).

## Psychological Correlates of Prenatal Development

The prenatal period, although taking up only a limited amount of time in our growth and development, is linked to physical and psychological functioning across the life span. Gestational age at birth and birth size, both a result of the prenatal environment, have been associated with numerous characteristics and behaviors in childhood and adulthood such as cognitive abilities, temperament, personality, depressive symptoms, and stress reactions. For example, birth weight, length, and head circumference are associated with children's visual-motor integration, verbal competence, and language comprehension at 4 and one-half years of age (Heinonen et al., 2008). Small body size is linked to temperament at 5 years of age in terms of children's anger, discomfort, and proneness to sadness (Pesonen et al., 2006). Individuals who had a low birth weight are less likely to experience sexual intercourse, to leave home, and to cohabit with an intimate partner in early adulthood (Kajantie et al., 2008). Furthermore, young adults who had a very low birth weight, or who were born prematurely, score higher on personality traits such as conscientiousness and agreeableness, and lower in openness to experience. They also report fewer hostile and impulsive behaviors and are less assertive on average (Pesonen et al., 2008). Gestational length also predicts depressive symptoms, with shorter gestational lengths predicting more depressive symptoms, and those with lower gestational ages showed higher blood pressure levels in older adulthood (Feldt et al., 2007). Much of what we present about the links between prenatal development and functioning across the life span is from the Helsinki Health Study that examined a sample of midlife adults and obtained data not only on their current mental and physical health, but also on indicators of their health at birth (Lahelma et al., 2012). It is important to keep in mind, though, that these findings are not based on experimental studies that can determine cause and effect. There may be many other factors that drive the associations between early development and later functioning.

# External Changes and Influences

**LO 2-7** **What physiological and psychological changes does a woman experience during pregnancy?**

**LO 2-8** **Which health behaviors in a woman promote healthy fetal development? What are some of the harmful toxins that a fetus may be exposed to?**

Although the changes that the fetus undergoes are seemingly endless, the woman may experience many physiological and psychological changes, as well. Morning sickness may be among the most well known, but not every woman experiences morning sickness. In the early days of pregnancy, symptoms may also include general fatigue, breast changes and soreness, and painful constipation. Other symptoms during pregnancy include heartburn and indigestion, swelling, hemorrhoids, varicose veins and stretch marks, frequent urination, and dizziness. These changes are linked to fluctuating levels of hormones circulating through the woman's body, such as progesterone that helps manage the woman's immune system response to the fetus so that the pregnancy can be maintained. Estrogen is another hormone and is responsible for uterine and placental functioning that promotes the development of the fetus.

**FIGURE 2-8** Changes in hCG, progesterone, and estrogen over the course of a typical pregnancy.

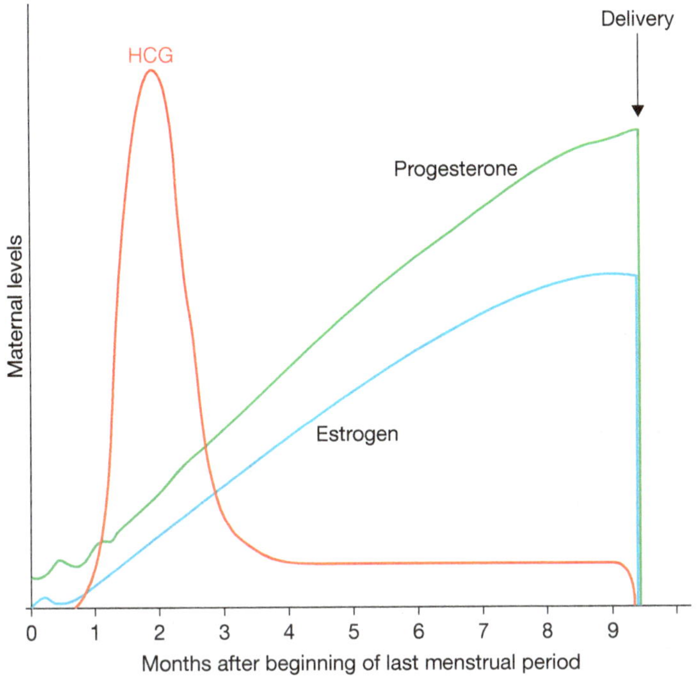

*Source*: http://www.medicine.mcgill.ca/physio/vlab/other_exps/endo/reprod_horm.htm.

# Maternal-Fetal Attachment

There are other changes that occur for many pregnant women apart from the more apparent physiological changes. Many women develop an attachment to the fetus that often grows stronger as gestational age progresses (Yarcheski et al., 2009). **Maternal-fetal attachment** includes maternal thoughts and behaviors involving affiliation, protection, and interaction with the unborn fetus (Cranley, 1981). There are many prenatal attachment behaviors that both women and men engage in, such as reading, singing, talking, and playing music that may be beneficial to the developing fetus; they also provide bonding opportunities for those on the outside.

Gestational age is the strongest predictor of maternal-fetal attachment, but other factors, such as social support, can contribute to the type of attachment a woman feels toward the fetus during pregnancy. Symptoms of anxiety and depression, self-esteem, planned pregnancy, marital status, income, ethnicity, and education are only minimally associated with maternal-fetal attachment (Yarcheski et al., 2009), whereas factors such as in vitro fertilization do not play a role in women's maternal-fetal attachment once risk for miscarriage decreases after the first trimester (Hjelmstedt et al., 2006). Expectant partners also show attachment behaviors toward the fetus, although on average not to the extent that pregnant women do (Mercer et al., 1988). Research on non-maternal-fetal attachment is limited, as is attachment for those who utilize various methods of ART or who adopt. Undoubtedly, these individuals feel attachment-related emotions toward their unborn children, but more research is needed to better understand these processes.

## Health Behaviors

The greater the level of maternal-fetal attachment, the more likely women are to engage in beneficial health practices such as prenatal care, a healthy diet, and regular exercise (Abrams et al., 2000; Lowry & Beikirch, 1998; Walker et al., 1999). The American Academy of Pediatrics (AAP, 2019a) emphasizes the importance of these types of health behaviors during pregnancy. Folic acid is crucial (400 micrograms per day) to reduce the risk of certain neural tube defects such as spina bifida. The AAP also recommends docosahexaenoic acid (DHA) supplements, or fish oil capsules for pregnant women, as research shows the infants of women who took fish oil capsules during pregnancy had fewer colds and shorter illnesses through their first 6 months (Imhoff-Kunsch et al., 2011). Caloric intake should be increased by roughly 300 calories per day, depending on the woman's health and diet prior to pregnancy, as the fetus requires additional nutrients. Regular, light exercise such as walking, swimming, or yoga (activities that do not involve any jumping or jarring movements) is also recommended (American Academy of Pediatrics, 2019a). However, women enter pregnancy in different states of health and are affected in different ways by pregnancy, so in all cases it is important that she consult a doctor about vitamins, diet, and exercise during pregnancy.

Two messages are universal and clear from the AAP: Don't smoke and don't drink alcohol (American Academy of Pediatrics, 2019b). Smoking can lead to premature birth and low birth weight, and it may be linked to sudden infant death syndrome (SIDS), learning disorders, respiratory disease, and heart disease. Alcohol consumption during pregnancy is linked to countless birth defects and developmental disorders in infants. Although there are many anecdotal stories of women drinking alcohol during pregnancy who go on to give birth to seemingly healthy infants, research has yet to identify any truly safe level of prenatal alcohol consumption or a time during pregnancy when it is safe to drink. Therefore, the AAP recommends that no woman drink any amount of alcohol during pregnancy (American Academy of Pediatrics, 2019b).

## Teratogens

Toxins that cigarette smoke and alcohol expose to the fetal environment are called **teratogens**. Teratogens are any agent introduced prenatally that can cause birth defects or health and developmental problems across the life span. A teratogen can be the result of something to which the mother is exposed, for example, X-rays, viruses like rubella, parasites that cause toxoplasmosis, or health risk behaviors of the mother, such as smoking and drinking alcohol. Much of what we know about teratogens is based on the differences we see in those infants who are exposed to them. Table 2-7 provides a listing of just a few.

**TABLE 2-7** Teratogens and Their Risks

| Teratogen | Potential Risks |
|---|---|
| Varicella Virus (Chickenpox) | Blindness, low birth weight, mental retardation, seizures |
| Tobacco | Heart defects, low birth weight, placenta previa |
| Alcohol | Fetal alcohol spectrum disorders, abnormal facial features; attention span, communication, and central nervous system problems; growth deficiencies; hearing, learning, memory, and vision problems |
| Accutane | Build-up of fluid in the brain, cleft lip and palate, facial deformities, heart defects, mental retardation |
| HIV | Spontaneous abortion, HIV |
| Radiation | Childhood leukemia, and cancer in later life, impaired brain development, severe mental retardation |
| Toxoplasmosis | Cerebral palsy, hydrocephalus ("water on the brain"), mental retardation, pneumonia, seizures |
| Phenytoin (or Dilantin) | Fetal hydantoin syndrome, cleft palate, heart defects, mild developmental disabilities |
| Mercury | Disruptions of mitosis, cell mutations, brain damage, hearing loss, learning disabilities, nervous system defects |

Other risks may be more difficult to avoid, such as influenza (the flu) and persistent fever. One study linked the two to autism (Atladóttir et al., 2012). Furthermore, gestational diabetes can lead to glucose intolerance and obesity in adolescence (Silverman et al., 1998). There are also certain cases in which avoiding teratogens may mean a trade-off between the woman's health and fetal health. Treatments for bone marrow, blood, and lymph node cancers may now be done safely to avoid risk to the pregnancy, even during the first trimester (Aviles & Neri, 2001). However, women with epilepsy may face a difficult choice in controlling their symptoms with medications given that some anti-epileptic drugs are associated with birth defects (Bromley et al., 2009). Reports on the safety of antidepressants taken during pregnancy are not necessarily straightforward, as some studies have been shown certain antidepressants cause no risk to a pregnancy (Stephansson et al., 2013), whereas other studies say there are increased risks for birth defects, preterm birth, and miscarriage (Domar et al., 2012). There are certainly some antidepressant treatments a woman should avoid altogether during pregnancy, but she should always weigh the risks and benefits with her doctors before making any decisions about changes in medications.

## Socioeconomics and Pregnancy

Research shows that some socioeconomic factors such as education, employment, income, and access to resources such as health care can affect prenatal development, risk for miscarriage, as well as physiological and psychological health and development across the life span (Conroy et al., 2010; Hackman et al., 2010; Norsker et al., 2012). Globally, poor socioeconomics influence a woman's exposure to prenatal teratogens and ability to maintain a nutrition-rich diet, which, in turn, are associated with fetal growth and premature birth. Studies have also shown that pregnant women from low socioeconomic status backgrounds have increased depressive symptoms, stress, and high blood pressure, each of which can affect the developing fetus (Goyal et al., 2010). Other established health risk behaviors, such as smoking, are more common among women of low socioeconomic status backgrounds, which contribute to prenatal risk. They are also more likely to have challenges in accessing health care resources (Norsker et al., 2012). It will be interesting to see in coming years how programs such as the Affordable Care Act in America will influence findings like these. However, research on women from low socioeconomic status backgrounds in the United States indicates a strong sense of communalism, in which there is support and interdependence among community members, which can alleviate some of the risks associated with socioeconomic status (Abdou et al., 2010).

## Myths and Misconceptions

A pregnant woman should avoid fish because it contains high levels of mercury. **Misconception**

Fish is part of a healthy diet. There are certain types of fish to avoid and certain amounts to avoid while pregnant. The American Academy of Pediatrics recommends that pregnant women avoid shark, king mackerel, tile fish, and swordfish, along with any raw or seared fish. They should limit consumption of fish like albacore white tuna and local fresh fish to no more than 6 ounces per week. **Fact**

A pregnant woman should get rid of her cat because it carries the virus that causes toxoplasmosis. **Misconception**

A pregnant woman should avoid changing a cat's litter box, because cat feces may contain particles that carry the virus. **Fact**

# CHAPTER 3

# Labor, Delivery, and the Newborn

Childbirth is an experience that varies from person to person and culture to culture. It is a phenomenon of life span development that is open to personal and cultural opinions and beliefs. Many, especially those who have not experienced childbirth, find it hard to believe that a woman's body is capable of delivering an infant. However, this capability is reflective of our human physiological adaptation as a species. The opening of the female pelvis is wider than the male's, and during labor **contractions** allow the cervix to open, while the fetus engages in a series of specific movements to appropriately align its head and shoulders to make its way through the birth canal.

# Labor and Delivery

**LO 3-1** **What happens during the first, second, and third stages of labor and delivery?**

**LO 3-2** **What types of complications may arise during labor and delivery?**

Labor and delivery are broken down into three stages. The first stage is labor and involves changes to the woman's cervix, followed by the descent and birth of the fetus through the birth canal, resulting in delivery of the infant, and lastly the delivery of the placenta. Common childbirth practices vary widely from culture to culture and preferences for how childbirth will unfold can vary from woman to woman, but the physiological aspects of these stages are, for the most part, universal.

The first step of childbirth is typically the onset of labor, when the woman's body and the fetus are ready for birth. For some labor may be relatively quick and last for only a few hours or less. For others it can be a process that occurs over days. It typically lasts longer for women who have never given birth before (**primipara**), but it is shorter for women who have (**multipara**). However, whether it's the woman's age, the gestational age of the fetus, or the number of previous births the woman has had, there is no way to accurately predict the course of most women's labor experiences.

## What Would You Do? Scarlett's Story

I wanted a natural childbirth, no drugs, minimal intervention, just my body telling me what to do. About half the women I talked to reported wonderful experiences of natural childbirth. For a long time I thought about having a home birth, but my partner wanted to have our baby in a hospital where, if something happened, intervention would be possible. So I agreed and began searching for a hospital that had a history of low intervention. I looked at statistics for number of cesarean deliveries and number of natural births, took anecdotal evidence from mothers in the area, and decided on a hospital that had a "birthing center." I signed us up for childbirth classes, one at the hospital where I was going to have the baby and another that specifically taught natural childbirth techniques. My partner and I thought this course was wonderful, teaching us about things such as the cycle of pain, ways to mentally deal with the pain, and physical techniques to manage the pain. I also practiced yoga throughout my pregnancy to maintain flexibility, breathing, and labor techniques.

We felt well prepared when my water broke at 9:36 a.m. on a Thursday. Our baby was nearly a week overdue, and we were scheduled for induction on Friday because of her size (she was estimated at 9 pounds, 14 ounces earlier that week). We didn't call our doctor right away because we already had an appointment for the afternoon, and I was not feeling any contractions. When we went in to the doctor at 2:30 p.m., they hooked me up to the monitor and the baby's heart beat was fine, and I was indeed having contractions. I was ecstatic; maybe this birth was going to be incredibly easy. I had been 3 centimeters the week before. and now I was having contractions and was completely unfazed by them. We went home and were able to spend some time laboring there, relaxing, and having dinner. By the time we went back to the hospital at 9:30 p.m., I was feeling moderate contractions; they were very uncomfortable but I could manage the pain through breathing and walking.

The nurses asked me if I was aiming for a natural childbirth and checked me in to a large room with plenty of tools for laboring (a birthing ball, a birthing bar, and a whirlpool tub). My contractions were then moderate to severe, but again manageable for me through walking and breathing. The doctor examined me and said, "You aren't going to have this baby tonight, you are going to have this baby tomorrow, so you should get some sleep, we can give you Ambien or morphine, neither of which is harmful to the

# First Stage: Labor—Latent Phase, Active Phase, and Transition

**FIGURE 3-1** Changes in the cervix as it dilates and effaces (A and B—tightly closed; C—60% effaced, 1 to 2 cm dilated; D—90% effaced, 4 to 5 cm dilated).

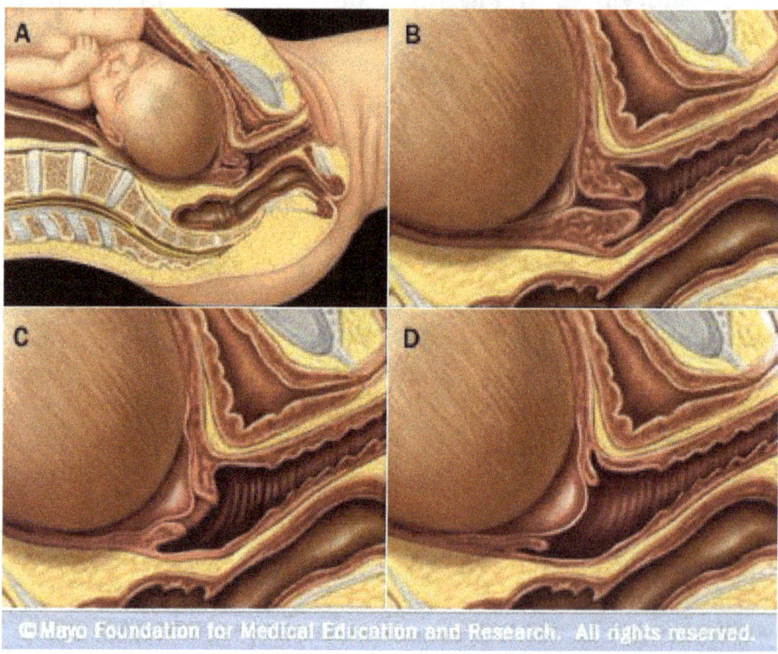


*Source*: https://www.mayoclinic.org/healthy-lifestyle/labor-and-delivery/in-depth/stages-of-labor/art-20046545.

baby; morphine will help slow the contractions, and you will be able to sleep."

I opted for morphine, but my contractions did not slow down. I did sleep but woke up every 2 minutes with a contraction, and at that point I couldn't control the pain using the techniques I had learned. After a while the nurse asked if I wanted to get into the tub, and I said yes. Although the tub really helped manage the pain, it was a challenge because I was still going in and out of sleep.

By 6 a.m. I was ready to push and was feeling less groggy from the morphine. The nurses checked my progress and said that I was fully effaced and at 9 centimeters on the cusp of 10 and that pushing would get me there. I went to the bed and got on my hands and knees and pushed with

The first stage of labor lasts the longest and is broken down into two phases: the latent phase when contractions begin and the active phase when contractions become more intense. The main physiological process that occurs in the woman's body during this stage is the **dilation**, or the widening of the cervix to make room for the fetus during delivery. and **effacement** of the cervix, or the elongation of the cervical muscles of the uterine wall. At the end of pregnancy, the cervix begins to dilate or expand, as well as efface or thin out and become elongated. Dilation is measured in centimeters and effacement is measured in percentages. Effacement occurs when the uterine muscles contract, causing the upper part of the uterus to shorten and the lower part of the uterus to shift so that the cervical muscles become incorporated into the uterine wall. Women may be 1 to 2 centimeters dilated for 1 to 2 weeks at the end of the pregnancy without being in labor. The goal of the first stage is for the cervix to become 100% effaced and to fully dilate to 10 centimeters so the fetus can descend down the birth canal.

During the first stage of labor and delivery, the fetus positions itself in preparation for birth and makes a series of movements, known as **cardinal movements** (see Figure 3-2) to fit through the woman's pelvis. This journey down the birth canal may temporarily change the shape of the newborn's head—usually without harm—causing it to look more elongated; this changes soon after birth.

**Latent phase. The latent phase** may also be referred to as the "prodomal phase," "prelabor," or "early labor." The women may begin to feel regular contractions between 30 and 90 seconds in duration that occur at time-able intervals, usually every 5 to 20 minutes. The latent phase may be as short as a couple of hours for some women, or it can last several days (especially for primiparae women). The mucus plug, which we will discuss shortly, may discharge and the uterine membranes may rupture during this phase, or these may occur later on in the first stage. Labor is typically much faster if the membranes rupture during this phase. It is not until the cervix is 3 to 4 centimeters dilated that the woman enters the next phase of the first stage, the active phase of labor.

**Rupture of the membranes.** When the amniotic sac that surrounds the fetus ruptures, we often refer to this as the moment the woman's water breaks. The sac may leak or break on its own prior to the onset of labor or not until the later on during the labor process. Amniotic fluid may leak from the vagina slowly or in a more apparent gush.

the next contraction. But the pain I felt was the wrong kind of pain. The pain I was having before felt extremely uncomfortable, but it felt right to me, like, "Wow this is painful, but that is what labor is supposed to feel like." This pain felt like something was wrong. At this point, I gave up on the idea of natural childbirth and asked for an epidural. I just needed that pain to go away. The nurse and my partner tried to convince me otherwise, telling me I was doing such a great job and not to give up. The doctor said to give it time. However, there was a shift change, and the new nurse called the doctor and the anesthesiologist to give me an epidural and Pitocin. As soon as they did my labor stopped.

I was crying, and my partner went into the hall to update my parents and talk to the doctor. The doctor said I needed to deliver the baby via cesarean because the baby was not in the correct position, but was facing up toward my abdomen, and would never be able to correctly position in my pelvis for birth. I asked my doctor if I could try positions so that the baby could engage in my pelvis. But I knew what was coming. My baby was going to be delivered via C-section. My partner told them to give me some time, and I grieved because in the end we went from my ideal—having a home birth—to having my baby in an operating room. I wasn't able to see her being born as I had hoped, and my first contact with her was her cheek next to mine. It was an hour before I could hold her and have her latch on to me. Although in the end my daughter was born healthy and latched easily, the birthing process was agonizing for me and added to the stress and emotions of being a new parent.

Think about what you would do in this situation after reading the chapter, and then decide the following:

- In the end, do you think the correct decision was made to deliver the baby via cesarean?
- If you were Scarlett, are there ways you could have prepared differently for childbirth? How would you cope with your emotions after childbirth?
- If you were Scarlett's partner, would you feel differently about deciding against a home birth? How would you support her during the transition to cesarean delivery?
- If you were Scarlett's nurse or doctor, how would you counsel her on this transition? What kinds of emotional support would you provide during the process and afterward?

'**FIGURE 3-2** Cardinal movements of delivery.

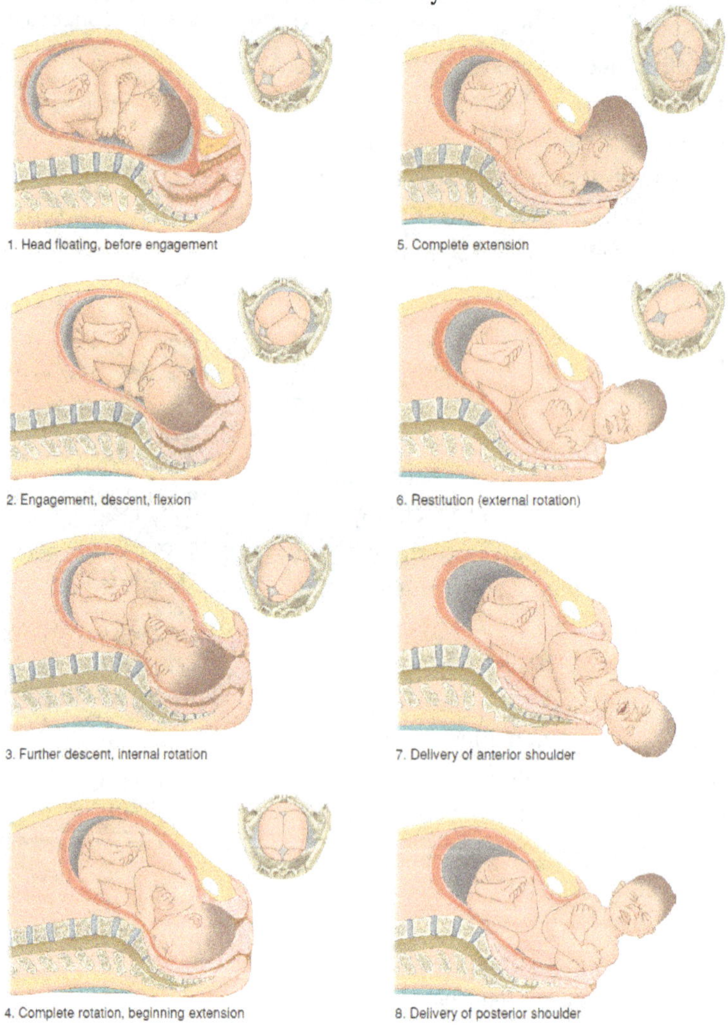

*Source*: http://www.med.cmu.ac.th/dept/obgyn/2011/images/stories/Lectures/MedSTD5/Kasemsri/NL04.gif.

If a woman's water breaks prior to the active labor phase, it is likely that she will go into labor within 24 hours. A woman's membranes may also rupture prior to the 37th week of pregnancy. If this occurs, it is important that she be evaluated right away by a health care provider to evaluate the health of the fetus and determine next steps, whether it be bed rest for a limited time prior to delivery or immediate delivery. Alternatively, the membranes or amniotic sac may be ruptured by a health care provider to facilitate the progression of labor once it has already begun. Although uncommon, some infants are born with the amniotic sac still intact. In this case, the sac is ruptured upon delivery. Although this poses no risk to the infant, membranes are now typically ruptured by the health care provider if they have not ruptured prior to delivery.

**Braxton Hicks contractions.** Before labor beings, many women experience contractions that are not indicative of the start of labor. These are called **Braxton Hicks contractions**. Braxton Hicks contractions involve the tightening of the muscles in the uterus, and the reason for these contractions is unknown. It is thought that Braxton Hicks contractions may be one of the body's ways of preparing for labor by promoting the expansion of the cervix. They may also be caused by factors such as dehydration or even a full bladder.

Braxton Hicks contractions may occur as early as 6 weeks into a pregnancy but typically occur during the second and third trimesters. They last about 60 seconds and can be felt as a painless sensation or mild cramping, but can also be more painful in nature. These "false labor" contractions are different from true labor contractions in that they are irregular and infrequent. We will discuss in a moment how true contractions occur at more regular intervals that persist until the baby is born.

If the woman experiences these contractions, rhythmic breathing, changing positions, or lying down on the left side may alleviate or stop the contractions all together. Although Braxton Hicks contractions may be part of a normal pregnancy for some, a woman should monitor these contractions and report them to her health care provider when they occur (MacKinnon & McIntyre, 2006).

**Why are contractions painful?** Labor pains and contractions are often the most intense pain a woman will ever feel (Niven & Gijsbers, 1984). The physiological causes of contractions are not 100% known, although it's believed that layers of the uterine wall being deprived of oxygen, compression of the nerves in the cervix, the stretching of the cervix, and the stretching of the membrane that lines the abdominal cavity over the fundus (the top of the uterus) all contribute to the pain that's experienced. Endorphins are release by the body in an attempt to cope with the intense pain.

Factors such as personal expectations, anxiety, fear, and support from others all impact a woman's experience of and ability to cope with labor pains. Cultural norms and learned behaviors regarding what's expected during childbirth also appear to affect a woman's pain perception and expression. In some cultures, pain expression during childbirth is suppressed, whereas in others it's perfectly acceptable to vocalize these pains. Having a first or subsequent birth may be the root of differing pains during childbirth, but not necessarily the experience of pain itself. During a first birth, the descent of the fetus is more gradual, as the structures in the pelvis shift to accommodate the fetus, which may cause one type of pain. However, in subsequent births, the fetus moves more quickly down the pelvis that may cause more sudden and intense pain (Callister et al., 2003; Lowe, 2002).

Women may opt for a variety of strategies to cope with the intensity of the pain as labor progresses. Inhaled analgesic drugs and spinal epidurals are very effective in helping with pain management. However, there is a documented trade-off. Those who use inhaled analgesics are more likely to experience nausea and dizziness, and those who receive epidurals are more likely to require instrumental vagina births, although these approaches pose no long-term risks to the fetus. Many women opt for "natural childbirth" and use no pharmacological interventions to cope with labor pains. Other strategies that may reduce pain include acupuncture, relaxation, breathing techniques, varying positions and postures, water baths, and massage. Cognitive strategies such as distraction and self-efficacy also appear to impact the experience of pain during childbirth (Escott et al., 2009). Women may also use aromatherapy and hypnosis, but there is little scientific evidence to support their effectiveness (Jones et al., 2011).

**Cervical mucus plug.** The cervical mucus plug blocks bacteria from entering the uterus. As labor approaches and the cervix begins to dilate, the mucus plug becomes dislodged and is released either all at once as a lump, or gradually resulting in an increase in vaginal discharge over the course of a few days. Just as a cervix can be dilated to varying degrees prior to labor and delivery, a woman may discharge the mucus plug a few hours or a few weeks prior to the onset of labor. Intercourse or vaginal examinations may also dislodge the mucus plug. It's also referred to as "bloody show" because blood released into the cervix gives the mucus a pink, red, or blood color.

**Active phase.** During the **active phase** of the first stage of labor, contractions will likely become longer and stronger and occur more frequently, with little time in between each contraction. The cervix dilates faster, from 3 to 4 centimeters to 8 to 9 centimeters. The duration of this phase lasts approximately 5 hours if the woman is primipara and approximately 2 hours if the woman is multipara. Breathing and other relaxation techniques are often used by women to circumvent the pain during the active phase. However, some women opt for pain reducers to manage pain during this phase.

**Transition.** Some refer to the last part of the active labor phase as "transition" or "deceleration" when the cervix dilates at a slower rate from 8 to 10 centimeters and the fetus begins to descend more rapidly into the lower pelvis and on into the birth canal. Pain is most intense during this phase, and there is often pressure in the lower back and pelvis, similar to the sensation of a bowel movement, and the urge to push.

## Second Stage: Delivering the Fetus

The second stage begins when the cervix is fully dilated, contractions continue to increase, and the fetus is fully engaged in the pelvis in a position to be birthed. This stage can last anywhere from 15 minutes to several hours (again, longer for primiparae women), often depending on the size of the fetus. The woman may be in a variety of positions to deliver the fetus, including lying on her back, sitting, standing, squatting, kneeling, or on her hands and knees. Some contend that squatting or standing reduces the duration of the second stage, the need for an assisted delivery, as well as pain severity (Ness et al. 2005). A woman will feel pressure in the rectum as the fetus descends. She will likely have the urge to push and be instructed to do so in timing with contractions to aid the continued descent of the fetus. The fetus will crown (its head will begin to show), which can be accompanied by a very strong stinging or burning sensation for the woman. This stage ends with the birth of the baby's head, the clearing of its airway, and the birth of the rest of its body.

## Third Stage: Cutting the Cord and Delivering the Placenta

This stage begins with the clamping of the umbilical cord. This typically occurs between 30 and 60 seconds after delivery of the infant. In countries where poor nutrition is a problem, there may be some benefit to delaying the clamping of the cord to increase the level of iron in the infant's blood. However, in other scenarios, delayed clamping is associated with increased risk for jaundice in infants, resulting in the need for phototherapy (Neilson, 2008). Once the umbilical cord is clamped and cut, the infant is fully independent of the woman's body.

During this stage the placenta separates from the uterine wall and is expelled from the woman's body, along with the attached umbilical cord that joined the fetus and the placenta. Health care providers will often give the woman medication and massage the abdomen, and she will continue to have mild contractions and may be asked to push to facilitate this process. The delivery of the placenta typically occurs within 15 minutes of the delivery of the baby, and the uterus begins the process of contracting in size. It is important that the placenta is intact and completely expelled from the uterus to prevent bleeding and infection. The World Health Organization (WHO, 2009) recommends that this stage of labor be managed by health care providers to reduce risk for hemorrhaging and retained placenta in the woman, which both can be life threatening. Finally, as some women experience vaginal tearing during the birthing process, stitches may be required after the placenta has been delivered.

**Hormones.** During pregnancy, labor, and delivery, there are high levels of oxytocin present in the woman's bloodstream to promote contractions and endorphins to suppress pain. There also appears to be a rise in adrenaline during the transition phase. **Oxytocin** also helps the uterus shrink after the placenta is delivered. Another hormone, prolactin, peaks during labor and delivery and remains high for a few days following. Prolactin, along with oxytocin, supports a woman's ability to breastfeed. There are also high levels of oxytocin in the baby after childbirth. Oxytocin in both the mother and the infant promote bonding and attachment. Table 3-1 shows a few of the hormones that are activated to promote bonding behaviors.

**TABLE 3-1** Hormones Involved in Parental Bonding Behaviors (Anestis, 2010)

| Hormone | Target tissues | Principal physiological actions | Principal behavioral actions |
|---|---|---|---|
| Oxytocin | Brain, uterus, mammary tissues | Responsible for milk letdown response, and uterine contraction during labor | The "bonding" hormone; associated with maternal and affiliative behaviors in mammals |
| Vasopressin | Brain, kidneys | Involved in water retention and regulation | Involved in pair bonding; often considered the male counterpart to oxytocin |
| Prolactin | Mammary glands, brain | Responsible for milk production in lactation | The "parenting" hormone; associated with parental behavior in females and males in some mammals |

The hormones that are released during labor and delivery may have long-term benefits as well. A recent study suggests that they may alleviate any long-term pain a woman would otherwise feel as a result of the physiological changes that happen during pregnancy and childbirth (Eisenach et al., 2013).

Men who become fathers experience hormone changes, too. Animal studies across many species of primates show an increase in prolactin, whereas both human and other male primates show a decrease in testosterone after childbirth. Men also show hormonal responses to infant cries much like women do (Anestis, 2010). Lower levels of testosterone appear to be somewhat stable, as testosterone levels tend to be lower for men who are fathers compared with those who are not. In addition, fathers who are involved in daily caregiving of their young children, and whose daily caregiving is valued by their partners, show lower levels of prolactin, compared with fathers who spend less time involved in daily caregiving (Gettler, McDade, Agustin, & Kuzawa, 2011; Gettler, McDade, Feranil, & Kuzawa, 2011).

## Fourth Stage: Labor and Delivery Complications

"Failure to progress" is a general term used when the mother does not progress at any time during the first stage of childbirth (Ness et al., 2005). "**Dystocia**" is a more specific term that means abnormal or difficult labor and delivery, when labor progress slows and eventually stops. Dystocia occurs when the latent phase lasts longer than 20 hours for women who are primiparae but 14 hours for those who are multiparae. Dystocia in the active phase of labor occurs in 25% of women giving birth for the first time and 15% of those who have given birth before (Ness et al., 2005). Dystocia may be caused by the maternal age (older than 35) and hypertension, fetal weight (more than 4 kg or roughly 9 pounds), labor induction, and fertility treatments.

"Active phase arrest" occurs when the cervix is at least 4 centimeters dilated but there is no change in dilation for 2 hours. In countries where medically assisted births are the norm, a health care provider may recommend the woman be given oxytocin and/or have her membranes ruptured (if they have not already done so) to facilitate labor progress. Some may recommend a **cesarean delivery** at this stage. In a study conducted on women who experienced active phase arrest, 33% went on to have a vaginal delivery, whereas 67% had a cesarean delivery. There were no differences between the two groups on infant outcomes (Henry et al., 2008).

Other common complications include breech births, when the head is not in an appropriate position to pass through the birth canal, and instances when the fetus fails to descend through the birth canal. If the fetus is under stress from a prolonged labor, or because of certain health problems the woman may experience during pregnancy (gestational diabetes, high blood pressure), they are at a higher risk for expelling meconium during the delivery process and inhaling it along with amniotic fluid. When this occurs, intervention may be necessary immediately following birth to clear the infant's airway.

Many obstetricians do not allow the second stage of childbirth to last longer than 1 to 3 hours, depending on whether the woman has previously given birth and whether she received an epidural. Complications during the second stage should be addressed as they can lead to increased risks, both short and long term, and in rare cases may result in the death of the woman or the fetus (Ness et al., 2005).

**A partner's birth experiences.** Much of what we know about a partner's experiences of childbirth focuses on male partners in opposite-sex relationships. Partners are much more likely to be present during childbirth now, especially in many industrialized areas of the world. A partner's role in the childbirth process varies considerably, from a more passive observer to an active birth coach.

Researchers and health care providers tend to view the partner as a support for the woman and are less concerned with the partner's experience of the birth process. Likewise, the focus of childbirth both prior to and during the event is largely on the woman who is giving birth. Given this, some men feel their needs go unmet or are underprioritized (Plantin et al., 2011). Nevertheless, most men who are present during childbirth report that it is a positive experience. They feel they are able to support the woman and that she benefited from the their presence (Porrett et al., 2013).

# Variations in Childbirth

**LO 3-3** **What are some of the procedures commonly used to facilitate birth if complications arise?**

**LO 3-4** **What are common maternal and fetal complications?**

There are many ways that a woman can give birth, from the person who performs the delivery and where it is performed, to techniques for facilitating the birthing process. For example, in the United States, even though less than 1% of births happen in the home, it is a growing trend among women. In the 1960s, when many of your parents were born, partners were not allowed in the birthing room at a hospital, but now that is the norm.

In most industrialized societies, women and their health care providers come up with a preliminary birthing plan that is dependent on the health of the women and the fetus. However, not all labors go according to plan, and sometimes adjustments must be made for the health of the woman and the fetus. A few of these variations are discussed next.

## Health Care Providers and Environments

There are a variety of health care providers who may aid in childbirth, including obstetricians, obstetric nurses, midwives, and doulas. Obstetricians hold medical degrees and are trained to provide care for the woman throughout the pregnancy and during delivery. They are typically affiliated with a hospital where the woman receives care and will deliver the infant. Some may specialize in high-risk pregnancies or certain conditions such as gestational diabetes. Obstetrical nurses receive obstetrics training and provide care in a hospital or clinic setting during pregnancy, labor, and delivery. Midwives are health care providers who are typically certified and licensed and are trained to provide basic care in low-risk situations for pregnant women and during childbirth. Midwives tend to intervene less with the natural processes of childbirth but are trained to recognize when medical attention is necessary. Nurse-midwives have training in both obstetrical nursing and midwifery and are typically affiliated with hospitals, much like doctors and nurses. However, they provide care more in line with the practices of midwifery. A doula is yet another practitioner who may work with a woman during pregnancy and be present during childbirth and who provides continuous, nonmedical, and emotional support.

**Hospital births.** Prior to the 20th century, childbirth typically occurred at home, which is currently the practice in many countries worldwide. However, most women in industrialized parts of the world now give birth in hospitals. In the United States, when a woman should go to the hospital once labor begins varies based on the health care provider's recommendations, the woman's medical history, and how the beginning stages of labor progress (for example, how much discomfort she's feeling, how far apart and how long the contractions are, or how dilated she is).

The length of a hospital stay after childbirth has also changed. In the 1950s, women in the United States would be hospitalized for anywhere from 8 to 14 days after childbirth (Weiss et al., 2004). The American Academy of Pediatrics (AAP) now recommends that "the hospital stay of the mother and her healthy term newborn infant should be long enough to allow identification of early problems and to ensure that the family is able and prepared to care for the infant at home" (Committee on Fetus and Newborn, 2004). In the United States, it is advised that a woman with a routine labor and delivery stay in the hospital for at least 48 hours. The purpose of this is to allow the woman adequate recovery time, to perform necessary tests, to ensure the infant is feeding and that the woman feels confident and capable of returning home, as well as to ensure that an appropriate support system is in place for the woman. A woman who delivers via cesarean should be allowed adequate surgical recovery time and will likely stay for an additional 48 hours.

In the United States, certain women are more likely to be discharged from the hospital early (prior to 48 hours). And it appears that some of the most vulnerable are sent home the earliest. Multiparae women tend to leave the hospital earlier. Young women, those from low socioeconomic status backgrounds, and those insured through publicly funded health insurance programs are most likely to be discharged from the hospital between 18 and 30 hours after giving birth. Meanwhile, a woman who is White, married, and who lives with the infant's father is likely to have a longer hospital stay (Weiss et al., 2004). Researchers have found that women who were not ready to go home when they were discharged were more likely to return to the hospital with their infant for medically necessary reasons within the 1st month after childbirth and believe that this accounts for added, unnecessary health costs and potentially avoidable risks to the woman and infant (Bernstein et al., 2013).

Being born is the most common reason for a child's hospitalization in the United States. It is also the most expensive childhood condition. A newborn's stay in the hospital, without complications, costs roughly $1,700. With complications, the expense jumps to $13,600, on average. However, 92% of newborn stays in United States are billed to either publicly funded or private health insurance (Podulka et al., 2011), minimizing the out-of-pocket expenses that need to be paid.

**Birthing centers.** Birthing centers are facilities that provide an atmosphere more similar to the home than a hospital for women experiencing normal pregnancies. They are staffed by obstetricians, nurses, midwives, and doulas who may assist a woman during labor with more varied practices, including water births. Doulas allow more people, including friends and family, to be present during the birth. Should complications arise, a birthing center is prepared to transport the woman to the hospital for more advanced care. Research shows that there is no increase in mortality rates for the woman or infant at birthing centers. In addition, those who utilize birthing centers are less likely to have medical intervention (for example, epidurals, episiotomies, the use of vacuum extractors or forceps), tend to be more satisfied with the birth experience, and tend to be discharged earlier (often around 6 hours after the infant's birth) than those who give birth in hospitals (Wax et al., 2010).

**Planned home births.** Worldwide, most births occur outside a hospital setting and typically inside the home. In industrialized areas, where hospital births are now the norm, another option for those who would prefer a more natural experience is a planned home birth. Midwives typically supervise home births. During the labor and delivery process, midwives periodically check the vital signs of the woman and the fetus. Midwives may also provide basic care and treatment such as oxygen or certain homeopathic remedies. After delivery, both the woman and infant are examined to determine whether either needs to be evaluated in the hospital. As in birthing centers, if there are complications with the labor, the woman will be advised to go to the hospital. Of course, there are risks that coincide with home births. However, research shows that for many women with good medical histories, without pregnancy complications, and without labor complications, who can also be quickly transported to a hospital should complications arise, the risk for neonatal complications including death is only slightly higher than those who have hospital births (van der Kooy et al., 2011).

In industrialized areas, there are a number of factors that influence where a woman will give birth and the practices employed during labor and delivery. In other places, however, where a woman gives birth can influence how birth complications are addressed and is associated with certain socioeconomic and social justice factors such as women's access to education and access to care (Stephenson et al., 2006).

**FIGURE 3-3** Harry was the last born of his mother's three children. He was delivered via a planned home birth after only 1 hour and 20 minutes of active labor and less than 10 minutes of "pushing." He came out so fast that he didn't get a good "squeeze" passing through the birth canal, leaving a bit of fluid in his lungs. He was born at 9 p.m., loud and red with a perfect Apgar score. Around 11 p.m. the midwife and family noticed that he wasn't breathing properly. They arrived at the hospital at 11:30 p.m., where he was intubated and his lungs were suctioned over the next several hours. By morning, the tube was removed; he was breathing fine and nursing.

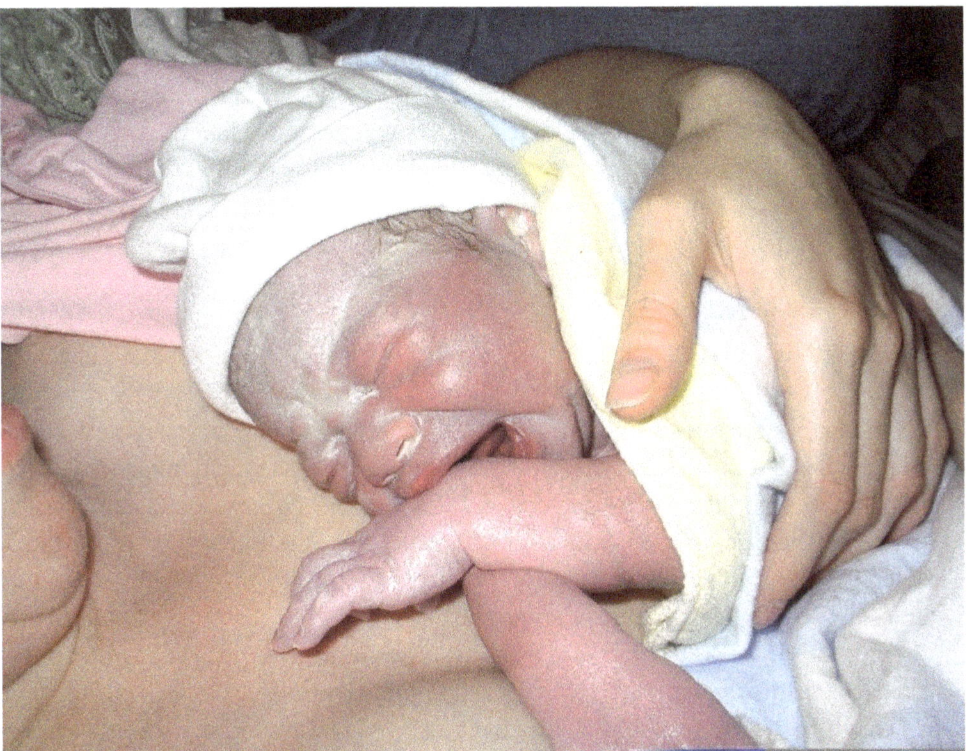

*Source*: Copyright © Jenney Cheever. Reprinted with permission.

## Labor Induction

**Labor induction** may occur through the use of medication or various procedures to promote the onset of labor and is most often done in cases where a woman is more than 2 weeks past her due date or there is risk to the woman or the fetus. However, there are some who opt for medically induced labor out of convenience. Two of the most common ways to induce labor are through the administration of Pitocin (a form of oxytocin) and through artificial rupture of the membranes. Current statistics suggest that 22% of hospital births are medically induced, and the jury is still out on the risks and benefits of labor induction (Janakiraman et al., 2010; Mozurkewich et al., 2011). However, in cases where it is not medically necessary, the practice is linked to increased risk for a cesarean delivery and infant treatment in neonatal intensive care. Labor is often more painful when artificially induced, and because of this, women who have induced labor are more likely to receive epidurals (Lancaster et al., 2012). Given this, health care providers agree that nonmedically necessary labor induction should be avoided (Grivell et al., 2012; Thorsell et al., 2011). Although, it seems that many factors, most importantly gestational age, play a role in outcomes for women whose labors are medically induced.

A less invasive procedure that can be done in a health care provider's office is stripping the membranes that connect that amniotic sac to the uterine wall, causing the body to release hormones that may help induce labor. Lastly, there is little scientific evidence demonstrating the effectiveness of other ways to induce labor, but some suggest that sexual intercourse, walking, herbs, and certain types of food may increase a woman's likelihood of going into labor.

## Cesarean Delivery

Cesarean deliveries, also known as cesarean sections or C-sections, are performed when there is a preexisting medical condition or a pregnancy complication that may further complicate labor and delivery. It is the most common major surgery for women in the United States (MacDorman et al., 2011). Alternatively, it is performed when problems arise during labor and delivery that may put the woman's or the fetus's life in danger. It requires a surgical incision in the abdomen of the woman to remove the fetus and the placenta from the uterus and is accompanied most often by local anesthesia so that the woman is fully conscious.

Globally, the World Health Organization (WHO) estimated that in 2008, of the approximate 129 million births worldwide, roughly 18.5 million cesarean deliveries were performed. This report also found that some countries underutilized the procedure to the detriment of women and children (Gibbons et al., 2010). In fact, countries that underutilized the procedure had higher infant and maternal mortality rates (Volpe, 2011). However, many countries around the world overused the procedure, and the WHO reported that 6.2 million cesarean deliveries were unnecessary. Of the countries assessed, Chad and Burkina Faso, both located on the African continent, had the lowest rates (.4% and .7%, respectively), whereas Brazil and Italy had the highest rates (46% and 38%, respectively) (Gibbons et al., 2010). In 2010, approximately 33% of all childbirths in the United States were via cesarean deliveries (Hamilton et al., 2011). The risk for maternal and fetal mortality is low in cases of cesarean delivery in developed countries, especially when the gestational age of the fetus is greater than 39 weeks. However, a risk for surgical complications remains that doesn't exist for women who give birth vaginally (Delbaere et al., 2012). Because of this, experts caution against nonmedically necessary cesarean deliveries.

## Adoption

> **Myths and Misconceptions**
>
> Roman emperor Julius Caesar was born via cesarean section. **Myth**
>
> Cesarean sections were practiced in ancient Rome prior to the birth of Gaius Julius Caesar. They were part of Roman law so that the fetus could be cut from a woman who had died during childbirth. **Fact**
>
> There are many myths and legends across cultures worldwide related to cesarean sections. However, the first modern cesarean section was performed in 1826 in South Africa. Both the mother and the child survived. In 1996, roughly around the time many of today's young college students were born, the rate of C-section births was almost 21%, and in 2010 it was around 33% (Martin et al., 2011).

There are a number of reasons why a person, couple, or family may choose to adopt, including same-sex relationships, infertility, to help a specific child, or because of issues related to social justice (Child Welfare Information Gateway, 2010). Working in conjunction with an agency or a social worker, there is often a long waiting period. Along with this there is a rigorous screening process for the prospective adoptive parent(s) that includes motivations to adopt, family backgrounds, and personal and financial resources, as well as home evaluations.

For some adoptive families, the birth of a healthy child does not necessarily mean that baby will go home with the adoptive parents. Laws differ from state to state in the United States and from country to country to protect the best interests of the child, as well as those who are placing the child up for adoption. In many cases, those who are placing the child for adoption have the opportunity to change their minds about the adoption arrangement well after the infant is born, so long as legal documents have not been signed. If the prospective adoptive parent has already met the child, this can be devastating.

In the end, most adoptive parents are happy with their decision to adopt, regardless of the challenges they may face during the process. However, they may experience many of the same issues other new parents do, such as post-adoption depression syndrome (PADS), much like other new parents face postpartum depression, which we will discuss later (Child Welfare Information Gateway, 2010).

## Unexpected Outcomes

We've presented expected variations in childbirth experiences above. Now we turn to those cases that may require special planning prior to or during childbirth. Approximately 9 out of 10 births have some kind of complication, but they vary in their type and severity as well as outcomes for the woman and child.

**Twins.** In most cases, so long as there are no complications, nonconjoined twins can be delivered vaginally. However, there are some cases in which the first twin is born vaginally, but the second twin is born through cesarean delivery.

**FIGURE 3-4** Will and Katie's mom, Joanne went into labor at 38 weeks pregnant. Will was born first, vaginally, at 11:45 p.m. on August 1st. Then, while still in labor, Joanne's cervix closed. Katie, who was not born yet, was in distress—doctors lost her heart beat and then found that it was falling fast. Joanne was sedated for an emergency cesarean section. Katie was then born at 12:15 a.m. on August 2nd. Will was 7 pounds and 21 inches, and Katie was 4 pounds, 13 ounces, and 19 inches. Since then Will has always been 20 pounds heavier and 2 inches taller. Now, at 17, their mom says, "they have both grown into amazing young adults with hopes and dreams of the future!".

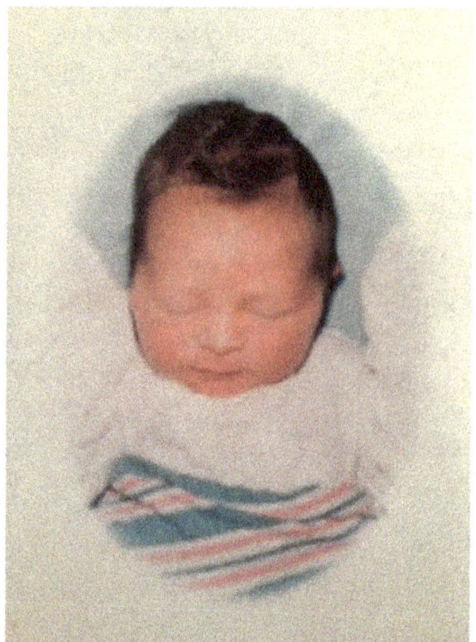

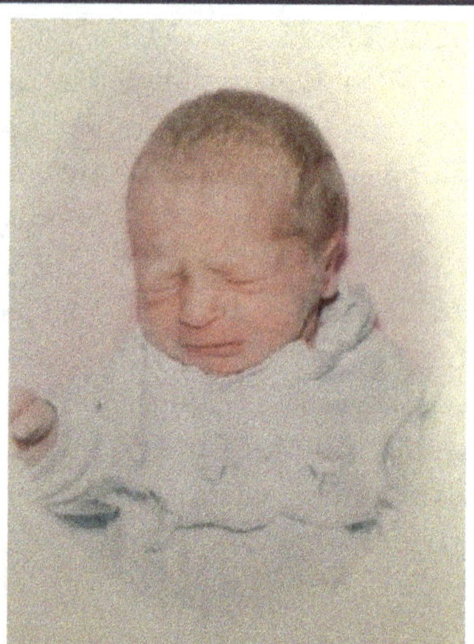

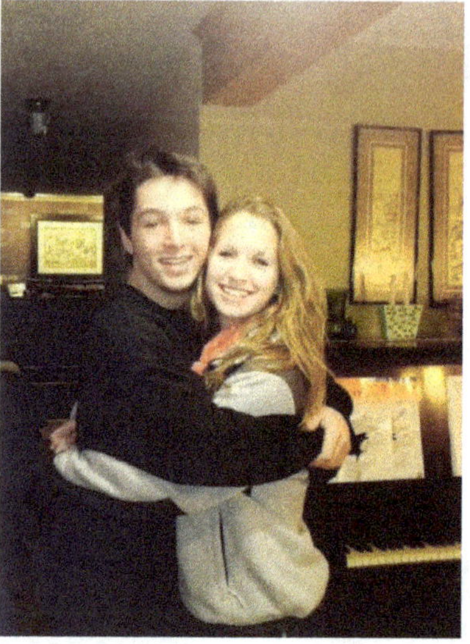



**Maternal complications.** Childbirth can lead to complications and injuries such as vaginal tears that may result in mild infections, long-term incontinence problems, and many other things. However, maternal infection and hemorrhage after childbirth are the major causes of maternal mortality, especially in developing countries. Infections can easily be treated with good hygiene and close monitoring to detect and treat a problem if necessary. If the normal bleeding that occurs after childbirth becomes severe, oxytocin can be administered to help stop blood loss. Virtually all maternal deaths (99%) occur in developing countries, and the disparities between developed and developing countries are staggering (16 maternal deaths per 100,000 births versus 240 per 100,000 births, respectively). Half of maternal deaths occur in sub-Saharan Africa whereas one third occur in South Asia. There are marked differences in maternal mortality rates within these countries as well, depending on factors such as maternal income and the location of the birth (urban versus rural) (World Health Organization, 2012).

**Fetal complications.** Most complications that result in fetal injuries do not have long-term implications for the infant. Like maternal complications, they can be relatively mild if treated properly, such as a laceration or hematoma due to instrument delivery. However, more severe complications can arise due to sexually transmitted infections in the woman, as well as neonatal death due to labor and delivery complications, such as a lack of oxygen to the fetus. Worldwide, four million infants die within 4 weeks of birth of the roughly 130 million infants born every year, with the majority of these deaths occurring within the first 24 hours. The most common fetal complication resulting in neonatal death is preterm birth (Centers for Disease Control and Prevention, 2019).

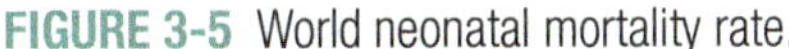

**FIGURE 3-5** World neonatal mortality rate.

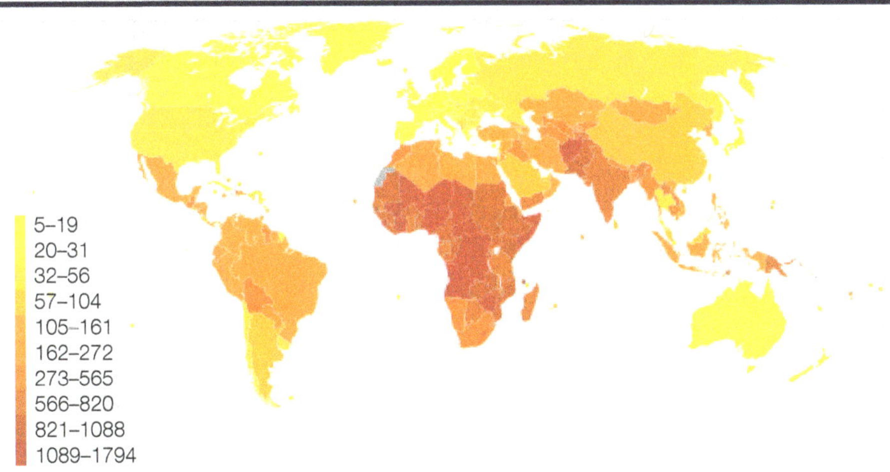


Statistics from WHO (2019) for neonatal conditions. Death per million persons grouped by deciles

The following groupings/assumptions were made:

- France includes the overseas departments as well as overseas collectivities.
- The United Kingdom includes the Crown dependencies as well as the overseas territories.
- The United States of America includes the insular areas.
- The Netherlands includes Aruba and the Netherlands Antilles.
- Denmark includes Greenland and the Faroe islands.

*Source*: Copyright © Chris55 (CC BY-SA 4.0) at https://commons.wikimedia.org/wiki/File:Neonatal_conditions_world_map-Deaths_per_million_persons-WHO2012.svg.

Like maternal mortality rates, there are great differences worldwide in neonatal mortality rates. For example, infant mortality rates for babies who are full term (37 weeks or after in gestational age) are higher in the United States than in many countries in Europe. However, this comparatively high rate of infant mortality is linked with the higher percentage of preterm births in the United States. For example, 1 in 18 births in Ireland and Iceland is preterm whereas 1 in 8 births in the United States is preterm (MacDorman & Mathews, 2010).

**Preterm births.** According to the Centers for Disease Control, **preterm birth** or premature birth is broadly defined as a birth that occurs before 37 weeks. It is further broken down into late preterm (between 36 to 37 weeks), moderately preterm (between 32 and 36 weeks), and very preterm birth (earlier than 32 weeks). Depending on gestational age the outcomes for preterm infants, including survival rate, can differ dramatically. Those born very preterm are at risk for intellectual disabilities, cerebral palsy, as well as breathing, digestive, feeing, visual, and hearing problems. Other highly treatable risks for those born preterm include jaundice and low blood sugar (Centers for Disease Control and Prevention, 2013e).

**Postterm births.** A **postterm birth** occurs after the 42nd week of pregnancy and are prevalent in up to 10% of all pregnancies (Gulmezoglu et al., 2006). The major concern for postterm births is that after time the placenta begins to degrade while inside the woman's uterus. There are some risks for the woman, mainly related to labor and delivery. One common feature of infants who are delivered postterm is noticeably cracked skin (Warren & Phillipi, 2012). This is due to placental aging, so the infant's skin is lacking vernix, an oily, cheesy-looking substance that surrounds the fetus prenatally to keep their skin moisturized. Postterm birth is associated with increased neonatal risks such as meconium inhalation, low Apgar scores, and mortality. One study recently found that postterm birth was also associated with problems in early childhood such as attention deficit hyperactivity and risk for obesity after the age of 12 (Beltrand et al., 2012; El Marroun et al., 2012). A relatively easy way to avoid postterm birth is through artificially induced labor. Research suggests that women should be offered this option between 41 and 42 weeks. Additionally, women who are postterm should have additional maternal and fetal monitoring as pregnancy progresses postterm and during labor (Gulmezoglu et al., 2012).

# The Newborn

**LO 3-5** **What kinds of reflexive behaviors do infants demonstrate?**

**LO 3-6** **What are the various methods that caregivers use for feeding infants?**

The months of planning and waiting are over and the baby is here. What should practitioners and parents expect? There are certain behaviors we expect from the newborn over the first few minutes, hours, and days that signal they are healthy and developing as expected.

# Infant Capacities and Behaviors

Next we describe the ways in which we evaluate the newborn immediately following birth and the reflexive behaviors we expect to see in the early months of his life.

**Apgar score.** An **Apgar score** is named after Dr. Virginia Apgar who developed a quick, standardized method for assessing newborn breathing and heart functions. The test is performed at 1 and 5 minutes after birth. The 1-minute score provides an assessment of how the infant tolerated the transition from the uterine environment through the birthing process. The 5-minute score provides an indication of how well the infant is adjusting outside the uterine environment. The infant is scored in five categories on a scale of 0 to 2 and the test yields a total score of 0 to 10, with higher scores indicating better functioning (see Table 3-2). Most infants score between 7 and 9. Infants with scores lower than 7 require immediate medical attention, including oxygen and physical stimulation to get the heart beating normally. Using an Apgar score may be difficult for infants who are premature, who have congenital defects, or who have been exposed to drugs. The Apgar score can also stand for appearance, pulse, grimace, activity, and respiration.

**TABLE 3-2** Apgar Scores

| | 0 | 1 | 2 |
|---|---|---|---|
| Color | Pale or blue all over | Body pink, extremities blue | Body and extremities pink |
| Heart Rate | Absent | Slow (<100) | Fast (≥100) |
| Reflex Irritability (response to stimulation of sole of foot) | None | Grimace/feeble cry when stimulated | Grimacing and strong cry, cough, or sneeze |
| Muscle Tone | Limp, loose, floppy | Some flexion of extremities | Active motion/well-flexed arms and legs that resist extension |
| Respiratory Effort | Absent | Weak cry, slow or irregular breathing, gasping | Strong, lusty cry |

**Reflexes.** The newborn comes into the world with a set of reflexive actions rooted in the central nervous system that may be spontaneous or in response to stimuli that have an immediate survival value to the infant (rooting to obtain food), whereas others are more primitive and are no longer useful for the contemporary human (the grasping reflex to hold on to a fast-moving mother). Table 3-3 provides a list of some well-known reflexes. Most reflexes diminish across early childhood as the frontal lobe develops, so they are no longer observable in healthy adults. However, they may still appear in cases where there is neurological damage (cerebral palsy, traumatic brain lesions, strokes, and dementia). It is believed the lack of some reflexes and the continuation of others after they would otherwise normally diminish may be indicators of autism spectrum disorder (Gallese et al., 2013).

**TABLE 3-3** Infant Reflexes

| Reflex and when it occurs | Behavior | Emerges | Declines | Adaptive Purpose |
|---|---|---|---|---|
| **Moro reflex/startle reflex/embrace reflex**<br>When the infant is startled by a loud noise, sudden change in head position, or temperature change | The infant will extend his arms, legs and head, then pull back in his arms and legs, clench his fists and cry | Birth, peaks in the 1st month | Up to 6 months | Helps infant cling to a caregiver for safety |
| **Positive support reflex**<br>When the infant is held upright with the soles of the feet touching a solid surface | The infant will straighten his legs for 20 to 30 seconds | Birth | Around 4 months | Remerges as a voluntary response around 6 months to promote standing |
| **Step reflex/walking reflex/dance reflex**<br>When the infant is held upright with the soles of the feet touching a solid surface | The infant will appear to "walk" or "dance" | Birth | Around 4 months | Remerges as a voluntary response around 8 months to promote walking |
| **Rooting reflex/search reflex**<br>When the infant's mouth or cheek is stroked or touched by something | The infant will turn his head in the direction of the stimulus and open his mouth to search for the object | Birth | Around 4 months | In combination with the sucking reflex it helps the infant breastfeed and gradually becomes a voluntary response |
| **Suck reflex**<br>When the roof of the infant's mouth is touched | The infant will begin to suck | Birth | 2 months | In combination with the rooting reflex it helps the infant breastfeed and gradually becomes a voluntary response |

| Reflex and when it occurs | Behavior | Emerges | Declines | Adaptive Purpose |
|---|---|---|---|---|
| **Asymmetrical tonic neck reflex/fencing reflex**<br>When the face is turned to one side | The infant will extend the arm on the side to which to head is turned while the arm on the other side bends and the fist clenches | Birth to 1 month | 4 months | Promotes the development of hand-eye coordination and the ability to voluntarily reach |
| **Tonic labyrinthine (inner ear) prone reflex**<br>When the infant is placed on his stomach | The infant will tuck his head toward the chest and pull his knees in and under | 1 to 2 months | Up to 4 months | Promotes muscle development |
| **Palmar reflex/grasp reflex**<br>When the infant's hand is stroked | The infant will strongly grip the object in his hand | Birth | 6 months | Helps infant cling to a caregiver for safety |
| **Plantar reflex**<br>When an object touches the sole of the infant's foot (when CNS pathology is present, this is called the Babinski reflex) | The infant's foot will point down and his toes will curl or the foot will point up and the toes will fan | Birth | 1 year | Due to underdeveloped parts of the CNS |
| **Galant reflex**<br>When the side of the infant's back is stroked | The infant will flex toward the side that is stroked | Birth | Around 6 months | Promotes muscle development |
| **Swimming reflex**<br>When an infant is placed faced down in a pool of water | The infant will paddle and kick | Birth | 6 months | Potential survival mechanism prior to terrestrial life |

**Other behaviors.** The newborn infant possesses a range of capacities beyond reflexive behaviors to engage and disengage with the environment (see Table 3-4). Newborn infants can show alertness and attention to their surroundings by widening the eyes and focusing on a stimulus such as an object or a noise. They can react to objects in close proximity to the face, along with voices and sounds in the environment. However, they can also become accustomed to and relatively unaffected by certain stimuli after repeated exposure, say to a loud noise such as a dog barking or a vacuum cleaner. They can also move spontaneously and in response to what they perceive in the environment. The newborn also possesses capacities for cuddling and being consoled by nestling into the contours of a caregiver's body and to lower their state of arousal. They also possess self-soothing behaviors that include moving their hands to their mouths, sucking on objects, or changing positions to alleviate any distress (March of Dimes, 2003).

**TABLE 3-4** An Infant's Signals for Engagement and Disengagement (Hotelling, 2004)

| Engagement Cues | Disengagement Cues |
|---|---|
| Your infant wants to communicate with you when they: | Your infant wants a rest from brain activity when they: |
| • Stop moving | • Turn head away |
| • Gaze intently at your face | • Cry, become fussy |
| • Have smooth arm and leg movements | • Burp, hicup, pass gas |
| • Reach out to you | • Have droopy eyelids |
| • Turn head or eyes toward you | • Arch their back |
| • Stretch fingers or toes toward you | • Fall asleep |
| • Slow or stop sucking activity | • Squirm or kick |
| • Smile | • Have pale or red skin |
| • Coo | • Turn eyes away |
| • Begin babbling/talking | • Exhibit fast breathing |
| • Have eyes wide open | • Yawn |
| • Exhibit a brightened face | • Wrinkle forehead |
| • Raise head | • Have dull-looking eyes |
| | • Frown |
| | • Place hand to mouth |

Source: Barbara A. Hotelling, from "Newborn Capabilities: Parent Teaching Is a Necessity," The Journal of Perinatal Education, vol. 13, no. 4. 

# Infant Feeding

Advice on infant feeding in Western countries has varied over the past century. In the 1940s and 1950s, formula feeding was widely popular in the United States. Breastfeeding declined until the 1970s when it experienced a resurgence a steady increase ever since (Fomon, 2001). The standard recommendation by most health care providers is to encourage the mother and infant to breastfeed within the 1st hour of birth, and have the infant sleep in the same room as the mother, as opposed to in a nursery room (Warren & Phillipi, 2012). The AAP reports that roughly 75% of women in the United States breastfeed initially (Section on Breastfeeding, 2012). However, rates vary according to sociodemographics and cultural norms. Eighty percent of Hispanic and Latino women breastfeed after the birth of their child, yet only 58% of African American women do. Lower-income mothers breastfeed at a rate of 67%, whereas higher-income mothers breastfeed at a rate of 84%. Mothers who are younger than 20 breastfeed at a lower rate than mothers who are older than 30, and single women are less likely to breastfeed compared with married women (Brand et al., 2011).

**Breastfeeding.** Many health care providers, along with the AAP, now recommend exclusive breastfeeding through 6 months of age without the use of supplemental formula or foods, as research demonstrates a link between formula feeding and the development of allergies, type II diabetes, and obesity (Stevens et al., 2009). Additionally, the WHO (2002b) recommends breastfeeding for the first 2 years of a child's life. Because of this, hospitals and health care providers make extensive efforts to promote breastfeeding among new mothers in their care.

The benefits of breastfeeding appear to be far-reaching. Not only is it cost effective, depending on the duration and exclusivity of breastfeeding, it is associated with lower risk for hospitalizations due to respiratory tract infections, lower risk for gastrointestinal tract infections, and inflammatory bowel disease, leukemia, type I and type II diabetes, celiac disease, asthma, eczema, obesity, and sudden infant death syndrome (SIDS) in young children. There are benefits for the mother as well, such as better recovery after birth, decreased postpartum depression, and weight loss (Section on Breastfeeding, 2012).

**Alternatives to breastfeeding.** Of course, there are some who cannot breastfeed because their bodies do not produce enough breast milk to sustain the infant. There are also women who should not breastfeed for a number of health reasons, including untreated tuberculosis, H1N1 influenza, HIV, and drug addiction. Mothers who drink should use caution when breastfeeding and should wait 2 hours after having an alcoholic beverage before breastfeeding, and those who smoke should not breastfeed as it is associated with SIDS. There are certain medications that mothers may take that are not safe for the baby while breastfeeding, such as aspirin in high doses and certain cholesterol-lowering medications (Section on Breastfeeding, 2012).

There are other barriers to breastfeeding. Adoptive parents have a more obvious barrier as breast milk is typically not an available resource for them. It is also the case that some women never start to breastfeed, whereas others stop after a short time for a variety of reasons, such as challenges with the baby's ability to latch on to the nipple or potential allergic reactions to breast milk. Some women do not to breastfeed out of personal choice. Researchers and health care providers acknowledge that there are circumstances when a mother cannot breastfeed and that a parent's well-informed opinion should be respected (Committee on Fetus and Newborn, 2004).

One study on a diverse sample of American women showed a number of reasons why they did not initiate breastfeeding, including preference for bottle feeding, job schedule, physical or medical problems, refusal by the infant, and not knowing how to breastfeed. Similar reasons were given for why others stopped, including the mother's milk supply being inadequate, difficulty latching, and pain (Brand et al., 2011;

Taylor et al., 2003). Other factors, such as social support from family, partners, and health care providers, along with cultural norms on breastfeeding, influence a mother's decision whether to breastfeed and when to stop (Hofvander, 2003). However, what is less well understood is the interaction of these decisions with demographic, economic, social, and psychological factors. For example, self-efficacy and social support (both personal and professional support) combined may impact a mother's reluctance to start breastfeeding and decision to stop early (Brand et al., 2011). Likewise, the need to return to work for some mothers may necessitate bottle feeding.

**FIGURE 3-6** A picture of baby Rowan being bottle fed by his big sister Charlie. Rowan is the third of three children, and his mother, a married, 44-year-old White/European American woman who holds a doctorate in child and family policy, did not breastfeed any of them. She tried breastfeeding with her oldest son but was only able to produce small amounts of milk during feedings. After a month of trying, and struggling with postpartum depression made worse by her failed efforts at breastfeeding, she finally gave up. Given this, she did not try to breastfeed at all with her second and third babies.

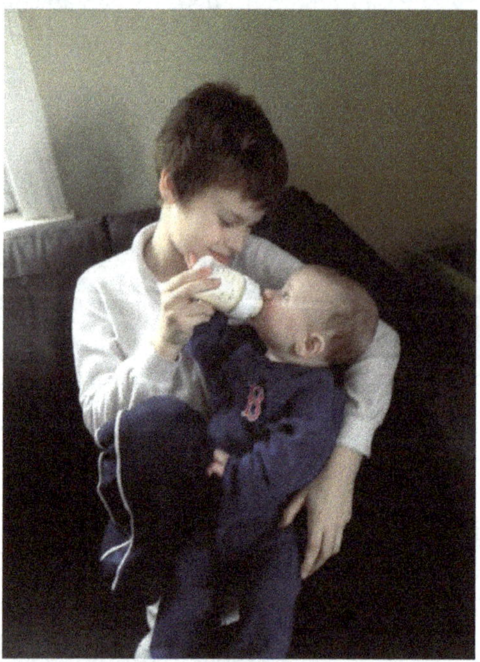



Current laws in the United States say women may breastfeed anywhere. It is forbidden, however, in some countries and cultures, and it is not uncommon for people to object to women breastfeeding in public. For example, in 2012 a mother was asked to move when she began breastfeeding her 7-month-old child outside a popular mall store known for advertisements with bikini-clad young women and shirtless young men in low-hanging pants (Huffington Post, 2013).

**Voiding.** The infant will void a meconium stool and urinate typically within the first 24 hours. Meconium stools are blackish in color, and as the infant begins to feed, stools become a mustard yellow color (Warren & Phillipi, 2012).

## Infant Sleep

One of the first adjustments to the routines of new parents is their sleep schedules. Newborn babies can sleep between 10 and 18 hours a day, that are typically broken up into smaller chunks lasting anywhere from 30 minutes to 3 hours. Some infants sleep more during the day and less at night, which can cause stress for any new parent. There is little we can do to predict how a baby will sleep early on, but patterns begin to emerge between 4 and 6 weeks. At the same time, a new parent shouldn't be alarmed by variations in these patterns even well beyond the first few months of life.

The National Sleep Foundation recommends that daily sleep schedules be established between 2 and 3 months to coincide with the child's natural sleep/wake rhythms as best as possible. Bedtime rituals such as baths, stories, or songs can help establish a routine and signal that it is almost time for bed. The National Sleep Foundation recommends infants be put into their cribs when they are drowsy and not fully asleep as much as possible to develop self-soothing skills to put themselves to sleep. They also recommend that an infant should be in her permanent sleeping arrangement by 3 months and transitioned from a crib to a regular bed between 2 and 3½ years to avoid sleep problems. The sooner the baby develops a normal sleep pattern, the sooner the parent will be able to return to a normal sleep pattern (Mindell, 2020).

There are many factors that play a role in parent and infant sleep in the early days, including biological rhythms, environmental cues, cultural practices, parental beliefs and emotions, and infant behaviors. However it is important to remember that these links are bidirectional, so as much as parental and environmental factors influence the baby, the baby herself is affecting her parents and her environment (Sadeh et al., 2010).

**Cosleeping.** **Cosleeping** is when the parent(s) and infant sleep in close proximity (either in the same room "**room sharing**" or the same bed "**bed sharing**"). It is routinely practiced in many cultures worldwide. In the United States, roughly 60% of new mothers report bed sharing with their infant at least once 1 month after leaving the hospital, but only 9% of mothers did so by 3 months (Krouse et al., 2012).

The prevalence of cosleeping and bed-sharing practices vary worldwide. Data show that 91% of children in India cosleep at some point prior to age 6 and 80% of infants in Japan cosleep. The practice of cosleeping in these and similar countries is rooted in notions of interdependence and the belief that the child is too young to sleep alone. Mayan infants cosleep with their mothers for the 1st year of life to promote closeness between the mother and baby. In Turkey, roughly 72% of new mothers anticipate room sharing with their infants as it is a normative cultural practice. In Egypt cosleeping rates are 70%, with family members regularly sharing beds with up to four other family members. Whether this is done out of belief or necessity or both is unclear, though.

The United States and certain other Western countries have different ideas of autonomy and individualism. Therefore, solitary, self-sleeping arrangements are often promoted. In fact, the AAP recommends cosleeping in the context of room sharing, but cautions against bed sharing, which can lead to accidental suffocation of the infant. However, a recent review of the literature on bed sharing and SIDS found that parents who smoke, consume drugs or alcohol, or sleep with a baby on a sofa put their children most at risk in bed-sharing arrangements (Ball, 2009).

Still, there are many parents in America who room share or bed share with their children for a period of time. Most mothers who cosleep feel it is a positive experience of physical and emotional closeness to share with their young children (Giannotti & Cortesi, 2009). In addition to providing mothers the opportunity to bond with their infant, cosleeping may allow the parent to get more sleep, especially those mothers who are breastfeeding. Alternatively, cosleeping may lead to sleep disturbances.

**Sudden infant death syndrome (SIDS).** The most important guidelines a parent can follow for establishing a sleep routine are those related to **sudden infant death syndrome**. SIDS is the sudden death of an otherwise healthy child under the age of 1. It's most likely to occur between the ages of 2 and 4 months, in boys rather than girls, and in the winter time. The exact cause of SIDS is unknown, but many believe that it is related to sleep and a build-up of carbon dioxide in the blood (Kaneshiro & Zieve, 2011). There are several factors that increase the risk of SIDS, including sleeping on the stomach, exposure to cigarette smoke, and soft bedding. There are also several recommendations from the AAP for parents to help prevent SIDS, including putting a baby to sleep on her back, keeping the room at a low but comfortable temperature, and offering a pacifier at nap or bedtime (Task Force on Sudden Infant Death Syndrome, 2005).

## Common Procedures After a Hospital Childbirth

### LO 3-7 What types of practices, tests, and procedures do newborns typically experience in the hospital?

A pediatrician will conduct a complete examination of the infant within the first 24 hours of childbirth. Another common practice is to weigh the infant and measure both the length of the infant and his head circumference. Tracking growth at birth and throughout childhood is one of the most important indicators of newborn health. These measurements are compared with norms and rated on a percentile scale. Infants born at term who fall below the 10th percentile at birth are considered "small for gestational age," whereas those at the 90th percentile and above are considered "large for gestational age." A 10 to 12% weight loss is not uncommon during the 1st week, and healthy infants should return to their original birth weight by the first 2 weeks of life. Head circumference is measured to indicate micro- or macrocephaly, which are indicators of preexisting genetic conditions, environment toxins, or poor nutrition (Warren & Phillipi, 2012).

The AAP recommends that a core panel of 31 treatable congenital conditions be screened for just after birth (Newborn Screening Authoring Committee, 2008). Newborns will also likely receive a hearing test to check for any potential problems (Warren & Phillipi, 2012). Infants of women who use drugs during pregnancy, such as opiates, may experience, and should be monitored for, signs of withdrawal. If symptoms of withdrawal are serious, the infant is often treated in neonatal intensive care (Warren & Phillipi, 2012).

## Skin-to-Skin Contact

**Skin-to-skin contact,** or kangaroo care, is a common practice used for a variety of reasons. Skin-to-skin contact releases oxytocin in both the infant and the parent and the benefits of skin-to-skin contact are well documented. For example, researchers believe that skin-to-skin contact aids the infant following what is likely the stressful experience of being birthed (Bystrova et al., 2003). It reduces infant crying and promotes breastfeeding, interaction, and affection between the parent and infant and reduces postpartum depression and stress (de Alencar et al., 2009; Moore et al., 2007).

Skin-to-skin contact has been widely studied in preterm infants. It helps with the bonding experience, reduces potential pain experiences, and aids in their development (Feldman & Eidelman, 2003; Johnston et al., 2003; Uvnäs-Moberg, 2012). It also allows women with preterm infants to produce more breastmilk (Conde-Agudelo et al., 2003). However, there are some situations in which the benefits of skin-to-skin contact are less understood. For example, the impact that skin-to-skin contact can have on adoptive parents and infants is notably understudied (Parker & Anderson, 2002).

Newborns are prone to heat loss, which can be both stressful for the infant and cause her to deplete fat stores, therefore, skin-to-skin contact can also keep a newborn warm (Warren & Phillipi, 2012). A radiant warmer may be used in the event that skin-to-skin contact is not possible, or not sufficient to keep the infant warm. Likewise, many infants are swaddled after childbirth to keep them warm.

## Vaccinations and Medications

There has been much controversy in recent years about potential risks of vaccinations in the early weeks, months, and years of a child's life. However, there are no scientific studies that show evidence for the harm of vaccines on children's medical, psychological or behavioral outcomes. The Centers for Disease Control and Prevention recommends that young children receive a series of immunizations to protect against hepatitis A and B, tetanus, whooping cough, polio, influenza, chicken pox, measles, mumps, and rubella (among others) during the period between birth and the first 15 months, as contracting any of these can be life-threatening. It is also standard procedure among hospitals to administer certain medications such as vitamin K to promote blood clotting in the infant, given that they do not possess an adequate amount of gut flora to produce vitamin K, and eye ointments to prevent potential infection (Warren & Phillipi, 2012).

## Male Circumcision

**Male circumcision**, a surgical procedure in which the foreskin of the penis is removed, occurs in 59% of male newborns, making it the most common procedure for newborns, with vaccinations and immunizations the second most common medical procedure performed on newborns (Owens et al., 2003). Male circumcision is less common in Europe and Asia, whereas in the United States, male circumcision rates have declined roughly 10% over the past 30 years (Owings et al., 2013). The medical benefits of male circumcision are debated and the American Academy of Pediatrics recommends that parents make their own decision based on cultural and religious beliefs. However the World Health Organization (2013b) encourages male circumcision in developing countries, as it helps reduce the spread of infectious diseases including HIV.

# Adjusting to Caring for a Newborn

### LO 3-8 What types of experiences might new parents encounter?

The first few days and weeks of an infant's life vary from family to family and across cultures. New parents can likely expect changes in routines, sleeping patterns, and stress levels, as well as uncertainty about their abilities as parents and the baby's well-being. Nevertheless, these often occur alongside enriching opportunities for bonding and enjoyable interactions with the infant.

In the United States, infants will undoubtedly have their first well-visit with a pediatrician to ensure their health and to assess their behaviors. Certain cultures have other standards that correspond with religious traditions, such as circumcision, naming ceremonies, and baptisms. For many parents, the first few weeks and months will signal a return to work. Regulations on parental leave vary from state to state within the United States, and often depend on the employer. Family leave in other countries is often of far greater duration and is often publicly subsidized.

## Postpartum Depression

**Postpartum depression** is not uncommon. It typically emerges within the first 6 weeks after childbirth and is associated with a past history of depression, marital status, and socioeconomic status. It occurs in approximately 15% of women and 10% of men, and despite some opinions it is not more common in women who have cesarean deliveries (Marcus, 2009; Paulson & Bazemore, 2010; Sword et al., 2011).

Postpartum depression symptoms are similar to those of major depressive disorder. However, there are also symptoms of anxiety and self-doubt in parenting abilities. If postpartum depression goes untreated it can put the child at risk for poor quality parent-child interactions and disrupted feeding and sleep routines at a minimum. Parents who do not seek treatment may go on to develop more long-term psychological difficulties as well. Health care providers, including pediatricians, should be trained how to spot signs of postpartum depression, as beneficial treatments exist for those with PPD, including counseling, parent education, and parent-child interaction therapies (Field, 2010).

Postpartum depression is different from postpartum blues or "baby blues" that are more temporary symptoms, including mood swings, fatigue, irritability and tearfulness. Postpartum blues occurs in as many as 70% of women. Unlike postpartum depression, symptoms tend to go away within 10 days or so, without the need for any treatment or intervention (O'Hara & Segre, 2008). Whether the symptoms are mild or moderate, they are part of the adjustment to parenthood for both men and women, and sharing these with a health care provider can be beneficial in promoting the health and well-being of the parent as well as the child.

## Parent-Infant Attachment

During these early days, most parents will continue to develop an attachment bond with their child. **Attachment** is broadly defined as an emotional connection between individuals who share intimate relationships. It appears to serve an adaptive purpose in promoting optimal social, emotional, and physical development and well-being in the child, thus promoting the survival of the species (Ainsworth, 1967; Bowlby, 1969, 1973). Although mothers have historically been viewed as the first and primary attachment figure for infants and young children, in many cultures (and across many different species) children can become meaningfully attached to fathers, siblings, grandparents, or other critical caregivers in their lives as well (Hrdy, 1999; Tronick et al., 1992). We'll talk more about attachment in later chapters, as it becomes more fully developed and observable in infants roughly around 9 months old, and because it plays a role in a person's behaviors and well-being across the life span. For now, it is important to realize that in these early days the attachment between an infant and his caregiver(s) continues to grow and there are many newborn and parental behaviors that can promote this attachment.

# CHAPTER 4 Infancy

It can be exciting for new parents to discover what their babies can do as they grow through the first few weeks and months of life. Tables like 4-1 that describe "what most babies do" at a particular age or stage of development are often helpful for new parents as they discover the individual their child is becoming and the accomplishments she makes from week to week and month to month. However, for parents of children with documented and uncertain developmental delays or differences, reminders of these milestones can be frustrating and distressing.

This chapter will focus on infancy, broadly defined as the period from birth through the 1st year of life, in typically developing children. Although important changes occur in neurological, motor, and social development across childhood, development and change occur within each of these domains throughout the life span. Additionally, progressions, regressions, and growth across these domains can happen simultaneously, and in some cases, development in one domain can trigger normative progression

### What Would You Do? Chelsea's Story

When I was pregnant and planning on having a child, I thought about the little things: what their name would be or who they would look more like. I never thought about the scary stuff, so it was hard for me to comprehend what was going on when my child was born early.

I went into labor when I was 32 weeks pregnant. I got to the hospital before the contractions progressed too far, and when I arrived the doctors were able to stop them. They chose to admit me to the hospital, gave me the steroids to help the baby's lungs grow faster, put me on bed rest, and closely monitored me and the baby. Three days later I went back into labor, and this time they could not stop it. Twelve hours later my son was delivered via natural childbirth. I hadn't decided on a birth plan yet, so I didn't know when I could ask for medications for the pain and by the time I did, the hospital staff said it was too late.

Logan was born weighing 3 pounds, 14 ounces, and he was the smallest baby I had ever seen. We were lucky. Like other preterm babies, he had medical issues, such as apnea, so he would stop breathing. He was in the neonatal intensive care unit (NICU) at the hospital for 2 months before he was healthy and stable enough to come home. As a new mother it was the scariest time of my life. While in the hospital I focused on getting by one day at a time. It was hard, but I tried not to worry about some of the things the doctors were telling me regarding the potential long-term effects of his premature delivery. And I made it a point not to do research on my own, like on the internet, because I felt like that would just make me worry more.

I was 23 when I had Logan. He was my first child, and I didn't have any other babies around in my life, so I didn't know about timelines and what babies are supposed to do and when. How old should he be when he smiles? How old should he be when he crawls? I was clueless to the many questions that all new mothers have, but I had another hundred questions. Most importantly, how did Logan compare because he was preterm and not full term?

Given that Logan was as premature as he was, he received early intervention services when he was 3 months old. This meant that someone came to my house weekly to play with him and to see how he was progressing. They would provide me with some tips and tricks on how to teach him and how to get him closer to his developmental milestones. I also went to a weekly "Mommy and Me" class they offered so I could meet other mothers and children who were going through similar situations. The early intervention was great because they helped me understand the different

or normative regression in other areas. Because of this, it is often difficult to break down aspects of "biological," "psychological," and "social" development into distinct categories. The three are in constant interaction with one another. For example, neurological development and increased capacities in motor functioning can set the stage for development and change in psychological development. Likewise, developing psychological capacities and increasingly sophisticated social contexts can stimulate neurological development. They often influence each other and rarely work in isolation.

# Biological Development

Infants make tremendous developmental strides during the 1st year of life. The brain creates neurological connections that will be the basis of the more sophisticated thinking, behaviors, and social interactions we see as the year progresses. At first glance, the infant begins this year with limited motor capabilities, but even the uncontrolled movements we see early on serve an important purpose in facilitating the development of more complex motor behaviors such as sitting, crawling, and walking.

**LO 4-1** **How does the nervous system develop early in life?**

**LO 4-2** **Describe how motor control and development typically progresses during the 1st year of life.**

## Neurological Development and Functioning

Although a significant portion of neurological growth and development occurs prenatally and in the first few months of life, it is not until we reach approximately age 30 that the **nervous system**, which houses the brain and our nerves, reaches its full adult configuration (Hadders-Algra, 2004).

The development of the nervous system begins early in the prenatal period with the growth of **neurons** near the structures that ultimately become part of the ventricular system of the brain. Ventricles produce cerebrospinal fluid that surrounds the brain inside the skull and the spinal cord inside the spinal column. From here the development of neurons occurs in specific locations in the brain. The individual parts of the neuron, such as the axon and dendrites, differentiate from one another and begin to produce the **neurotransmitters** that are responsible for communication from neuron to neuron. Brain development then moves to the occipital and motor regions, then to the temporal and parietal regions, and then to the lateral cortices and the prefrontal cortex.

**Myelination** of the axon also occurs prenatally and is predominant during the 1st year of life. Myelination is the production of the myelin sheath that surrounds the axon of a neuron. This sheath increases the speed at which signals travel from the cell body down to the synaptic terminal. Myelination of neurons begins in the base of the brain in the pons, then moves to parts of the corpus callosum (1 to 3 months), and then to the frontal, parietal, and occipital lobes (8 to 12 months) (Paterson et al., 2006).

developmental stages—where Logan should be and where he actually was. Logan always seemed to impress the doctors and early invention team because he was right where other babies his age should be. He was just a lot smaller than them! I was able to enjoy milestones as they came, his first laugh, the first time he rolled over, sitting up on his own, and all the other wonderful things that babies do as they grow.

Logan was evaluated at 9 months to see if he still qualified for early intervention. He passed all areas but one. He had minor developmental delays in his language skills. Logan was a late talker but not by much. Although, I personally think he didn't talk because he was too busy running around like a mad man. Logan does things in his own time. He even climbed a ladder before he was comfortable standing without support. When he had his second evaluation 6 months later, he passed with flying colors; Logan had no developmental delays.

Logan is a year and a half now and is a walking and talking bundle of joy with a big personality. No one would know that he was premature unless I told them about it. And whenever I do tell people they are always surprised. Occasionally when I see a child who is the same age as Logan and can do something that he can't yet, I can't help but have the thought, is this because he was premature? Then I brush it off because at this point it is a silly question for me to have. My son is doing great and we're all so lucky that being a premature baby doesn't seem to have had a huge impact on him.

Think about what you would do in this situation after reading the chapter, and then decide the following:

- If you were Chelsea, what questions would you have for the doctors and nurses while Logan was in the NICU, and how would you prepare yourself for any potential challenges? Now that Logan has no developmental delays, would you still have feelings of worry or anxiety?
- If you were Chelsea's nurse, doctor, or early intervention specialist, what types of information would you share with her about the effects of premature deliveries? What kinds of support would you provide?
- If you were Chelsea, how would you counsel other mothers with children who may have more significant challenges due to premature delivery?

**FIGURE 4-1** The structure of a neuron.

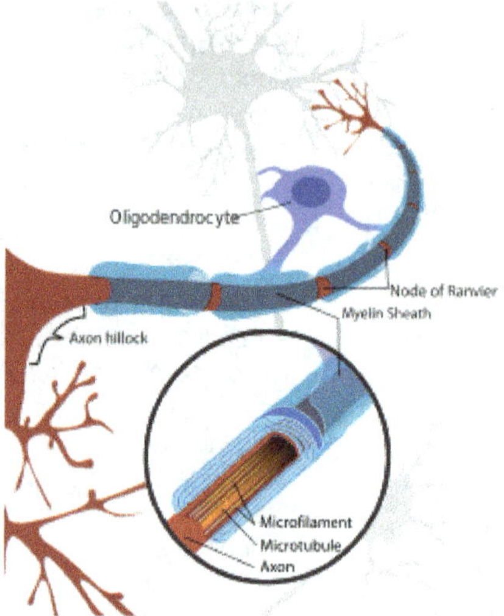


*Source*: https://commons.wikimedia.org/wiki/File:Neuron_with_oligodendrocyte_and_myelin_sheath-2.svg.

**TABLE 4-1** What most babies do at ... (Centers for Disease Control and Prevention, 2012)

| Age | Movement/Physical Development | Cognitive (learning, thinking, problem solving) | Language/ Communication | Social and Emotional |
|---|---|---|---|---|
| 2 months | • Can hold head up and begin to push up when lying on tummy<br>• Make smoother movements with arms and legs | • Pay attention to faces<br>• Begin to follow things with eyes and recognize people at a distance<br>• Begin to act bored (cry, fussy) if activity doesn't change | • Coo, make gurgling sounds<br>• Turn head toward sounds | • Begin to smile at people<br>• Can briefly calm themselves (may bring hands to mouth and suck on hand)<br>• Try to look at parent |
| 4 months | • Hold head steady, unsupported<br>• Push down on legs when feet are on a hard surface<br>• May be able to roll over from tummy to back<br>• Can hold a toy and shake it and swing at dangling toys<br>• Bring hands to mouth<br>• When lying on stomach, push up to elbows | • Let you know if they are happy or sad<br>• Respond to affection<br>• Reach for toy with one hand<br>• Use hands and eyes together, such as seeing a toy and reaching for it<br>• Follow moving things with eyes from side to side<br>• Watch faces closely<br>• Recognize familiar people and things at a distance | • Begin to babble<br>• Babble with expression and copy sounds they hear<br>• Cry in different ways to show hunger, pain, or being tired | • Smile spontaneously, especially at people<br>• Like to play with people and might cry when playing stops<br>• Copy some movements and facial expressions, like smiling or frowning |

**TABLE 4-1** Continued

| Age | Movement/Physical Development | Cognitive (learning, thinking, problem solving) | Language/ Communication | Social and Emotional |
|---|---|---|---|---|
| 6 months | • Roll over in both directions (front to back, back to front)<br>• Begin to sit without support<br>• When standing, support weight on legs and might bounce<br>• Rock back and forth, sometimes crawling backward before moving forward | • Look around at things nearby<br>• Bring things to mouth<br>• Show curiosity about things and try to get things that are out of reach<br>• Begin to pass things from one hand to the other | • Respond to sounds by making sounds<br>• String vowels together when babbling ("ah," "eh," "oh") and like taking turns with parent while making sounds<br>• Respond to their name<br>• Make sounds to show joy and displeasure<br>• Begin to say consonant sounds (jabbering with "m," "b") | • Know familiar faces and begin to know if someone is a stranger<br>• Like to play with others, especially parents<br>• Respond to other people's emotions and often seems happy<br>• Like to look in a mirror |
| 9 months | • Stand, holding on<br>• Can get into sitting position<br>• Sit without support<br>• Pull to stand<br>• Crawl | • Watch the path of something as it falls<br>• Look for things they see you hide<br>• Play peek-a-boo<br>• Put things in her mouth<br>• Move things smoothly from one hand to the other<br>• Pick up things like cereal between thumb and index finger | • Understand "no"<br>• Make a lot of different sounds like "mamamama" and "bababababa"<br>• Copy sounds and gestures of others<br>• Use fingers to point at things | • May be afraid of strangers<br>• May be clingy with familiar adults<br>• Have favorite toys |
| 1 year | • Get to a sitting position without help<br>• Pull up to stand, walk holding on to furniture ("cruising")<br>• May take a few steps without holding on<br>• May stand alone | • Explore things in different ways, like shaking, banging, throwing<br>• Find hidden things easily<br>• Look at the right picture or thing when it is named<br>• Copy gestures<br>• Start to use things correctly; for example, drinking from a cup, brushing hair<br>• Bang two things together<br>• Put things in a container, take things out of a container<br>• Let things go without help<br>• Poke with index (pointer) finger<br>• Follow simple directions like "pick up the toy" | • Respond to simple spoken requests<br>• Use simple gestures, like shaking head "no" or waving "bye-bye"<br>• Make sounds with changes in tone (sounds more like speech)<br>• Say "mama" and "dada" and exclamations like "uh-oh!"<br>• Try to say words you say | • Are shy or nervous with strangers<br>• Cry when mom or dad leaves<br>• Have favorite things and people<br>• Show fear in some situations<br>• Hand you a book when they want to hear a story<br>• Repeat sounds or actions to get attention<br>• Put out arm or leg to help with dressing<br>• Play games such as "peek-a-boo" and "pat-a-cake" |

The "condition" of neurological functioning (for example, optimal, nonoptimal, delayed) shows some stability over the course of infancy. It appears to be highly stable in infants who are born full term (93% of infants), but much less so in preterm infants (30% of infants). In other words, brain development and functioning are quite changeable for those born preterm. Some may have serious deficits across the life span, whereas others may be indistinguishable from their peers who were born full term.

Neurons and neural connections not only grow, but many unnecessary neurons and connections between synapses die off through a process called "**pruning**" throughout the life span. After structures and connections are in place, the potential for **brain plasticity** across the life span remains, as some behaviors and characteristics are stable, whereas others have the potential for both minute and monumental changes (Hadders-Algra et al., 2010).

When comparing the infant brain with the adult brain, it is clear that their structures and associated functions are indeed very different. Developmental science typically uses the adult brain as a rough guide to pinpoint where the early origins of certain behaviors and characteristics lie within the brain (Paterson et al., 2006). As we've highlighted earlier, it is difficult to know exactly whether and when it is brain development that causes particular behaviors, or if it is developing behaviors that cause brain development. There are even those times when the brain and behaviors develop simultaneously (Paterson et al., 2006).

## Motor Development and Functioning

Motor development and cognitive development are very much tied together. For example, cognition and motor activity, along with all of our behaviors, thoughts, and physiological functions, have their roots in neurological development and functioning. Each transition a child makes in his motor development, whether it be sitting, crawling, standing, or walking, affects how he interacts with the world and his capacity to gather new information, learn, and develop.

FIGURE 4-2 As is true for many skills we develop across childhood, there is a "normal range" of ages at which that skill first appears. These images represent the average age (in months) when typically developing children reach that particular milestone.

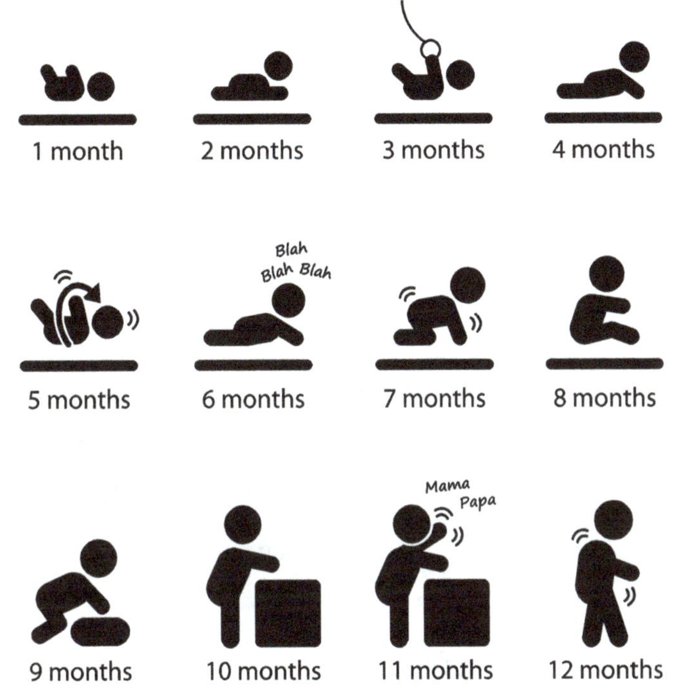


*Source*: Copyright © 2014 Depositphotos/leremy.

## Myths and Misconceptions

The configuration of the brain does not change once you reach adulthood. **Myth**

There is great potential for brain plasticity across the life span. We see this, for example, in cognition and the ability for older adults to respond to cognitive training. This suggests that brain structures and communication among neurons have the potential for development and change across the life span. **Fact**

Motor development begins with spontaneous actions based in reflexive behaviors, such as turning the head or kicking, that slowly develop into controlled behaviors such as gaining head control, rolling over from stomach to back then from back to stomach, sitting independently, standing while holding on, standing alone, and walking independently (see Figure 4-2). Most of these accomplishments follow a forward, linear sequence. However, there are times when the sequence of skills is out of order, when there are jumps, such as an infant who walks without ever crawling. There can also be regressions, such as an infant who could previously sleep through the night but all of a sudden cannot. The exact timing of motor development depends on many factors, including body mass, interest level, and practice. When an infant will progress from one milestone simply cannot be predicted. One thing is clear, for the typically developing child, these abilities happen largely without prompting or encouragement.

Early on, infants exhibit self-generated and spontaneous movements that seem to have no rhyme or reason, but really they are of great importance for the developing brain and are evidence of optimal neurological development. These **general movements** (GMs) that young infants exhibit have their beginnings in utero, but continue into the first few months of life. More controlled motor functioning starts in the head and neck, then moves to the shoulders and torso, then to the hips, legs, and feet. And once the infant's shoulders are stable, control extends from the arms to the wrists, fingers, and thumbs. The ability to reach and grasp is an important progression as well. Between 4 and 7 months, infants are typically able to pick up an object with one or both hands, then become better able to use the thumb and fingers to grasp. The ability to use the thumb tip and the finger tip for a more precise grip, known as the **pincer grasp**, develops around 11 months (see Figure 4-3) (Kopp, 2011).

**FIGURE 4-3** The pincer grasp.

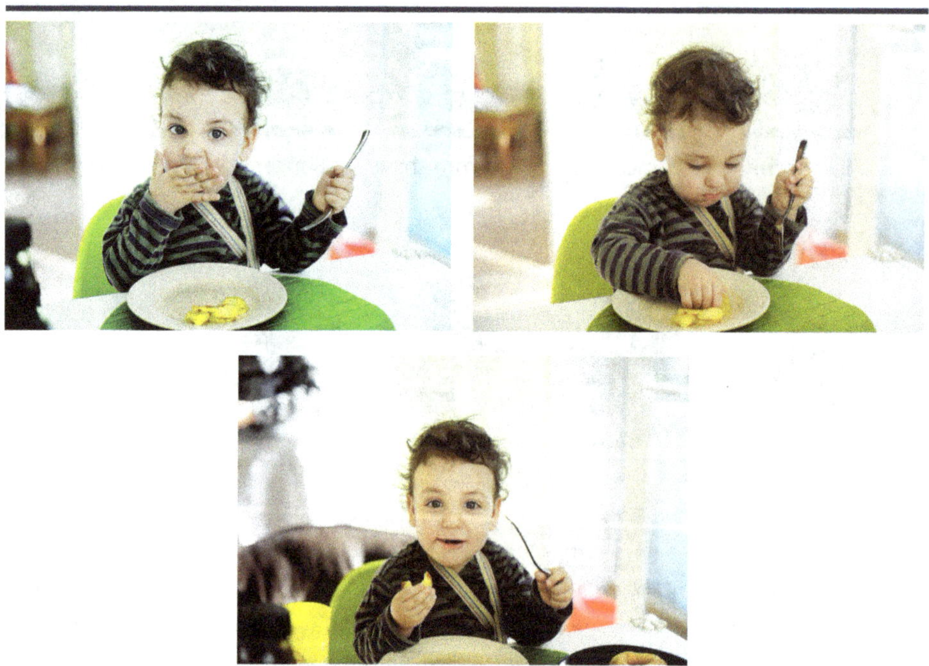

*Source*: Copyright © 2016 Depositphotos/alinute.

Motor development certainly occurs within a social context. Although there is no way to actually teach an infant how to sit, the ways we hold and care for an infant facilitate motor development, such as the head support we provide in the early days, the way we carry an infant upright, or prop him up against a solid surface, among others. Some motor skills are socioculturally dependent, such as learning a particular type of precision grip. For example, learning to grip chopsticks requires different skills compared with learning to grip a spoon (Kopp, 2011).

Motor development also facilitates communication for infants and young children. You may find yourself questioning how this could be possible, but think about a preverbal child who is crying and pointing to his cup of milk on the counter. The ability to point (a motor skill indeed) helps the child communicate information about his distress. Some researchers also believe that an infant's ability to point as a communication tool is a marker of developing social interaction skills and an awareness of other individuals as independent thinkers (Tomasello, 2009).

**FIGURE 4-4** An infant can communicate by reaching.

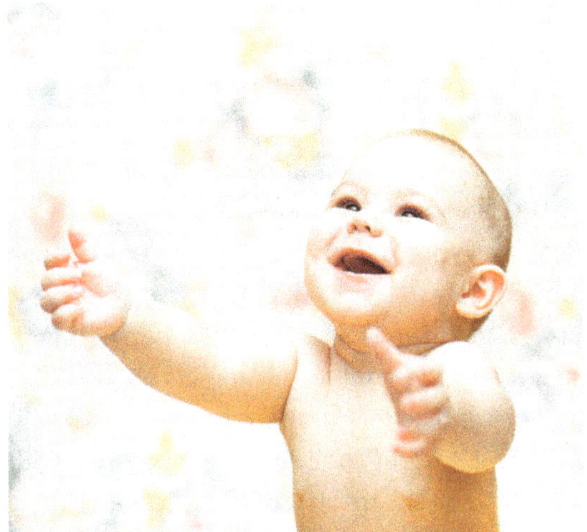

*Source*: Copyright © 2013 Depositphotos/asayenkaa.

# Psychological Development

Many of the seemingly ordinary, but still important psychological capacities of the young child are a reflection of very complex neurological, social, and cognitive processes. These ordinary abilities, such as knowing that the dolly you just hid is behind your back and not gone forever, or the ability to pay attention to the story you are reading her, require tremendous skill. They also lay the ground work for more complex psychological processes related to thinking, interacting with the world, and developing social relationships.

**LO 4-3** **How do the senses develop during the 1st year?**

**LO 4-4** **What is joint attention and why is it an important cognitive process?**

**LO 4-5** **What types of memories do infants have?**

**LO 4-6** **How does the infant's temperament affect her environment?**

**LO 4-7** **Why are caregiver-infant attachment relationships important for survival and development?**

## Perceptual and Sensory Capabilities

As discussed in the previous chapter, an infant's preferences for familiar tastes and smells have roots in the prenatal period. In general, and not surprisingly, infants prefer sweet tastes to sour and bitter, and pleasant smells over foul odors. Across the 1st year, they will have their first foods, and will likely show preference for some over others. Research shows that of the five major tastes, sweet, sour, bitter, salty, and savory, more infants at 6 months prefer sweet, salty, and savory and are indifferent toward sour and bitter. However, the longer an infant is breastfed, up to 12 months of age, the greater the preference she will have for savory. At 12 months, more infants prefer sweet and savory and are indifferent to salty and bitter tastes (Schwartz et al., 2013). In addition to prenatal exposure, a willingness to try and accept new foods is moderately to strongly heritable (Harris, 2008). However, factors such as early and repeated exposure to certain foods can also influence taste preferences (Faith, 2010). For example, in animal studies, prenatal exposure to alcohol is associated with increased alcohol consumption in infant rats (Arias & Chotro, 2005).

The sense of taste and the sense of smell are very closely linked. Although our taste buds perceive the five major tastes, it is our nose and our sense of smell that perceive the nuanced differences between chocolate and vanilla ice cream, and between plain potato chips and sour cream and onion. Compared to other mammals, such as your dog or your cat, the human sense of smell is rather underdeveloped. However, we can still differentiate between thousands of different smells. For example, we know the difference between burning wood and burning plastic, or the differences between lilacs and roses and lilies. As previously mentioned, newborns are sensitive to smells. Research shows they can locate their mother's nipple by smell, and by age 3 children tend to have the same likes and dislikes for smells as adults have. Our ability to smell is a developmental process that plateaus around age 8 with olfactory sensitivity declining with age. Females, on average, are more sensitive to smells than males. Given the proximity of the olfactory bulb (where the brain processes smell) to the amygdala (a major brain structure involved in memory and emotions), smells can be extremely powerful in eliciting emotional memories (Fox, 2009).

Both distance vision and color vision develop postnatally. Given this, much of what the newborn sees appears blurry with minimal color differentiation. During the first 3 months infants can only track objects that are between 9 and 12 inches from their face. Coincidentally this is approximately the distance from a woman's breast to her face—the optimal range of vision for being held or fed. By roughly 3 months, infants can recognize familiar faces, even at a distance.

**TABLE 4-2** Visual Development Across the First Year (American Optometric Association, 2013)

| Age | Visual Capacity |
|---|---|
| Birth to 4 months | • Vision is abuzz with visual stimulation. Infants may look intently at a highly contrasted target, but do not have the ability to easily tell the difference between two targets or move their eyes between the two images. Primary focus is on objects 8 to 10 inches from their face or the distance to the parent's face.<br>• The eyes start working together and vision rapidly improves. Eye-hand coordination begins to develop as the infant starts tracking moving objects with their eyes and reaching for them. By 8 weeks, infants begin to more easily focus their eyes on the faces of a parent or other person near them.<br>• For the first 2 months, an infant's eyes are not well coordinated and may appear to wander or be crossed. This is usually normal. However, if an eye appears to turn in or out constantly, an evaluation is warranted.<br>• Infants should begin to follow moving objects with their eyes and reach for things at around 3 months of age. |
| 5 to 8 months | • Control of eye movements and eye-body coordination skills continue to improve.<br>• Depth perception is not present at birth. It is not until around 5 months that the eyes are capable of working together to form a three-dimensional view of the world and begin to see in depth.<br>• An infant's color vision is not as sensitive as an adult's. It is believed that good color vision develops by 5 months.<br>• Crawling helps further develop eye-hand-foot-body coordination. |
| 9 to 12 months | • At around 9 months, infants begin to pull themselves up to a standing position, and by 10 months should be able to grasp objects with thumb and forefinger.<br>• By 12 months of age, most babies will be crawling and trying to walk.<br>• Babies can now judge distances fairly well and throw things with precision. |



The sense of touch is the first to develop prenatally, and skin-to-skin contact during the postnatal period is vital. Tactile stimulation of the infant, in the form of rubbing, rocking, touching, and holding, plays a central role in physical and psychological development. It helps soothe and regulate the infant, and supports infant communication and exploration. A greater amount of postnatal touch is associated with more smiling and less crying as the infant develops in the 1st year. Research has also shown that touch is very effective in alleviating distress during otherwise stressful situations using the "still-face" paradigm (a scenario designed to elicit stress in infants in which a caregiver gazes at the infant with a still face; see Figure 4-5) (Stack & Jean, 2011). The still-face paradigm is used in research to simulate the experience of maternal depression and depressive episodes. Note the changes in the infant's expressions from panel to panel. Turning the head away from the mother is thought to be a sort of coping mechanism, to block out the unwanted stimulus (the mother's still face).

**FIGURE 4-5** Note the infant turning away in frame D of the still-face paradigm. Turning away is a self-soothing behavior that infants exhibit in times of distress.

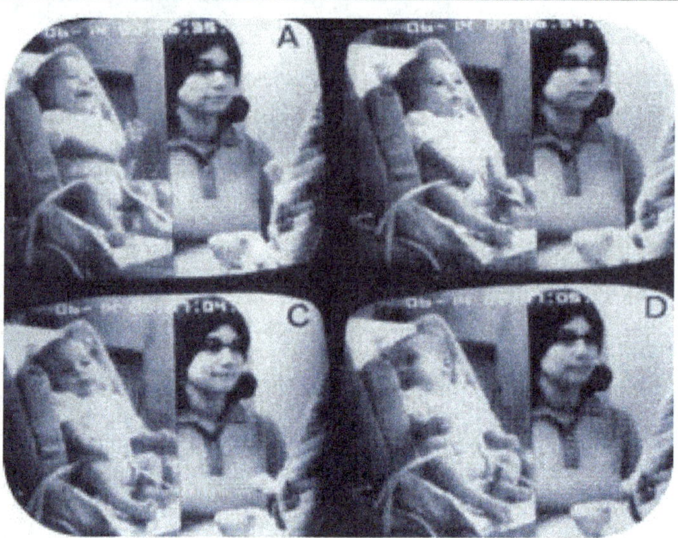


*Source*: http://www.adbb.net/gb-echelle.html.

The development of the brain and corresponding senses and perceptions during the 1st year is unlike any other period of development. In fact, some researchers argue for "a rare sensory phenomenon that has been associated with exuberant neural connectivity and that is characterized by strong arbitrary associations between different sensations" (Wagner & Dobkins, 2011, p. XX). They argue that this phenomenon leads to "infant synaesthesia" in which stimulation of one sense perception (such as hearing) produces perception in a seemingly unrelated sense perception (such as smell). They also contend that failure to eliminate certain neural connections may lead to synaesthesia in adults (Wagner & Dobkins, 2011). Figure 4-6 provides an example of synaesthesia in which the sight of letters elicits the perception of certain colors.

FIGURE 4-6 Synaesthesia can cause the sight of certain letters to elicit the perception of certain colors.

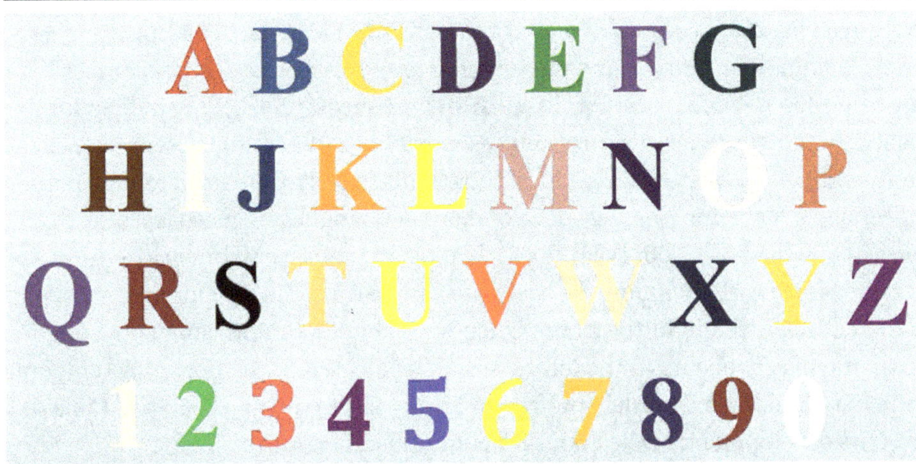


*Source*: https://www.psychologyinaction.org/psychology-in-action-1/2011/01/28/synesthesia-when-ordinary-activities-trigger-extraordinary-sensations.

## Hearing, Language, and Communication

Infants are born with a fully developed capacity to hear sound. It is our preferences for familiar sounds, certain tones, and ultimately our ability to interpret language through sound that develop and change over time. Younger infants prefer the higher-pitched tones that are characteristic of **infant-directed speech**, also referred to as motherese or parentese, which includes exaggerated tones and simplistic language (Fernald, 1985). There has been some debate over whether infant-directed speech is culturally relative, in other words, if it's found in some cultures but not others. Recent research suggests that infant-directed speech may be a "species-specific adaptation" or a universal phenomenon for the human species, but that its manifestations may be hard to detect for those who do not belong to the cultural community being studied (Broesch & Bryant, 2013; Bryant et al., 2012). Infant-directed speech also extends to hearing-impaired parents and their hearing-impaired infants. Hearing-impaired parents tend to sign at a slower tempo, with repeated and exaggerated signs, when interacting with their hearing-impaired infants in comparison with their friends. These types of exaggerated movements when interacting with infants is called "motionese." In addition, hearing-impaired infants tend to prefer motionese, as demonstrated by their attention and emotional response, over faster-paced sign language (Dunst et al., 2012; Masataka, 1996). A child's response, and more specifically nonresponse, to infant-directed speech can be indicative of psychopathology, because orientation to and preference for infant-directed speech is impaired in children with autism spectrum disorder (O'Connor, 2012).

Our early capacity for hearing and our ability to interpret sounds are vital to the development of our communication skills, from crying to be fed or comforted, to recognizing the voice of our primary caregiver, to clearly articulating our needs, wants, opinions, and so on, and understanding those of others. In this process, we must develop a capacity for **rapid auditory processing** (RAP), which is fundamental for language acquisition, and responsible for detecting shifts in vocalizations, particularly related to the use of consonant sounds. Deficits in rapid auditory processing affect later language development and language-baased learning disorders (Benasich et al., 2006; Tallal, 2004). It appears that several brain structures are responsible for RAP, including the thalamus and parts of the temporoparietal areas in the left hemisphere of the brain. Once we reach adulthood, language comprehension typically occurs in the left hemisphere, located in the posterior temporal cortex, alongside areas in left prefrontal cortex (Paterson et al., 2006). Table 4-3 presents developmental milestones for communication during infancy.

**TABLE 4-3** Infant Communication (American Speech-Language-Hearing Association, 2013)

| Hearing and Understanding | Talking |
|---|---|
| **Birth to 3 Months**<br>• Startles to loud sounds<br>• Quiets or smiles when spoken to<br>• Seems to recognize your voice and quiets if crying<br>• Increases or decreases sucking behavior in response to sound | **Birth to 3 Months**<br>• Makes pleasure sounds (cooing, gooing)<br>• Cries differently for different needs<br>• Smiles when sees you |
| **4 to 6 Months**<br>• Moves eyes in direction of sounds<br>• Responds to changes in tone of your voice<br>• Notices toys that make sounds<br>• Pays attention to music | **4 to 6 Months**<br>• Babbling sounds more speech-like sounds, including *p*, *b* and *m*<br>• Chuckles and laughs<br>• Vocalizes excitement and displeasure<br>• Makes gurgling sounds when left alone or playing with you |
| **7 Months to 1 Year**<br>• Enjoys games like peek-a-boo and pat-a-cake<br>• Turns and looks in direction of sounds<br>• Listens when spoken to<br>• Recognizes words for common items like "cup" or "book"<br>• Begins to respond to requests like "Come here" or "Want more?" | **7 Months to 1 Year**<br>• Babbling has long and short sounds such as "tata upup bibibibi"<br>• Uses speech or noncrying sounds to get and keep attention<br>• Uses gestures (waving, holding arms to be picked up)<br>• Imitates different speech sounds<br>• Has one or two words (hi, dog, dada, mama) around first birthday, although sounds may not be clear |

Source: Adapted from "How Does Your Child Hear and Talk?" ASHA.org. Copyright © by American Speech-Language-Hearing Association.

Table 4-3 outlines communication in typically developing children. However, many infants may experience delays in speech and language. Causes of speech delay may include hearing loss, bilingualism, psychological deprivation, autism, and cerebral palsy, or they may be a sign of underlying language processing and speech disorders. The American Academy of Pediatrics recommends that a child be evaluated by a child development specialist if she does not responsively coo (makes soft, murmuring sounds like "ooo-") by 6 months, does not babble (makes sounds like "bah- bah- bah" but not words) by 10 months, and/or shows no basic gesturing (waves goodbye, reaches to be picked up) by 12 months (Macias & Twyman, 2011).

## Cognitive Development

Infancy is a remarkable time for cognitive development. From the very young infant who smiles for the first time at the sight of his father, to the almost 1-year-old who may listen and follow along with a story that is being read to her, each of these behaviors and many others represent the endless cognitive processes that the infant is beginning to develop and refine. In this section, we will focus on some that are critical to thinking, learning, and becoming an active social being.

**Object permanence.** Most famously investigated by the renowned psychologist Jean Piaget and part of his stage theory of cognitive development, **object permanence** has been the focus of extensive research in infant cognitive development. Object permanence is the capacity to keep track of and search for an object, even when it is not within view. It can be seen in some basic forms in infants as young as 3 months of age but becomes solidified as a skill typically between 7 and 9 months of age. Some researchers believe that object permanence, with its links to working memory, attention control, and inhibitory skills, is a precursor to **executive functioning** skills, which we will discuss in the next chapter in more detail. Object permanence requires a number of higher-order mental and cognitive processes that incorporate past experiences with current behaviors (Diamond, 2002; McCandliss et al., 2003). Animal studies have demonstrated that the emergence of this capacity coincides with the development of the brain's frontal lobes and the prefrontal cortex, as well as increases in glucose metabolism (Paterson et al., 2006).

**Face processing.** Face processing is a critical skill that informs social behaviors and facilitates social interactions. Even though face processing and a preference for human faces can be seen at birth, it is a capacity that develops over time. We go from preferring faces presented in our peripheral vision, that are perceived as specific objects using subcortical structures in early infancy, to using cortical structures as faces become their own category of objects to be perceived. In other words, faces become "faces" and are recognized as such, rather than being one of many objects that exist in the infant's environment. The cortical regions of the brain responsible for face processing also appear to change in adulthood as our understanding of and exposure to social interactions becomes more neurologically sophisticated.

**Joint attention.** **Joint attention**, when attention to a stimulus or task is shared by two social partners, regardless of the initiator, is an important cognitive function that plays a role in social skills and language development. It is also associated with traditional measures of intelligence. Scientists believe, like object permanence, the development of joint attention may be attributed to glucose metabolism. Links between joint attention and certain brain regions depend on whether the joint attention experience is being initiated or being responded to. In other words, does the infant want you to respond to her or is the infant responding to your bids for joint attention? Areas of the orbitofrontal and temporal cortices of the brain are activated during initiated joint attention experiences, and responding to bids for joint attention seems to occur in the parietal lobes. As infants become better social partners, it appears that the mechanisms for joint attention move from the posterior of the brain to the anterior (Paterson et al., 2006).

It may not seem like a complex task, but joint attention is really quite challenging. It requires a shift in one's attention and focus to disengage with a stimulus (that involves inhibitory processes) and to engage with a social partner. The implications for joint attention are clear. If the infant can engage with the world and with social partners, then he's likely to gain rich learning and experiential knowledge that will promote development. It appears that those with autism may have impairments in their capacity for joint attention, which has implications for both social cognition and language development (Mundy & Neal, 2001).

**Memory.** Assessing memory development in infancy can be a challenge, particularly given that parts of memory are assessed largely through verbal communication—a skill that infants clearly lack. It is not until roughly age 3 that children become reliable communicators of events they have experienced in the past, which coincides with the average age of adults' earliest memories. Just because most of us cannot remember what happened prior to that age (a phenomenon known as **infantile amnesia**) it does not mean that memory doesn't exist in infancy and early childhood. In fact, infants have robust memory capabilities, as evidenced by their ability to learn from and therefore benefit from past experiences.

Before we go on to discuss memory development further, let's stop for a minute to distinguish between different types of memories. **Implicit memories** are typically beyond our awareness. These include memories associated with the ability to learn, to develop skills, and to become conditioned. For example, "this is how I hold a spoon" or "stoves are hot." **Explicit memories** require some level of conscious awareness and include recognition and recall of past experiences, for example, "We colored at Jenney's today" or "I was a dinosaur for Halloween this year."

The capacity for implicit memory appears to be largely functional at birth. However, explicit memory becomes more sophisticated starting late in the infant's 1st year of life. The parts of the brain responsible for memory are well documented.

The hippocampus and areas surrounding the amygdalae in the brain help us form the long-term memories that are associated with explicit or declarative memories of past events, with assistance from temporal and cortical structures that develop later in infancy. Those long-term memories that are associated with skill learning are housed in several places elsewhere in the brain, such as the neocortex and cerebellum (Bauer et al., 2011; Rovee-Collier & Cuevas, 2009).

We use research tools that examine infants' responses to novel and familiar visual stimuli and other techniques as windows into infant memory and its development. In assessing infant memory, we see that "at 6 months of age, infants can remember an average of one action of a three-step sequence (taking a mitten off a puppet's hand; shaking the mitten which, at the time of the demonstration, held a bell that ran; and replacing the mitten) for 24 hours" (Bauer et al., 2011; Rovee-Collier & Cuevas, 2009). This capacity increases substantially across infancy and beyond (see Table 4-4).

**TABLE 4-4** Capacity for Remembering in Young Children

| Age | Memory Retention |
|---|---|
| 6 months | 24 hours |
| 9 months | 24 hours to 5 weeks |
| 10–11 months | 3 months |
| 13–14 months | 4–6 months |
| 20 months | 12 months |

**Developmental timing.** In this book we point out roughly when infants, children, and even adults achieve important developmental milestones, whether it is a neurological, motor, cognitive, or social milestone. Many variations in timing are perfectly normal and attributable to a multitude of factors working together in ways that are difficult to fully understand. However, researchers have isolated some key factors, including gestational age at birth, that impact developmental timing. Perhaps not surprisingly, overweight infants and those with greater amounts of subcutaneous fat are more likely to experience motor delays (Slining et al., 2010). The patterns an infant shows in her early motor development, alongside factors such as birth weight and less infant weight gain, predict adult physical strength, endurance, and aerobic fitness in adulthood (Ridgway et al., 2009).

Many causes of developmental differences are unknown, but we do know some are associated with delayed functioning in infancy. Minor neurological dysfunction is associated with gestational age at birth, lower parental education, and younger maternal age (Hadders-Algra et al., 2010). Women who are characteristically anxious have a greater chance of having infants who show nonoptimal reaching, grasping, and sensorimotor dysfunction. This may be due to increases in levels of maternal **cortisol**, a stress hormone that disrupts fetal neurological development (Kikkert et al., 2010). Other studies have shown that the timing of certain spikes in a woman's anxiety level is an important factor to consider when examining cognitive and motor development. Elevated cortisol early in pregnancy can have a negative impact on children's development through the 1st year, whereas elevated cortisol levels later on in pregnancy may accelerate cognitive development in infants (Davis & Sandman, 2010). Lastly, reaching milestones early, specifically walking, has been associated with slight differences in IQ scores (one-half point for every 1 month earlier). They speculate that this may be due to suboptimal cortical-subcortical connectivity that may delay walking and impact IQ simultaneously (Murray et al., 2007).

## Temperament

We've demonstrated that interaction with the environment is fundamental to a developing child. At the same time, the child is now able to take part in social interactions. Many researchers believe children are born with innate characteristics that shape how they interact with the environment and how those within their environment react to them. These characteristics, first detected in infancy, can often be seen across the life span as well. In child psychology, these innate characteristics are referred to as **temperament**. Researchers Alexander Thomas and Stella Chess were among the first psychologists to acknowledge that the infant is an active agent in the environment and within their caregiving experience.

Thomas and Chess were also the first to classify infants into one of three temperament categories, "easy," "slow to warm up," and "difficult," based on behavioral characteristics, as noted in Table 4-5. They took into consideration interview data, questionnaires, and observations to document infant behaviors such as activity during diaper changing, movements during sleep, feeding and sleep schedules, and behaviors toward unfamiliar objects (e.g., puts a new toy in his mouth to explore it). When examining the classifications, note that these behaviors are measured on a 9-point scale—no one infant is measured as "either/or," but rather in terms of their degree on a continuum. In one of their original papers they also noted that whereas 65% of infants fit into one category or another, 35% did not, as they displayed a mixture of the classifications ( for example, difficult or easy) depending on the situation and the behavior being studied (Thomas et al., 1970).

Thomas and Chess argued for a "goodness-of-fit" approach to the caregiving environment and the fit between the caregiver's behaviors and the child's behaviors. For example, a difficult child may not fit well with a flexible parent. It could be the flexible parent gives in too often to the difficult child, resulting in nonoptimal behaviors. In addition to the caregiving environment, temperament can influence and be influenced by other aspects of the environment such as culture and socioeconomics (Chess & Thomas, 1999).

**TABLE 4-5** Temperaments and Their Associated Characteristics (Thomas et al., 1970). Distractibility, or the degree to which extraneous stimuli affect behavior, varies across types, attention span, and persistence, or the amount of time devoted to an activity, and the effect of distraction on the activity can be high or low across types and threshold of responsiveness, or the intensity of stimuli required to evoke a discernible response can be high or low across types.

| Type of Child | Activity Level | Rhythmicity | Approach/ Withdrawal | Adaptability | Intensity of Reaction | Quality of Mood |
|---|---|---|---|---|---|---|
| Easy | Varies | Very regular | Positive approach | Very adaptable | Low or mild | Positive |
| Slow to warm up | Low to moderate | Varies | Initial withdrawal | Slowly adaptable | Mild | Slightly negative |
| Difficult | Varies | Irregular | Withdrawal | Slowly adaptable | Intense | Negative |

Jerome Kagan (2005), a well-known expert on the study of temperament, argues for the biological underpinnings of temperament and defines it as "a distinctive profile of feelings and behaviours that originate in the child's biology and appear early in development" (p. XX). Kagan suggests that both genetic influences and prenatal events, which affect hormones and neurotransmitters in the brain, can lead to the differences we see in temperament. You may wonder what prenatal events could possibly affect someone's temperament. One recent study examined women who used assisted reproductive technologies (ART) to conceive and found that the pregnancy-focused anxiety that often accompanies ART was unrelated to infant temperament. However, a mother who is more anxious by nature is more likely to have an infant with a difficult temperament (McMahon et al., 2013). And although it is well documented that a fetus's exposure to alcohol in utero is associated with cognitive and behavioral difficulties and delays, researchers also found that women who binge drank in early pregnancy (that is, consuming more than five drinks in one sitting at least

## Myths and Misconceptions

The infant is a sponge that passively soaks up his environment. **Misconception**

The infant brings something of his own to the environment and his experiences from day 1 and perhaps even earlier. These behaviors and characteristics may be innate and biologically based. **Fact** once a week during weeks 0 to 6) were more likely to have infants with difficult temperaments (Alvik et al., 2011).

The infant and his characteristics have a substantial impact on the environment, which, in turn, has an impact on the child. For example, infant temperament has been associated with maternal sleep during infancy (Goyal et al., 2009). In addition, infants and young children with difficult temperaments are exposed to greater amounts of television prior to 18 months of age (Thompson et al., 2013). An easy temperament may also be advantageous for children growing up in adverse environments. Generally speaking, those who grow up in higher-risk environments are more likely to experience behavioral problems and nonoptimal language development. However, those with easy temperaments who grow up in these environments are less likely to display nonoptimal behaviors and functioning (Derauf et al., 2011). This supports the idea that the infant is an active social being who can have a meaningful impact on others and his environment, thus altering his own development.

## Developing Attachments

As we mentioned last chapter, attachment is an important social bond. It develops during infancy and across the life span and also serves a biological purpose. It is an emotional connection between individuals who share intimate relationships. Forming a secure attachment to a primary caregiver provides an infant or young child with the safety and security necessary for them to explore and engage with the world. Thoughts and behaviors that affect the type of caregiver-child attachment that develops can be observed very early on in development, and we can begin to see clear attachment patterns in infants from 6 to 12 months of age (Ainsworth, 1967; Bowlby, 1969, 1973).

Although the mother has historically been viewed as the first and primary attachment figure for infants and young children, in many contexts and cultures (and across many different species) children become meaningfully attached to fathers, siblings, grandparents, or other critical caregivers in their lives (Hrdy, 1999; Morelli & Tronick, 1992). These attachment figures act like a safety net that protects the child from danger. When the child may be crying, crawling toward, or clinging to the caregiver in response to a perceived threat in the environment, the caregiver may move closer to the child or be smiling at her, calling, following, or carrying her to make her feel safe.

A child's attachment behaviors reflect the quality of care experienced by the child, which influences her confidence that the caregiver is someone who can be called on in times of stress and danger (George & Solomon, 2008). Over time, as experiences become less stressful or a strange environment becomes familiar, the child doesn't need to be as physically close to the attachment figure to gain a sense of security and protection. This allows her to explore her environment more fully and leads to growth and development (Marvin & Britner, 2008). We typically measure attachment behaviors in young children via the "strange situation" (Ainsworth & Wittig, 1969). The strange situation is an observational assessment that includes a brief separation of the young child and caregiver while a stranger (usually a member of the research team) remains with the child, thus introducing a strange situation and potential perceived threat. The caregiver returns to the room and reunion behaviors between he or she and the child are examined. Table 4-6 presents well-studied attachment classifications alongside child and caregiver behaviors.

**TABLE 4-6** Attachment Pattern Classifications and Their Associated Behaviors (adapted from Davis et al., 2014)

| Attachment Classification | Attachment in Childhood and Associated Caregiving |
|---|---|
| **Secure classification** | Caregiver is available, sensitive, cooperative, and responsive. Child will seek out caregiver for help in times of danger or distress. Child is comforted by contact with caregiver. This allows the child to return to developmentally appropriate exploration of the environment. |
| **Insecure classifications** | Caregiving is nonoptimal but nontraumatic |
| **Insecure-anxious Avoidant classification** | Caregiver is often rejecting perhaps by pushing the child toward premature independence or self-soothing when they are under stress. Child then avoids caregiver when in distress, may turn away and appear calm, but internal arousal (anxiousness) is high. |
| **Insecure-anxious Ambivalent/resistant classification** | Caregiver is erratic and inconsistent, may be intrusive with the child when not needed or disengaged when needed. Child may approach and attempt contact with the caregiver when distressed but may be angry or resistant. Alternatively, child may show minimal approach behaviors when distressed while exhibiting passive, fussy, and helpless behaviors. In general, the child is not easily soothed. |

Adapted from Cynthia Davis, et al., Attachment and the Metabolic Syndrome in Midlife: The Role of Interview-Based Discourse Patterns,Psychosomatic Medicine, vol. 76, no. 8. Wolters Kluwer, 2014.

This early relationship creates an underlying, reliable understanding or mental representation of the world. These representations are what British psychiatrist and psychoanalyst John Bowlby (1969), the founder of attachment theory, called **internal working models**. In normative, adaptive parent-child attachment relationships, the child develops a representation or a sense that the caregiver is reliable and available, that relationships are safe, and that the world is a place for learning and exploration, in which the child will be protected from harm if necessary (Main et. al., 1985). These early attachments with primary caregivers and the development of internal working models set the stage for the characteristics and quality of future attachment relationships, such as the relationship we have with a spouse (Bowlby, 1973, 1980; Hazan & Shaver, 1987; Main, 1991; Sroufe & Fleeson, 1986). If an individual has a secure internal working model, they tend to process information about attachment relationships, whether it is positive or negative, in a flexible manner with a positive bias. If the internal working model is insecure, then an individual will process information defensively or in a negative fashion (Dykas & Cassidy, 2011).

Factors such as the child's temperament may influence the quality of the relationship between caregiver and child, but the caregiver's internal working model, which influences the perception of their infant and attachment relationships, seems to be far more critical than any particular characteristic of the child (van Ijzendoorn, 1995; George & Solomon, 2008). Optimal caregiving also requires the parent's ability to be flexible, to view the child in relation to other needs and goals the parent may have, and to prioritize it accordingly (George & Solomon, 2008). Still, there are many other things that can affect attachment and parent-child relationships, including child maltreatment and certain socioeconomic risks (Cyr et al., 2010).

# Social Contexts and Development

Social contexts vary dramatically from infant to infant and from culture to culture. A parent may serve as the predominant social figure, but siblings, grandparents, other relatives, or close individuals can also play a role in socializing the infant. Likewise, important social interactions can take place in the home or other contexts where the child spends considerable time.

**LO 4-8** **How does time spent in formal childcare arrangements affect development?**

## Social Referencing

Infants can keenly interpret emotional signals through vocal tones as young as 5 months and through facial expressions of happiness, fear, and anger as young as 7 months. A byproduct of this understanding is **social referencing**, when the infant refers to the emotional reaction of another person to gauge and react to novel or ambiguous social stimuli (Kim, Walden, & Knieps, 2010). A parent or primary caregiver isn't necessarily the default social referencing figure. At times when it appears the parent or caregiver may not have the appropriate knowledge about a situation, the infant will seek out and look to the person who likely possesses the relevant information or "the expert" regarding the ambiguous stimuli in question (Stenberg, 2009). Social referencing along with the cognitive capacity for joint attention are critical in promoting a child's social learning (Pelaez, 2009). As with joint attention, deficits in social referencing appear to be present in children diagnosed with autism spectrum disorder (Brim et al., 2009).

As we've demonstrated, an infant's interaction with the environment and with caregivers is essential. Researchers often use free play interactions or teaching tasks to measure the quality of caregiver-child social interactions. We look for behaviors such as the caregiver's supportive presence or the quality of assistance they provide, as well as caregiver sensitivity, their structuring of interactions, their nonintrusiveness with the child, and nonhostility toward the child. We also look for child behaviors such as their responsiveness to the caregiver and their involvement of the caregiver during the interaction (Crowell & Feldman, 1988).

Several studies have demonstrated how the quality of parent-child interactions can stay with us across childhood and even into adulthood. Problematic parent-child interaction behaviors in the early years of a child's life are associated with nonoptimal attachment patterns, child behavioral problems, and child and adolescent depressive symptoms (Schmid et al., 2011). The good news is that interventions aimed at helping those at risk for poor parent-child interactions and even child maltreatment have been shown to improve parental sensitivity and reduce the potential for child abuse (Thomas & Zimmer-Gembeck, 2011).

## Social Contexts Outside the Family: Childcare

There has been some debate in the past over whether childcare, when started at an early age, can affect the social-emotional and cognitive-intellectual development of children. The U.S. National Institute of Child Health and Development, as well as other researchers worldwide, have focused significant efforts on this question for many years now.

The **formal childcare** experience (nonrelative, out-of-home care such as a home-based childcare provider, or larger, center-based childcare) may be somewhat stressful for young children, given that they show higher levels of the stress hormone cortisol in formal childcare arrangements than they do at home (Groeneveld et. al., 2010). However, it is now widely believed by the scientific community that it is not the type of care a child receives in his early years, but the quality of care that makes the difference, both for the infant and in terms of lasting effects across childhood. For example, in Norway, where high-quality childcare is essentially universally available, there is no evidence that a greater number of hours spent in childcare arrangements outside the home causes behavioral problems such as acting out (Zachrisson et al., 2013). In fact, there is evidence in the United States that high-quality childcare may actually be beneficial for children from low-quality home environments (Watamura et al., 2011). Formal childcare arrangements also can help academic readiness, vocabulary, and reading skills for children of mothers with low education levels (Geoffroy et al., 2010).

FIGURE 4-7 It is not the type of childcare setting, but the quality of care that makes the difference in development across childhood.

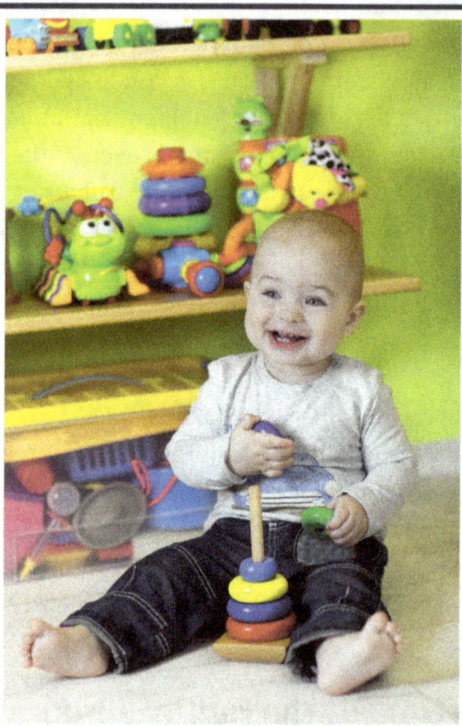

*Source*: Copyright © 2014 Depositphotos/pitrs10.

There appear to be differences between home-based childcare and center-based care as well. Caregiver sensitivity is an important predictor of cortisol levels for young children in home-based care, while overall quality of care is associated with cortisol for those in center-based environments (Groeneveld et al., 2010). The child also brings something to these social relationships. Infants with more difficult temperaments may be more greatly affected by childcare quality and show effects on social adjustment, even into late middle childhood (Pluess & Belsky, 2010).

**Shaken baby syndrome.** The leading causes of death among infants include heart defects, chromosomal disorders, disorders related to very preterm birth, and sudden infant death syndrome (Centers for Disease Control and Prevention, 2020). However, **shaken baby syndrome** (SBS) is the leading cause of traumatic death in infants. The injuries associated with SBS are caused by the violent trauma of an individual shaking a young child, typically because of infant crying or irritability. In cases that do not result in death, permanent damage is often apparent, including blindness, seizures, and severe brain damage that can lead to problems with learning, as well as problems with motor behavior and social skills (Committee on Child Abuse and Neglect, 2001). The following is taken from the Centers for Disease Control and Preventions (2013d) guide for preventing shaken baby syndrome:

# CHAPTER 5

# The Developing Toddler and Early Childhood

Toddlerhood (ages 1 to 3) and early childhood or preschool age (ages 4 and 5) mark great advances in children's autonomy that happen alongside equally great achievements in neurological, psychological, and social development. Table 5-1 presents a further overview of some milestones across toddlerhood and early childhood for typically developing children.

## Biological Development

**LO 5-1** **Why is chronic stress harmful to brain development and functioning?**

**LO 5-2** **What are some things that a child this age can do for himself?**

**TABLE 5-1** Further Developmental Milestones From the Centers for Disease Control and Prevention

| Age | Movement/Physical Development | Cognitive (learning, thinking, problem solving) | Language/ Communication | Social and Emotional |
|---|---|---|---|---|
| 18 months | • Walks alone<br>• May walk up steps and run<br>• Pulls toys while walking<br>• Can help undress herself<br>• Drinks from a cup<br>• Eats with a spoon | • Knows what ordinary things are for; for example, telephone, brush, spoon<br>• Points to get attention of others<br>• Shows interest in a doll or stuffed animal by pretending to feed<br>• Points to one body part<br>• Scribbles on his own<br>• Can follow one-step verbal commands without any gestures; for example, sits when you say "sit down" | • Says several single words<br>• Says and shakes head "no"<br>• Points to show someone what he wants | • Likes to hand things to others as play<br>• May have temper tantrums<br>• May be afraid of strangers<br>• Affectionate to familiar people<br>• Plays simple pretend, such as feeding a doll<br>• May cling to caregivers in new situations<br>• Points to show others something interesting<br>• Explores alone but with parent close by |
| 2 years | • Stands on tiptoe<br>• Kicks a ball<br>• Begins to run<br>• Climbs onto and down from furniture without help<br>• Walks up and down stairs holding on<br>• Throws ball overhand<br>• Makes or copies straight lines and circles | • Finds things even when hidden under two or three covers<br>• Begins to sort shapes or colors<br>• Completes sentences and rhymes in familiar books<br>• Plays simple make-believe<br>• Builds towers of four-plus blocks<br>• May use one hand versus the other<br>• Follows two-step instructions such as "Pick up your shoes and put them in the closet."<br>• Names items in a picture book such as a cat, bird, or dog | • Points to things or pictures when they are named<br>• Knows names of familiar people and body parts<br>• Says sentences with two to four words<br>• Follows simple instructions<br>• Repeats words overheard in conversation<br>• Points to things in a book | • Copies others, especially adults and older children<br>• Gets excited when with other children<br>• Shows more and more independence<br>• Shows defiant behavior (doing what he has been told not to)<br>• Plays mainly beside other children but is beginning to include other children, such as in chase games |

**TABLE 5-1** Continued

| Age | Movement/Physical Development | Cognitive (learning, thinking, problem solving) | Language/Communication | Social and Emotional |
|---|---|---|---|---|
| 3 years | • Climbs well<br>• Runs easily<br>• Pedals a tricycle (three-wheel bike)<br>• Walks up and down stairs, one foot on each step | • Can work toys with buttons, levers, and moving parts<br>• Plays make-believe with dolls, animals, and people<br>• Does puzzles with three or four pieces<br>• Understands what "two" means<br>• Copies a circle with pencil or crayon<br>• Turns book pages one at a time<br>• Builds towers of more than six blocks<br>• Screws and unscrews jar lids or turns door handle | • Follows two- or three-step instructions<br>• Can name most familiar things<br>• Understands words like "in," "on," and "under"<br>• Says first name, age, and gender<br>• Names a friend<br>• Says words like "I," "me," "we," and "you" and some plurals (cars, dogs, cats)<br>• Talks well enough for strangers to understand most of the time<br>• Carries on a conversation using two to three sentences | • Copies adults and friends<br>• Shows affection for friends without prompting<br>• Takes turns in games<br>• Shows concern for crying friend<br>• Understands the idea of "mine" and "his" or "hers"<br>• Shows a wide range of emotions<br>• Separates easily from mom or dad<br>• May get upset with major changes in routine<br>• Dresses and undresses self |
| 4 years | • Hops and stands on one foot up to 2 seconds<br>• Catches a bounced ball most of the time<br>• Pours, cuts with supervision, and mashes own food | • Names some colors and some numbers<br>• Understands the idea of counting<br>• Starts to understand time<br>• Remembers parts of a story<br>• Understands the idea of "same" and "different"<br>• Draws a person with two to four body parts<br>• Uses scissors<br>• Starts to copy capital letters<br>• Plays board or card games<br>• Tells you what he thinks is going to happen next in a book | • Knows some basic rules of grammar, such as correctly using "he" and "she"<br>• Sings a song or says a poem from memory such as the "Itsy Bitsy Spider" or the "Wheels on the Bus"<br>• Tells stories<br>• Can say first and last name | • Enjoys doing new things<br>• Plays "Mom" and "Dad"<br>• Is more and more creative with make-believe play<br>• Would rather play with other children than by himself<br>• Cooperates with other children<br>• Often can't tell what's real and what's make-believe<br>• Talks about what she likes and what she is interested in |

*(continued)*

**TABLE 5-1** Continued

| Age | Movement/Physical Development | Cognitive (learning, thinking, problem solving) | Language/ Communication | Social and Emotional |
|---|---|---|---|---|
| 5 years | • Stands on one foot for 10 seconds or longer<br>• Hops; may be able to skip<br>• Can do a somersault<br>• Uses a fork and spoon and sometimes a table knife<br>• Can use the toilet on her own<br>• Swings and climbs | • Counts 10 or more things<br>• Can draw a person with at least six body parts<br>• Can print some letters or numbers<br>• Copies a triangle and other geometric shapes<br>• Knows about things used every day, like money and food | • Speaks very clearly<br>• Tells a simple story using full sentences<br>• Uses future tense; for example, "Grandma will be here."<br>• Says name and address | • Wants to please friends<br>• Wants to be like friends<br>• More likely to agree with rules<br>• Likes to sing, dance, and act<br>• Shows concern and sympathy for others<br>• Is aware of gender<br>• Can tell what's real and what's make-believe<br>• Shows more independence (for example, may visit a next-door neighbor by himself [adult supervision is still needed])<br>• Is sometimes demanding and sometimes very cooperative |

## What Would You Do? Yoly's ("Jolie") Story

I had a good pregnancy—I wasn't too uncomfortable and my morning sickness didn't last that long. The delivery was also good, and I was able to have a vaginal delivery with no epidural, as I had planned. I was in heavy labor for 3 hours until I was ready to push, and Abby, my first child, came out in just three pushes. She was perfect and so beautiful. She was 7 pounds, 7 ounces, and 20 inches long, with a high Apgar score. Abby was a good baby, happy, laughing all the time, and she was always doing everything that a baby does at her age. She was doing great with all her milestones, but at about 13 months Abby started to lose her verbal skills. She stopped saying words that she knew but she also started getting a lot of ear infections, so she wasn't talking a lot any way. Her pediatrician said she had speech delay. That was fine I thought, because I'm originally from the Dominican Republic and my husband is from the United States, so we were speaking two different languages in the house, after all. When she was seen by the speech pathologist for the delay she asked us questions like "Is she very

We continue our discussion of biological development, focusing on neurological and motor development during this period. Remember, neurological development is deeply intertwined with the development of cognitive, emotional, and social functioning. Each of these areas provides clues into normal and abnormal development and functioning within the brain.

Although the brain is developing, so is the body. During the toddler years and early childhood, kids gain about 4 to 5 pounds and grow about 2 to 3 inches a year. By age 3 they will have all of their 20 "baby teeth" and 20/20 vision will develop by age 4. Across this developmental period, children slowly grow out of naps and require approximately 11 to 13 hours of sleep each day (Matricciani et al., 2012).

## Neurological Development and Functioning

A newborn's brain is roughly 25% of its adult weight, but by age 3 the brain is approximately 90% of its adult size. By this time, billions of neurons and hundreds of trillions of **synapses** have been formed. Synapses are areas where communication between adjacent neurons takes place. Neurological connections that are the basis for higher cognitive functioning are crucial. Stimulation from the environment is absolutely essential for promoting this growth and subsequent development.

Perhaps surprisingly, a 3-year-old has a brain with twice as many synapses as an adult's brain. After all, 700 of these neural connections are newly formed every second in the brain of a child (Center on the Developing Child). During these early years, and through roughly age 10, a child's brain is incredibly dense, jam-packed with billions of neurons and **glial cells** (Brotherson, 2009). Glial cells surround the neuron, provide insulation, and help support it. Remember from last chapter, though, our brain goes through a pruning process to get rid of any unnecessary synapses. The connections, used repeatedly and reinforced by the child's experiences, will become permanent, unless they are disrupted by illness or trauma. The ability to speak and our capacity for language development is a great example of this repeated reinforcement learning. Neural synapses in the brain become strengthened when babies and young children are repeatedly exposed to language, language patterns, and language rules. During this time, the development of sensory capabilities, such as vision and hearing, is also at its peak. This is one of many reasons why stimulation from the environment is so important for a child's developing brain. Without rich

active? Does she go to different toys?" and we told her yes. She did not seem so worried about it and we never went back for therapy, which now I think was a big mistake.

Eventually, Abby started losing all her words, and her eye contact was not what it should be. Her babysitter at that time told us something was wrong with her, but as a first-time parent I really thought it was because of the two languages we spoke at home. Then Abby got sick again, another ear infection. My husband, Mark, took her to the doctor, and the doctor said, "Did you take her to a specialist?" Mark told the doctor what happened at our visit with the speech pathologist, and the doctor said to Mark, "I think she has autism." You don't know how hard that is for new parents who want nothing more than that first child to be perfect (of course, she is, but it was painful). Looking back, we knew something was wrong, but there was some denial to a certain extent, and then we thought about what we may have done wrong, but we know we had done everything right.

Abby was age 2 when we met with a team of doctors, psychologists, and social workers. As soon as they saw her they said, "Oh she is so beautiful. I'm so sorry she has developmental delays." But it kind of felt like someone was saying, "She is beautiful and never going to have a life." Abby was initially diagnosed with Pervasive Developmental Disorder-Not Otherwise Specified (PDD-NOS), but 2 years later they changed her diagnosis to autism.[1] We cried a lot, but our main focus was getting help for Abby, and we did.

Having no language and no eye contact was difficult. In the early years there was no way to communicate with Abby, until we started teaching her to use sign language when she was about 3 years old. With Abby we also experienced the tantrums that went along with certain noises that bothered her and places with larger crowds where she didn't feel comfortable. I remember going to the mall with her when she was somewhere between age 5 and 7. She was having a tantrum on the floor and people were looking at us like "fix your child," but Mark and I have learned to ignore them. We've developed strategies for dealing with times like that, both with Abby and with strangers, and now there are no more tantrums.

---

[1] At the time of Abby's diagnosis, Pervasive Developmental Disorder-Not Otherwise Specified was a distinct classification in the DSM-4 to diagnose someone who met some, but not all, criteria for what was called autistic disorder (or autism). Rather than making separate distinctions, the DSM-5 now has one umbrella term for these types of disorders, including Asperger's disorder, called autism spectrum disorder.

It was hard, but when you have a child with special needs, you have to find a plan that works: having a routine with her, and teaching her what we are about to do, or where we are about to go, letting her know that it will all be fine. There was also the issue of school. Abby was in the care of our "Nana" (a great friend) since she was 3 months old. It was our Nana who told us there was something wrong with Abby. She was thinking Abby was deaf, because never looked or responded to her name. When Abby was in early intervention the decision was made to put her in a day care until her third birthday to try to build her social skills. She would also continue to get early intervention services at the day care but it was hard for her. Most of the time she was in her room, or she was in a corner on the floor. I told the people in the day care, that was not acceptable, and they agreed to make her go and play with other children. Day care in general was the hardest thing for us at the time because we did not know how Abby would take it, but after about a month, Abby was following directions.

When Abby turned 3, she went to preschool for almost 4 months, but things were not working there. She was regressing, instead of going forward. We had a very hard time with the school district to find the right match. They sent us to a few other schools around the area that were better equipped to address Abby's needs, but because Mark and I both worked, we needed a summer program and none of the programs we were looking at had one. By then we were angry and frustrated. That's when we heard about a place in our area that provides services for people with autism. We got an appointment; they did an evaluation, and she was accepted right away. There was a lot of red tape with our school district, and we had to commute to a center that was four towns away, but it was a great decision because that's where Abby needed to be.

The early years were harder than now (she's 13), but having a great team made a wonderful difference. I think she understands more now, and she is more aware of what is going on in her life (and we are very sure that she knows she is different from her sister). And her achievements—wow! The biggest one was that she learned how to communicate! At first she could sign, but now she can talk at the same time when she signs! That is the biggest. Why? Because we were always told she was going to be a very delayed child (I believe the exact words at the time were "very retarded") and she proved everyone wrong! As soon she started communicating, a different child came out!

Still all of these things took their toll. For example, I didn't want to have any more children for fear that they might have autism too, but Mark did. We eventually did, and Abby's younger sister Emma was born 4 years later. Having

stimulation, neural pathways do not become strengthened or reinforced, and because of this they can die off. This may be one of the many reasons why we see so many differences in physical health, emotional health, social skills, cognitive capabilities, language, and reading among children, and sometimes adults, based on how limited or how rich their early sensory environment was.

**Allostatic load.** Not only is lack of stimulation a problem for brain development, but **chronic stress** can negatively affect the development of certain structures in the brain and neural pathways). In times of stress the brain's natural response is to secrete hormones and neurotransmitters, such as cortisol and adrenaline, which leads to altered physiological states, such as sweating or a rapid heartbeat. When there is less stress, the brain adapts and returns to its normal state of functioning, known as **homeostasis**. When chronic stress affects the brain, the systems that regulate bodily functions, such as heart rate, metabolism, and gastrointestinal and immune functioning, are also affected. This wear and tear on the body is known as **allostatic load** (McEwen & Stellar, 1993). Research shows that allostatic load can have long-term impacts across the life span. For example, it can lead to obesity, high cholesterol, high blood sugar, and high blood pressure (Davis et al., under review; Seeman et al., 1997).

These hormones serve their purposes in times of stress, but they can also cause damage to the body if a person remains in a state of constant heightened arousal due to chronic stress. Heightened arousal states and the secretion of "stress" hormones can lead to increased blood pressure and changes in how the body finds and metabolizes food. If a person has experienced chronic stress from a young age, normal bodily processes are not properly regulated. This long-term condition can make it increasingly difficult for the body to return to homeostasis, which can affect cardiovascular and metabolic health and functioning.

Emma was the best decision I made, and we have a son, Sawyer, who is now 4 himself. When I was pregnant with Sawyer, I did not want to know the sex of the baby, because I thought of the higher risk of autism in boys. I also didn't want Emma or Sawyer to have vaccinations until their 1st year of school because of all the talk back then about potential links to autism. Sawyer did well until 15 months; still, he lost eye contact and some verbal skills, and like Abby he showed some repetitive behaviors. He was diagnosed with PDD-NOS, but with all of his therapy, play groups, and his social skills, he is doing great. On the surface you don't see autism.

In many ways, we treat Abby the same way we do Emma and Sawyer. There is no special treatment because she has autism. Everyone is the same. For example, she gets her things taken away and she has her "time-outs" when she's disobedient. I certainly do not regret my decision to have more children now. Both Sawyer and Emma know how different Abby is, but they love her a lot.

Think about what you would do in this situation after reading the chapter, and then decide the following:

- If you were the pediatrician who first identified the speech delay, what referrals would you have made?
- If you were the speech pathologist who made the first observation, would you have pushed for follow-up or would you have waited to see how Abby's behaviors progressed?
- If you were Yoly, would you have followed the advice of the first specialist? Would you have questioned some of the behaviors Abby continued to exhibit before she was diagnosed?
- If you were a doctor or specialist delivering an autistic spectrum disorder diagnosis to a parent, how would you be sensitive to their feelings and reactions?
- If you were a stranger seeing a child like Abby having a tantrum, what would your response be?
- If you were Yoly and Mark, would you want to have more children?
- If you were Yoly, what would your outlook be for Abby's future?

## Motor Development and Functioning

During the early toddler years, **fine motor skills**, or the control over small movements of the body such as fingers, hands, feet, and parts of the face and mouth, develop at the same time as the child's knowledge of the environment, what he wants to do, and what is necessary to go about doing it, for example turning a door knob. His motor skills are refined, so objects can now be used as tools, such as holding a spoon in an appropriate way to feed himself or adequately controlling a crayon to draw with it. Fine motor skills also become more precise, effective, and efficient, so acts can be carried out with increasing independence (Gerber et al., 2010). **Gross motor skills**, on the other hand, involve the activation and coordination of large muscle groups and include movements such as walking, running, and jumping. These too are accomplished with increasing coordination and refinement as the child grows older. Table 5-2 shows some fine motor skills and gross motor skills that develop across this time period.

The child's newly developing independence comes with some psychological challenges for both the child and parent. It is necessary for parents to set limits on what a child can and cannot do independently, such as going up and down stairs, slicing a tomato, or pushing a playmate. When a child is not allowed to or unable to perform an activity on their own, this can lead to frustration and anger that may result in crying, screaming, or tantrums. This limit and boundary testing that a child acts out is quite normal, and it is recommended that caregivers provide a safe and structured environment with well-defined rules for children to test their physical and emotional limits.

## Myths and Misconceptions

An adult's brain is more active than a child's. **Myth**

A 3-year-old has a brain twice as active as an adult's. **Fact**

**TABLE 5-2** Gross Motor Skills and Fine Motor Skills Across Early Childhood (Kaneshiro, 2014)

| Age | Gross Motor Development | Fine Motor Development |
|---|---|---|
| Generally | • Becoming more skilled at running, jumping, early throwing, kicking, catching a bounced ball | |
| At about age 3 | • Pedaling a tricycle | • Drawing a circle<br>• Drawing a person with three parts<br>• Beginning to use children's blunt-nose scissors<br>• Self-dressing (with supervision) |
| At about age 4 | • Becoming able to steer well<br>• Hopping on one foot and later balancing on one foot for up to 5 seconds | • Drawing a square<br>• Using scissors and eventually cutting a straight line<br>• Putting on clothes properly<br>• Managing a spoon and fork neatly while eating |
| At about age 5 | • Doing a heel-to-toe walk | • Spreading with a knife<br>• Drawing a triangle |

**FIGURE 5-1** A 3-year-old may be allowed to carry a younger sibling only with supervision, but a slightly older child may be allowed to help with younger siblings with increasing independence.

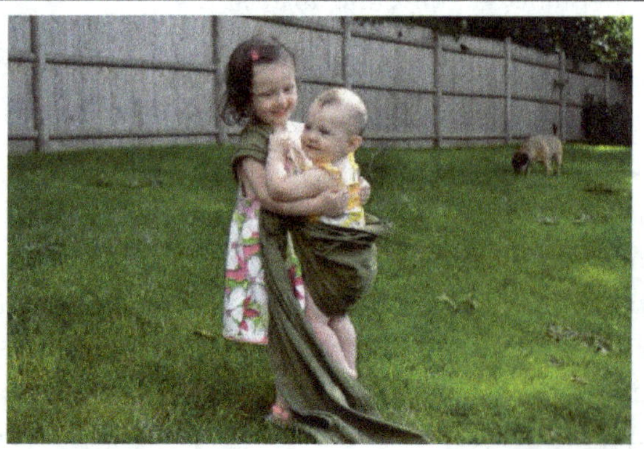

*Source*: Copyright © Jade D'Orsi. Reprinted with permission.

**FIGURE 5-2** Children with Down syndrome don't development motor skills in the same way or at the same rate as other children because of low muscle tone, greater flexibility in their joints, and less overall strength. They can receive physical therapy to promote the eventual development of more optimal posture, movement patterns, and a strong foundation for exercise across the life span (Winders, 2012).

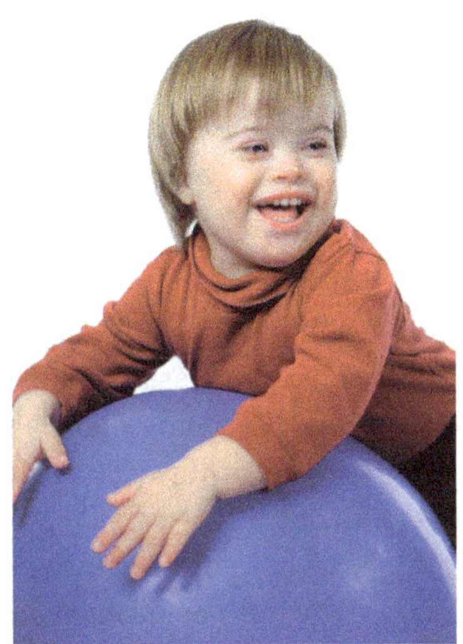

*Source*: Copyright © 2012 Depositphotos/ginosphotos1.

# Psychological Development

**LO 5-3** **What are some of the limitations of children's thinking during the toddler years and early childhood?**

**LO 5-4** **What sorts of cognitive processes are involved in executive functioning?**

**LO 5-5** **What is the role of the external environment in emotion regulation?**

**LO 5-6** **What are some of the characteristics of autism spectrum disorder?**

**LO 5-7** **How does gender development unfold across the toddler years and early childhood?**

A child's psychological development during early childhood is astounding. Not only are they developing physical and psychological independence in terms of what they can do and think for themselves, such as feeding themselves, or deciding that they don't like yellow t-shirts, but their newly developing cognitive abilities, such as their capacity for language or their ability to remember aspects of what has happened to them in the past, make them increasingly capable social agents who engage in a very active manner with their environment.

## Cognitive Development

The development of cognitive skills is still in its early stages, but young children begin to show their emerging cognitive capacities and memory capabilities and can demonstrate them as they become increasingly verbal.

**The preoperational stage.** Swiss psychologist Jean Piaget believed that during early childhood children were in the **preoperational stage** of cognitive development. This stage focuses on the limitations of a child's thinking because, according to Piaget, children have yet to develop mental operations—the ability to mentally manipulate information from the environment using organized, formal, and logical processes. The images that follow demonstrate this theory. In the first image, the child can identify that both rows contain the same number of coins. In the second image, she reports that the top row has more coins. The child concludes that the row with the coins spread apart has more coins because it appears longer than the other row. Piaget would argue that this child is lacking the mental operations necessary to manipulate the information in front of her to understand that the two rows have the same *amount* of coins even though the rows look different in *size*. The realization that objects or sets of objects remain the same even when they are moved, manipulated, or made to look different, is known as **conservation**. Children in the preoperational stage lack this cognitive ability. During this stage, children experience **egocentric thought**, meaning that they focus on their own thoughts alone and have a hard time understanding the thoughts and feelings of others. During free play, children with egocentric thought may talk in ways that simply reflect the verbalizing of their inner thoughts. Two children may be playing side by side, both talking, but the conversation may be confusing to an outside observer, because one child is verbalizing her thoughts, while the other is verbalizing his thoughts, which may have no relation to one another. On the other hand, while quietly playing with her toys, a child at this age may stop and ask a parent, "But Daddy, why did Elephant say that to Barbie?" It is likely that Elephant and Barbie were having a discussion in the child's mind, and the child assumed that the parent was also part of this inner conversation. According to Piaget, the child believes that everyone has the same inner thoughts and observations about the world as she does.

**FIGURE 5-3** A child in the preoperational stage could tell you that both rows have the same number of coins in the image on the left, but may think the top row has more coins in the image on the right.

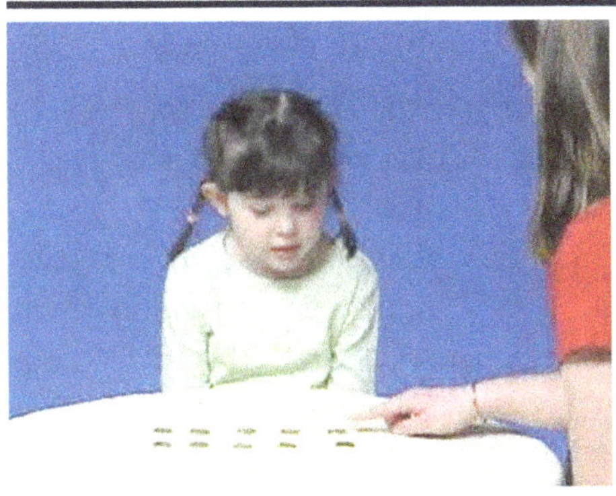

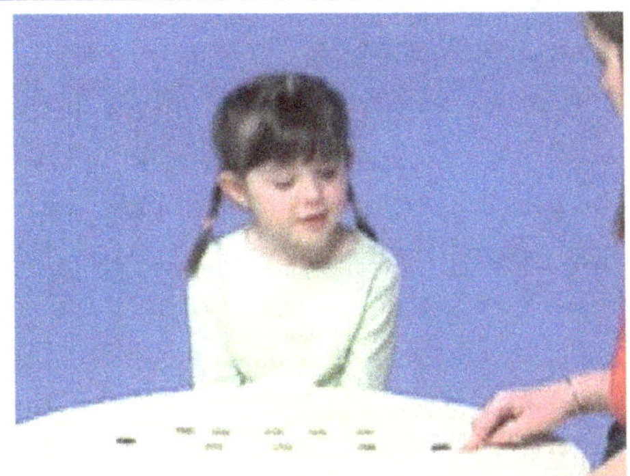

*Source*: https://www.youtube.com/watch?v=whT6w2jrWbA.

**Memory.** Around age 2, children begin to develop the ability to communicate their explicit memories. In other words, they can consciously recall and verbalize memories of events from the past. As we discussed in the previous chapter, this capacity is linked to their developing ability to understand and use language. Children can begin to talk about things they have done in the past or will do in the future. For example, a child may describe a special family event and say, "Remember when we went to California and we saw the fishies at the aquarium?" or if his birthday is tomorrow he might say "After this sleep then it will be my birthday." Some of these memories stay with us, as most adults can remember at least one event that occurred when they were 3 or 4 years old, whereas other adults can remember many events during this age period or one or two events from an even younger age (Strange & Hayne, 2013). Memories that are linked to particularly emotional events, like a trip to the hospital, are more likely to be remembered across the life span (Peterson & Whalen, 2001). Also, whether a parent continues to discuss these events with the child can make a difference on memory retention (Sales et al., 2003). When asked about important events, such as the birth of another sibling, we can typically provide greater detail about the event when we are adults, though. This is not because adults have better memories. It is likely because the details of the event are not necessarily memories from that actual time, but are pieces of information that have been provided by others over time (maybe a parent) who were also there (Gross et al., 2013).

**Executive functioning.** Executive functioning, a major component of cognition, involves mental processes that help "control, direct, or coordinate" cognitive functions such as memory, visual-spatial abilities, language, and motor skills. Executive functioning involves the ability to switch between various functions, to limit the influence of nonpriority functions and information, and to hold important information in working memory (Lee et al., 2013). Some suggest executive functioning emerges when infants can regulate their eye movement, and it becomes increasingly sophisticated during infancy as young children demonstrate joint attention (De Luca & Leventer, 2008; Johnson, 1995). During early childhood significant development occurs in areas of the prefrontal cortex, which is thought to promote executive functioning during toddlerhood and the preschool years. In young children, specifically, it appears to allow for the behavioral regulation of both thoughts and emotions (Espy et al., 2011).

The development of executive functioning is dependent on the characteristics of the child, the larger environment, and social experiences. Difficulties with executive functioning have been linked to genetic factors, increased activity in the frontal lobe during infancy (Kraybill & Bell, 2012), and a child's temperament characteristics such as negative emotionality (Leve et al., 2012). Caregiving behaviors can contribute to the development of executive functioning. For example, when a caregiver responds to a young child's cues it signifies to the infant that he has an impact on the environment. Parent-child interaction behaviors that promote a child's problem-solving abilities are also important, as are behaviors that interpret and verbalize the child's thoughts and feelings. These interactions provide the verbal skills needed to convey emotions and, in turn, help him understand and manage his feelings, or self-regulate (Carlson, 2003). The ability to interact with the environment, to problem solve, and to self-regulate are all important factors in executive functioning. It makes sense, then, that children who are raised in nonoptimal caregiving environments show deficits in executive functioning. For example, children who are adopted and experienced institutionalized care preadoption show reduced executive functioning. Researchers speculate that this is likely due to a lack of early caregiver attention and interaction, as well as poor physical care (Hostinar et al., 2012).

Executive functioning is measured by assessing several child behaviors, including delay of gratification and the ability to maintain rules in a variety of tasks when given conflicting information (Conway & Stifter, 2012). During toddlerhood and early childhood it can be linked with learning skills and behavioral difficulties across the life span (Fitzpatrick & Pagani, 2012; Leve et al., 2012).

## Emotion Regulation

**Emotion regulation** is the ability to self-regulate and adjust emotions and emotional expression in a way that is appropriate for a given social situation. It operates alongside executive functioning and many of the cognitive functions under its control. Emotion regulation is a cognitive task, primarily maintained by the caregiver at first who serves as an external regulator letting the child know what is acceptable behavior and what is not. Then gradually, over time, the child is able to self-regulate without the help of a caregiver.

Emotions are fundamental to organizing cognitive processes, learning, and behaviors. These cognitive processes help us interpret and regulate our emotions in a given social context so that emotions and cognition work together. In many cases emotions need to be calmed, but in other cases it is appropriate and sometimes necessary for a child to become excited or upset—for example, if they are hurt or in danger and need the help of a caregiver. Like many of our human characteristics and behaviors, think of emotion regulation on a continuum, as presented in Table 5-3. As you can imagine, the display of appropriate emotions is closely tied to cultural norms.

**TABLE 5-3** Characterizations of Emotion Regulation in Children (Carlson & Wang, 2007)

| | |
|---|---|
| Under-controlled | • Low in emotion regulation, impulsive, and high in emotional intensity<br>• Easily frustrated and prone to reactive aggression |
| Optimally regulated | • Controlled but flexible and use adaptive means of coping with emotions<br>• Described as relatively popular and socially competent |
| Highly inhibited | • Exhibit self-control but lack flexibility<br>• Tend to be socially withdrawn and sad or anxious |

**Emotion displays.** There is a long-held theory that six basic emotions are universal across the human species: happiness, surprise, fear, disgust, anger, and sadness. This theory, also known as a "universality hypothesis," argues that based on our evolutionary past and our biological make-up the expression of these emotions is universal because we all use the same facial movements to convey these states (Susskind et al., 2008). However, more recent research suggests that there are discrete variations in the ways different cultures convey these emotions. For example, in Westerners, these six emotions each have distinct facial movements. But among Easterners, there is some overlap in facial movements across emotions such as fear, disgust, and anger. Westerners use facial muscles to convey these different emotions, whereas Easterners tend to use eye movements of varying intensity to differentiate among certain basic emotions.

We need to consider what certain cultures deem appropriate for emotional expression in a particular social context. These learned behaviors are known as **emotional display rules** (Ekman & Friesen, 1969). Display rules often go hand in hand with the value a culture places on a particular emotion. If a culture values sadness over disgust, then the emotional expression of disgust is more likely to be repressed. Differences in emotional display rules according to cultural norms has been widely studied in a number of countries, including the United States, Japan, Hong Kong, South Korea, Italy, England, Russia, Costa Rica, and Canada; and studies have shown differences among certain ethnic groups within the United States.

**FIGURE 5-4** Note that countries with lower scores on individualism also tend to have lower scores on emotional expressivity, whereas countries with higher scores on individualism tend to have higher scores on emotional expressivity (adapted from Matsumoto et al., 2008).

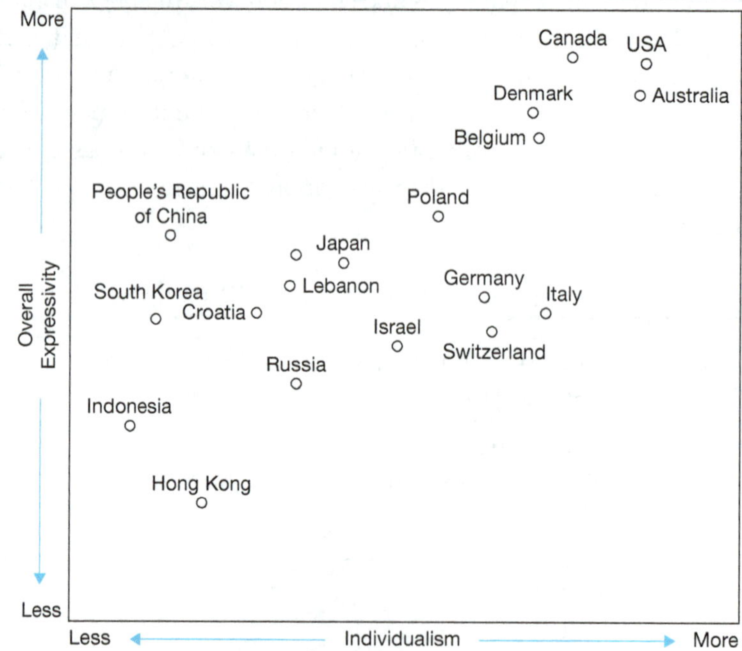


*Note*: Much of this relationship is carried by the relationship between individualism with happiness and surprise.
*Source*: "Mapping Expressive Differences Around the World: The Relationship Between Emotional Display Rules and Individualism Versus Collectivism." *Journal of Cross Cultural Psychology*, vol. 39, no. 1.

One could point to research showing that Japan does not permit expressions of anger, contempt, and, disgust as much as certain North American cultures (Safdar et al., 2009). However, culture and its display rules are not the only things that govern an emotional expression. There are also individual factors that lead to the display of emotions. Maybe you saw U.S. gymnast McKayla Maroney on the medal podium at the 2012 Summer Olympics. She thought her performance was better than the gold medalist's and made a face that perhaps conveyed her disagreement with the judges' decision. During the same year, silver medalist Kōhei Uchimura did not expect to do well going into the competition but his emotional expression conveys happiness and content.

Research also shows that even across different cultures men tend to express anger, contempt, and disgust more than women and women tend to express sadness and fear more than men do (Safdar et al., 2009). In a comparison of Dutch and Iranian children, researchers found that Iranian children used more display rules in their expression of emotions. They were more likely to do so with family members than friends. Dutch children were more likely to exhibit display rules with their friends rather than their families. Iranian children stated they used display rules with family members for the good of others and for self-protective reasons (Novin et al., 2009).

The same researchers also examined the strategies children of different cultures use for dealing with emotionally charged situations. Chinese children were more likely to be tolerant of an aggressor, whereas Dutch children were more likely to confront the aggressor to achieve their personal goals (Novin et al., 2011).

As with executive functioning, emotion regulation can be seen in infancy when in an effort to self-soothe an infant may suck a pacifier or her thumb, avert her gaze, turn her head, or seek proximity to a caregiver when distressed. Toddlers will engage in some of these and other behaviors in an attempt to regulate. For example, a toddler might be told they cannot play with a particular object, so they will distract themselves by playing with another toy. Typically developing children become increasingly better at emotion regulation as social demands become greater.

As one might expect, successful emotion regulation in preschoolers is associated with social competence and positive engagement with peers (Carlson & Wang, 2007). Emotion regulation has even been associated with pediatric obesity. Researchers believe this connection lies within the vagus nerve, a large **cranial nerve** that connects the brain directly to the abdomen to relay information between the brain and the body's organs. The vagus nerve is responsible for telling the brain when the stomach is full and is linked to physiological responses to coping, and thus emotion regulation. Therefore, it may be children who have a difficult time with emotion regulation also have challenges knowing when they are full. Another possible explanation is the notion of "emotional eating," or eating as a way of coping with stress or negative emotions. Emotional eating has been demonstrated in adulthood, but it is unclear whether children respond to stress in these same ways and whether they, too, are prone to emotional eating (Graziano et al., 2010). Another possibility for the link between emotion regulation and childhood obesity is that childhood stressors increase allostatic load and activate hormones from the hypothalamic-pituitary-adrenal axis. The body tries to prepare for a "fight-or-flight" response and seeks out high-fat, and high-energy food that can lead to fat storage and obesity (Davis, under review).

## Diagnosing Autism in Young Children

**Autism spectrum disorders**, sometimes called ASDs, are neurodevelopmental disorders that impair social instincts and include a set of disorders with symptoms that range from mild to severe (Lauritsen, 2013). These disorders include impairments with social interactions, communication abilities, and the capacity for imagination, and often coincide with certain repetitive behaviors. ASDs include autism, atypical autism, and Asperger's syndrome. Once a child has been referred for evaluation of a possible ASD based on behavioral symptoms, which would be noted in a medical history, and/or observed by parents or a trained clinician, the assessment should occur within 3 months, and should be done using the ICD-10 (*International Classification of Diseases*, 10th ed.) or the DSM (*Diagnostic and Statistical Manual of Mental Disorders*). There are also checklists, including the CHAT and the M-CHAT, that can identify if there is any risk early on, or if autism is suspected. However, these checklists should not be used for diagnosing autism (Allely & Wilson, 2011).

The number of diagnoses increased tremendously using the DSM-4 criteria, so the question arose of whether these were valid diagnoses. In response to this, revisions were made in the new version, the DSM-5 (see Table 5-4). In previous versions of the DSM, symptoms had to start prior to age 3, but this has since been removed, because it can often be hard to detect early signs of ASD and sometimes symptoms can be overlooked. This is also beneficial because there are some individuals who are not diagnosed until well into their adolescence or adulthood as environmental and social responsibilities increase (Lauritsen, 2013).

**TABLE 5-4** Revisions to of the *Diagnostic Statistical* Manual (DSM) for Autism Spectrum Disorder (DSM-5) (adapted from Lauritsen, 2013)

| To Be Diagnosed With Autism Spectrum Disorder, a Person Must Meet Criteria A, B, C, and D |
|---|
| A. Significant deficits in social communication and social interaction across contexts, including deficits in (1) social-emotional reciprocity (approach, back and forth conversation, reduced sharing of interests and emotions); (2) nonverbal communication behaviors (eye contact, body language, facial expression); (3) developing and maintaining relationships.<br>All three are required. |
| B. Restricted, repetitive patterns of behavior, interests, or activities including (1) repetitive speech, motor movements or use of objects; (2) excessive adherence to routines or behavior patterns or excessive resistance to change; (3) abnormally intense or focused, restricted, fixated interests; (4) extreme sensitivity or lack of sensitivity to sensory input or objects.<br>At least two are required. |
| C. Symptoms present in early childhood although may not be fully apparent until social demands are placed upon the individual. |
| D. Symptoms limit and impair everyday functioning. |

## Language Development

The capacity for speech and language development is innate in human, but it is also profoundly affected by the social environment. Groundbreaking case studies in the field of psychology demonstrate that speech and language suffer without input from an enriching social environment. One of the most famous case studies in the field of psychology involved a young girl names Genie who was almost entirely isolated from a social environment at a young age. It helped psychologists understand why speech and language cannot develop without input and interaction with others.

We know young children can readily communicate without using words. Crying, smiling, and gazing, among other things, signal what's happening in an infant's mind. These forms of communication, and the ability to put thoughts into words, are known as **expressive language**. As children grow, thoughts develop, or are conceptualized, in their minds. Children choose the words available to them to express a thought and sounds and speech are produced to vocalize that thought. Many caregivers experience toddlers who are very adept at expressing the word "no," either verbally with words, vocally with sounds, or nonverbally with actions. Another means of language communication in toddlers, **receptive language**, is children's ability to understand what is being communicated to them. A child's response, whether verbal or behavioral, most often indicates a capacity for receptive language. Table 5-5 shows a young child's capacity for language as it develops. At the same time, children and adults with certain motor impairments may be unable to respond to communication to indicate they understand what's being said.

## Theory Then and Now

**Theory then:** Noam Chomsky first proposed that humans have an instinctive capacity, called the language acquisition device, based in the brain that allows us to understand rules of grammar and to use language to communicate.

**Theory now:** He later put forth the notion of universal grammar, which states language development requires three components: (1) the innate ability to develop language based on humans' unique genetic makeup; (2) stimulation from the environment; and (3) factors independent of innate abilities and the environment.

Many contend that there are "critical periods" for the development of language. In other words, if we don't develop this ability during early childhood, our ability to develop it at all is in jeopardy. The longer a person goes without the tools for language development (based on the three requirements of universal grammar) the less likely they are to develop language. Those who don't develop this ability by the time puberty ends are unlikely to develop it at all (Pinker, 1994). Universal grammar, which proposes the principles of grammar are the same across all languages, has come into question in recent years, given what we know about the complexity of languages as well as developments in our understanding of cognition that have put forth new explanations for humans' capacity for language.

**TABLE 5-5** Language Milestones During the Toddler Years and Early Childhood (Wilks et al., 2010)

| Age | Language Milestone |
|---|---|
| 12 to 15 months | • Can point to body parts<br>• Can point to familiar objects when named<br>• Shakes head to communicate "no"<br>• Repeats words<br>• Mimics sounds (cat's meow) |
| 18 to 24 months | • Has approximately a 50-word vocabulary<br>• Understands pronouns<br>• Refers to self as "me"<br>• Can produce two-word sentences (noun + verb)<br>• Communicates wants (want dada)<br>• Communicates socially ("Hi Mama")<br>• 50% of speech is understandable by a stranger |

*(continued)*

**TABLE 5-5** Continued

| Age | Language Milestone |
| --- | --- |
| 2 years to 3 years | • Vocabulary increases<br>• Can produce three- to four-word phrases<br>• Can answer questions<br>• Communicates to learn (asks "what" questions)<br>• Understands concept of "one"<br>• Follows two-step commands |
| 3 to 4 years | • Communicates to learn ("why" questions)<br>• Becomes reliable reporter of events that occurred in the past<br>• Understands what's being communicated to her well<br>• 75% is understandable by a stranger |
| 4 to 5 years | • Can follow more complex instructions<br>• Speech is completely understandable to strangers |

Adapted from R. Jason Gerber, Timothy Wilks, and Christine Erdie-Lalena, Developmental Milestones: Motor Development, Pediatrics in Review, vol. 31, no. 7. American Academy of Pediatrics, 2010.

The social environment impacts many factors that contribute to a child's ability to communicate and possess language skills. Studies have shown that early cognitive stimulation is fundamental to language development. Caregiving behaviors such as reading, teaching, verbal interactions, and the availability of learning materials, including games and toys, all contribute to language development (Cates et al., 2012).

A child's gender is associated with early language development. Research shows that "females produce sounds at an earlier age, use words sooner, develop larger vocabularies, display greater grammatical complexity, spell better, and read sooner than males" (Lovas, 2011, p. XX). Nevertheless, female children show relatively small advances during early childhood over their male counterparts, and these differences typically disappear by the age of 5. It's believed that differences at the biological and social level contribute to these early abilities. Biologically speaking, during the prenatal stage females are exposed to different types and amounts of hormones that result in accelerated brain development, which leads to differences in perception and attention between the sexes. Socially speaking, on average, female infants tend to make more eye contact and participate in joint attention more often than males do. Because of these differences, females engage differently with the verbal and nonverbal behaviors of caregivers, leading to increases in language development during early childhood. Research also shows that parents tend to speak more and in more meaningful ways to their young daughters than to their sons (Lovas, 2011).

**Hearing impairment.** Two to three of every 1,000 children are born with some degree of hearing impairment, and most states in the United States perform mandatory newborn hearing tests to determine if some kind of hearing impairment exists (Natonal Institute of Health, 2013). Hearing impairments in young children may be a result of genetically inherited traits or environmental factors, including fetal alcohol syndrome and prenatal infections in the mother, such as chlamydia. Other environmental factors that could lead to hearing loss are mumps or meningitis, exposure to certain toxins, some types of brain tumors, or injuries that result in ruptured ear drums. Hearing impairment can range from mild to profound, to total deafness and is referred to as prelingual deafness if the impairment exists at birth or occurs prior to the child's acquisition of language.

Children with severe to profound hearing impairments spend less time communicating with their caregivers. In turn, children with hearing impairments tend to show greater language acquisition difficulties that may lead to attention difficulties and behavioral problems (Barker et al., 2009; Tasker et al., 2010).

Until recently children with hearing impairments relied on hearing aids, which amplify sound for ears that have been damaged in some way. Now it is somewhat more common for a person with a hearing impairment to receive cochlear implants. Rather than simply amplifying sound, cochlear implants artificially stimulate the cochlear (auditory) nerve and send auditory information directly to the brain bypassing the damaged parts of the ear all together. The "sounds" experienced are somewhat different, but for children under 2 years of age, cochlear implants can improve joint attention abilities, language skills, and speech, sometimes putting them on par with their peers without hearing impairments.

**Second language learners.** Young children are especially adept at acquiring language. Language acquisition is believed to have a critical period of development during early childhood as the brain undergoes the rapid production and pruning of neurons and synapses. It is a critical skill for the individual to obtain during this developmental period. Therefore, acquiring a second language during toddlerhood and early childhood can be easier than when it is learned later in life. In fact, second language learning is one area in which children are far superior to adults. Figure 5-5 shows that a person's ability to learn and speak a second language declines as they age.

The "critical" period for language development, however, depends on which aspect of language we're talking about. Phonetic language learning, how to say and make movements with the mouth to produce certain sounds, occurs during infancy and the 1st year of life. Syntactic learning, or learning various language rules to produce statements that make sense and sound correct for any given language, peaks from 18 months to 3 years of age. Many parents and caregivers describe (and research supports the notion of) an "explosion" of vocabulary starting at 18 months. Learning new vocabulary continues across the life span as we are always able to learn new words and terms in the languages we speak (Kuhl, 2010).

**FIGURE 5-5** The relation between age of acquisition of a second language and language skill (adapted from Johnson & Newport, 1989, as cited in Kuhl, 2010).

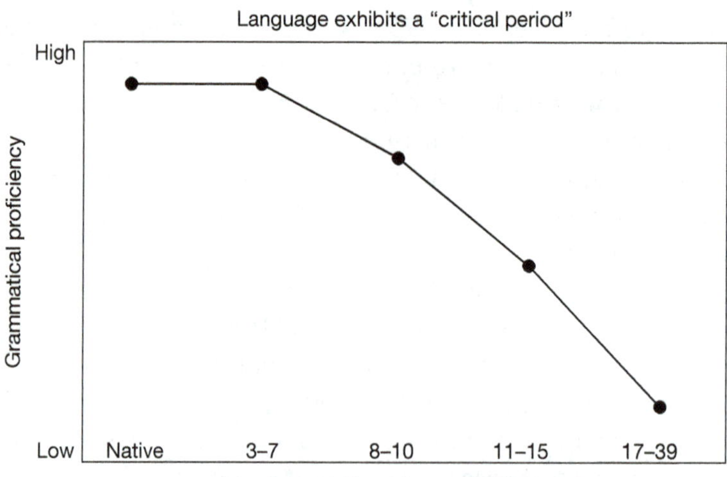


*Source*: "Critical Period Effects in Second Language Learning: The Influence of Maturational State on the Acquisition of English as a Second Language." *Cognitive Psychology*, vol. 21

## Theory Then and Now

**Theory then:** Language learning was due to the development of the corpus callosum, the area of the brain responsible for communication between the left and right hemispheres (Lenneberg, 1967).

**Theory now:** The way neurons develop early in infancy maximizes a child's ability to detect, process, and understand the basic language she is exposed to. Think about the simplistic ways in which many parents and caregivers speak to their children. Once the basics are established (in English, for example, the adjective "good" should come before the noun "boy"), they set the stage for learning the primary language completely, be it English or Arabic, and they delay the ability to learn language patterns that do not conform to those "basics" (Kuhl, 2010).

To put it another way, the brain, as it learns a language, is creating a pattern of neurons for English that is like a round hole, and the more complex rules for English that are learned across childhood are like a round peg. The rules (the round peg) fit the neuron patterns (round hole). However, the pattern for Arabic may be like a square hole. Trying to learn the language sounds and rules for Arabic (a square peg) if you are an English speaker would be like to trying to fit a square peg into a round hole! However, if you're learning both English and Arabic in early childhood, the brain will have created patterns to accommodate the learning of both languages.

**Speech and language delays.** Roughly 7% of children exhibit speech and language delays when they begin elementary school. These delays can include vocabulary, understanding grammar rules, interpreting meaning, sound production, and knowing how language is used in varying social contexts. There are some established risk factors for language delays. For example, did you know that by kindergarten children from higher socioeconomic status backgrounds have been exposed to roughly 32 million more words than children from lower socioeconomic status backgrounds (Wilks et al., 2010)? Learning English as a second language may contribute to delays in one or both of the languages a young child is exposed to. And as we've discussed, providing a rich cognitive environment is critical in supporting language development (Boyle, 2011).

If a language delay is not addressed, it can affect a child's ability to read, their social development and behaviors, as well as their mental health and well-being in adulthood. At the same time, it can sometimes be hard to tell whether a language delay is the sole or primary problem, or whether the language delay is the result of an additional or larger problem. Young children with language delays may also be within the range of a "normative" developmental timeline; therefore, the problem may be overlooked (Boyle, 2011).

**Myths and Misconceptions**

Educational videos promote children's language development (Wilks et al., 2010). **Misconception**

Educational videos often do not take into account and cannot provide the subtle interactive components necessary for speech promotion and language development. **Fact**

Reading to young children and interventions designed to increase the frequency and complexity of language exposure promote speech and language development. **Fact**

## Moral Development

Moral development, or our understanding of right and wrong, ethics, and contingencies, is rooted in our cognitive abilities and our social experiences. We see the beginning of moral development in early childhood. Psychologist Lawrence Kohlberg developed a theory of moral development that built on Piaget's work in cognitive development. Kohlberg believed the development of morals occurred in stages. Over the course of toddlerhood and early childhood, during the first stage of moral development, children begin to tell the difference between good and bad and have a firm understanding of these distinctions by the end of this developmental period. However, their morals and moral behaviors are based on obedience and punishment. Children have a certain sense of fear of authority, and they will act obediently to avoid punishment. The finer nuances of morals and ethics are far from developed, but they are based in an individual's ability to understand certain fundamentals of right and wrong that emerge during this period.

## Gender Development

Kohlberg also developed a theory about aspects of gender with regard to a child's ideas and feelings about being a boy or a girl that occurs in stages. The first stage is the development of **gender identity**, which usually takes place by age 2. The child labels themselves as a boy or a girl. They also know their anatomical parts. However, they do not understand that their sex and gender are, in general, stable across the life span. During this stage, a boy might say, "When I grow up, I want to be a mommy." Children are also motivated to behave in ways they believe their gender should. For example, a 3-year-old might say, "Girls don't wear gray shirts with trains on them because those are for boys." **Gender stability** is the next stage to develop, usually by age 4, when children realize that their gender is stable over time; they begin to understand that boys become men and girls become women. The last stage to develop is **gender constancy**, in which a child knows regardless of what they look like or what they do that their gender remains the same. In other words, wearing a gray shirt with a train on it does not make a little girl a boy.

**FIGURE 5-6A, B, and C** Aspects of gender are certainly influenced by the environment. What makes a girl a girl and a boy a boy is based on the roles that boys and girls and men and women play in that society. These thoughts, feelings, and behaviors can vary from family to family, from culture to culture, and from historical context to historical context.

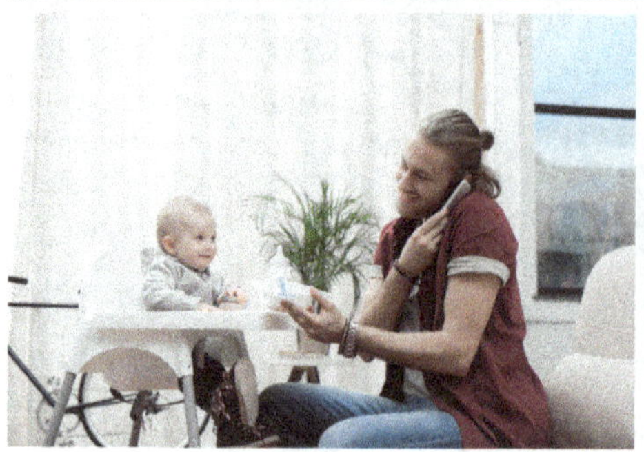

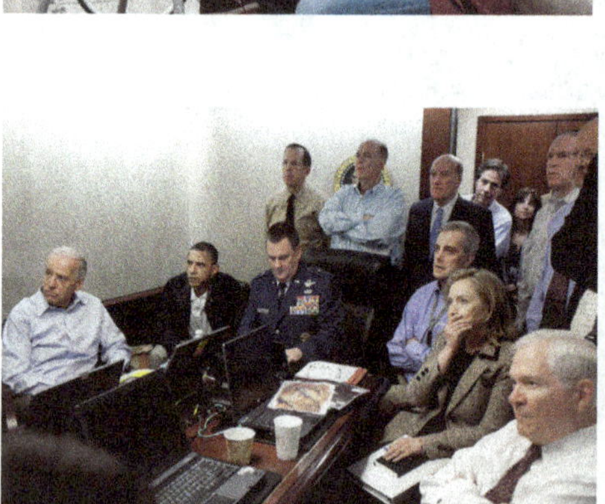

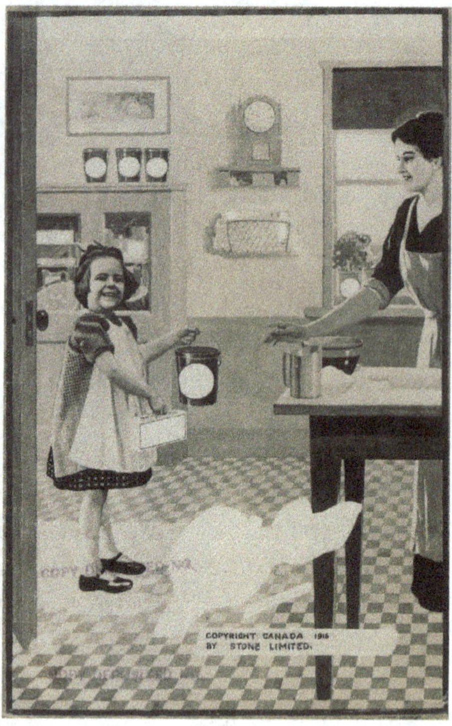


*Sources*: Copyright © 2017 Depositphotos/VitalikRadko.
Fig. 5.6b: https://commons.wikimedia.org/wiki/File:A_housewife_and_a_little_girl_in_a_kitchen_(HS85-10-32098).jpg.
Fig. 5.6c: https://commons.wikimedia.org/wiki/File:Obama_and_Biden_await_updates_on_bin_Laden.jpg.

Gender identity is also something we realize is not necessarily stable. Someone may realize early on that their gender identity does not match their sex, or this realization may come later in life. These issues are complex and are the focus of much debate in today's society and in the field of psychology.

# Social Contexts and Development

### LO 5-8 What are the goals of preschool?

Many aspects of development and functioning cannot be isolated from one another and they cannot be isolated from the social environment. Language and communication are necessary within a social context and are developed by an enriched social environment. Infants learn to point to or gaze at objects that hold their interest and engage their caregivers by gazing at them or uttering a sound or a word. As they grow, children show interest toward others to engage them in more complex exchanges and to share their experiences (Gerber et al., 2011).

# Play

Many young children will spend a considerable amount of their waking hours engaged in social interaction and play activities. Play can be a solitary or social activity, and it is a fundamental component of child development. In fact, play has been deemed a right of every child in the world by the United Nations High Commission for Human Rights (Ginsburg, the Committee on Communications, & the Committee on Psychosocial Aspects of Child and Family Health, 2007).

**Social play.** Children often engage in **solitary play** before they reach age 2 (Xu, 2008). In fact, some say that a child can play well in a group that is the same number as his age. For example, a 2-year-old can play well with one other child and a 3-year-old can play well in a group of three. After age 2, children typically play together with or near or next to one another by engaging in **parallel play**. However, there is limited social interaction in parallel play. They may look at each other or imitate the other's actions, but they're both doing their own thing, as they haven't quite mastered the skills necessary for **cooperative play**. Before a child learns the "rules" of cooperative play, emotional outbursts and aggression are usually the tools of choice for conflict negotiation. By age 3, most children are ready to engage in cooperative play with their playmates. Cooperative play between children involves joint goals and turn-taking, as they've learned the requisite skills for controlling outbursts and aggression (Gerber et al., 2011; Xu, 2008).

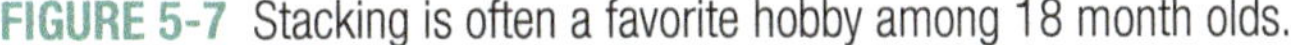
**FIGURE 5-7** Stacking is often a favorite hobby among 18 month olds.

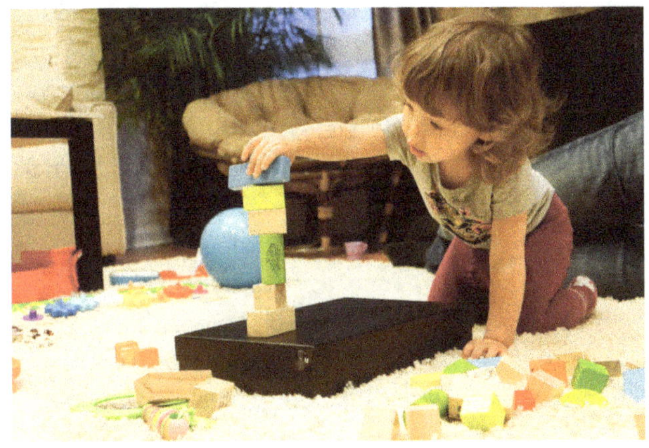

*Source*: Copyright © 2013 Depositphotos/ehaurylik.

**Pretend play. Pretend play** is a way for children to act out or create an imaginary object, scenario, place, or person. For example, a child may pretend her magic markers are a fairy wand, or her toy cow is going food shopping. A child can engage in pretend play on her own, through solitary play, or in the company of others through parallel play or cooperative play. Pretend play usually peaks between ages 3 and 5, but can occur well into middle childhood and beyond, and can be solitary or social (Lillard et al., 2013).

There is some debate about the importance of pretend play for child development. In the West, particularly in the United States, pretend play is strongly encouraged and promoted, and even written into the policies of some preschool accreditation agencies. However, the importance of pretend play is up for debate in other countries and cultures. A recently written review states that "in only five of 16 countries surveyed (the United States, the United Kingdom, Ireland, Portugal, and Argentina) do the majority of mothers say their children (ages 1 to 12) often participate in imaginative play" (Lillard et al., 2013, p. XX).

By 1 and a half years a child can engage in simple pretend play that often mimics behaviors he sees in his day-to-day activities, such as feeding a doll using a toy bottle. By 2 and a half pretend play becomes more complex, with more sophisticated "story lines," sometimes in which generic objects represent an item related to the story, such as laying a stuffed animal down on the table, using a napkin as a blanket, and putting it to bed. As the child grows older, these scenarios become increasingly complex and move into the realm of fantasy and imagination. They may start to pretend to be different people, animals, or objects (Gerber et al., 2011). Imaginary play is quite important at this age; imaginary fears are quite real for children because they have a hard time distinguishing between who and what is real versus imaginary. However, by the age of 4, children are typically aware of the difference between the two. As the child makes his way through early childhood, pretend play becomes even more complex. For example, at this age, they like to trick others and like to be tricked themselves. By age 5, pretend play is enjoyed while playing dress-up and acting out fantasies (Gerber et al., 2011).

Pretend play is not the only form of play. Think of a playground with swings and jungle gyms. Physical play, including rough-and-tumble play, has a role in a child's development; it assists with emotion regulation and promotes physical activity (Lillard et al., 2013). Current recommendations are that children have at least 60 minutes of structured physical activity (adult lead) and 60 minutes of unstructured physical activity (free play) each day (National Association for Sport and Physical Education, 2002). Regardless of its role in cognitive development, play is crucial to a child's daily life. In fact, methods that incorporate "playful learning" can be the best way to promote child development (Hirsh-Pasek, 2009).

## Preschool

In many Western industrialized nations, a common decision for parents is whether to send their children to **preschool**. Preschool typically starts around age 3. For some parents, especially those whose children have participated in formal childcare from an early age, the decision to enroll children in preschool may seem obvious. For others, it can be a difficult transition. Preschool means new caregivers, more children, more structure, and greater expectations. For some children, this is their first time out of the home and with caregivers other than parents or family members for an extended period of time. All these things, coupled with new schedules and routines, can cause worry or anxiety in children and parents.

### Theory Then and Now

**Theory then:** According to Vygotsky (1967), pretend play causes cognitive development, whereas according to Piaget (1962), pretend play is just one indicator that a child's cognitive development is happening.

**Theory now:** Depending on the domain of cognitive development (for example, creativity, emotion regulation, etc.), pretend play may be one of many factors that promotes cognitive development, or it may be something that goes hand in hand with cognitive development, but pretend play does not necessarily cause cognitive development (Lillard et al., 2013).

The goal of preschool education is to prepare a child for entry into primary or elementary school through enrichment of verbal, written, and mathematical literacy skills, as well as scientific thinking, communication, play, creativity, physical health and development, social skills including communication, one-on-one and group interaction (for example, sharing and taking turns), and personal, emotional, and self-help skill development. Teachers must recognize that children enter preschool with a range of experiences, knowledge, and capabilities that affect their cognitive, social, and behavioral skills; physical and motor development; and understanding of norms for social interactions. High-quality teachers and centers can help level the playing field for children from various backgrounds and promote school preparedness.

Preschools typically consist of structured classrooms where children are grouped based on their age. Variations in the structure may be the result of federal, state, or local regulations such as class size and student-to-teacher ratios, as well as variations related to teaching beliefs and teaching practices. For example, Montessori and Reggio Emilia are two types of preschools that both have origins in Italy, but they are different in terms of how they understand the developing child. The **Montessori approach** believes that the child learns through the structured use of specific materials. Montessori classrooms are often organized around core content areas, such as math and literacy, with physical spaces populated with materials specific to the content, such as counting blocks, or sand paper letters for tracing. The **Reggio Emilia approach** also touts the importance of a material-rich environment, but the materials and their uses are based on the interests of the child. In a Reggio Emilia school, teachers document and learn from how the children interact with their world. In turn, they offer guidance to the children in the form of materials and experiences to deepen the children's learning and development (Pufall-Jones, 2014).

**Preschool and children with special needs.** The transition to preschool can be particularly challenging for children with special needs. In the United States, many of these children have been provided early intervention services by the federal government from birth up to age 3. Preschool means not only transitioning *into* a new environment, but transitioning *out of* an established environment, routine, or caregiver that specifically addresses their unique needs. Parents and schools need to build solid partnerships before the transition takes place. These partnerships should continue throughout by understanding everyone's roles in the child's life and educational experiences and by maintaining good communication and meeting regularly to discuss the child and goals related to their preschool experience. Centers and teachers that have flexible programs and schedules can be beneficial (Walker, 2012). In addition, the National Association for the Education of Young Children (NAEYC) states that parent involvement in transition planning, as well as maintaining a level of continuity between early intervention and preschool environments and strategies, is vital for a child's success. For example, if a child experiences conflicting messages in terms of expectations for behaviors and skills from one caregiving context to the next, the child's ability to maintain their current skills and develop new skills falls into jeopardy.

**Cultural variations.** There is considerable variation in preschool experiences across cultures. For example, in Japan and China, as well as many countries in Europe, preschools are "universal." They are programs that are available to all children and are funded by the government. This is not the case in other countries such as the United States.

There are not only differences in the availability of preschools across cultures, but there is tremendous variation in the beliefs and the practices of centers and teachers. In the 1980s, a group of researchers set out to make cross-cultural comparisons of preschools in China, Japan, and the United States. They revisited these programs in recent years to examine what has changed and what has stayed the same. They found in each of these countries educators placed a high value on the influence of parenting and the importance of parental goals for each individual child's development. In China and the United States, the preschool curriculum focused largely on cognitive stimulation, and in the United States there was special emphasis placed on providing academically rigorous programs to meet accreditation and policy standards. In Japan, however, priorities included a focus on the moral development of the child, as it's considered highly important for a child's intellectual growth. In dealing with social interactions, China's preschools valued children's independence and creativity but balanced this with socialist values, such as connectedness to others and the interdependence of members of society. Preschool teachers in Japan took a nonintervention approach in which children were allowed to resolve conflicts independently while being closely monitored by teachers. In the United States, however, teachers played a direct role in children's social interactions through guidance and intervention (Tobin et al., 2009).

# CHAPTER 6 Middle Childhood

As children transition into middle childhood, their day-to-day lives continue to expand into larger social institutions such as schools. Middle childhood is typically considered the years between 6 and 11 (Centers for Disease Control and Prevention, 2011b). Many cultures believe that a child's entry into society should coincide with their entry into the formal education system. Although we will focus considerable attention on those populations throughout this chapter, we must not forget that vastly different practices exist in many other countries.

It may be hard to comprehend that children could be forced to work, to become soldiers, or be deprived of basic health care and education, but that is the harsh reality for many children throughout the world. The International Labor Organization estimates that 14.5% of children between the ages of 5 and 14 are part of the active labor force, and that globally around 215 million children are working, many full time. For these children there is no school, there is no play, and there are no activities, such as karate, lacrosse, or scouts. Many children in the world work in hazardous environments, some under conditions of forced labor and slavery, whereas others are used in drug trafficking, prostitution, or armed conflict, and most do not receive proper nutrition or health care (Diallo et al., 2010). Some children in the labor force work alongside their parents. However, the horrible reality is that others are abducted, then bought and sold, or rented to work as indentured slaves. Table 6-1 presents a ranking of the 10 countries with the worst child labor conditions, and Figure 6-2 shows a map of child labor risk worldwide. In Myanmar, where 40% of children never enroll in school, those who experience the most severe conditions commonly commit suicide. Note that in Figure 6-2, the United States represents a *medium* risk for child labor. This is because in the United States the agricultural industry is exempt from labor laws, and because of this, a considerable number of Latino children work long hours, sometimes under dangerous conditions, on a daily basis (McKenna, 2012).

Many children around the globe, however, are given the opportunity to explore their increasing independence, to learn, and to develop meaningful social relationships during middle childhood. These opportunities match the increasing expectations, demands, and responsibilities that are placed on them. As we will discuss, middle childhood is so much more than a "latency" stage, the relatively uneventful period between important stages of development that Freud described. On the contrary, contemporary theorists, such as Erik Erikson, whose eight stages of life span development we'll highlight later, recognize that there is a lot going on during this developmental period, as physical, cognitive, emotional, and social development domains continue to progress (see Table 6-2). We will continue to look at what's going on in each of these domains and begin to focus on development within traditional educational environments—a focus for many children around the globe during middle childhood.

## What Would You Do? Jenney's Story

I don't remember making a conscious decision to homeschool my children. I just never really considered any other options. When they were babies and toddlers, I was fortunate to be able to be with them full time, as I could bring them with me to my part-time job. I really enjoyed spending our days together, playing, working, and learning. Homeschooling just seemed like a natural extension of that. I'd heard it said that we are our child's first teacher: We teach them to walk and talk, feed themselves, and use the bathroom. Continuing to teach them beyond age 6 just felt like the right thing to do for our family.

In the beginning, a lot of people questioned our decision to homeschool, and we had certain relatives who felt that by making this choice we were depriving our kids of the socialization that comes with the school experience. I disagreed with this. I felt that by homeschooling I could provide not only a solid academic education, but also opportunities for socialization and real friendships, without some aspects commonly associated with school, such as peer pressure and bullying. And I am thankful to say that we have never experienced any bullying.

When my oldest child was preschool age, we joined a local homeschooling group. Ten years later, we are still close friends with many of the families we met then, and we've met many more throughout the years. My kids have friendships with kids and adults of all ages, and they have developed strong bonds with others based on common interests and values. Because we tend to hang out in groups of parents and kids, where the adult-to-child ratio is around two to five kids to each adult, there is consistent modeling of appropriate social behaviors.

**FIGURE 6-1 (A)** A young garment worker in Kolkata, West Bengal, India **(B)** A child soldier in Vietnam.

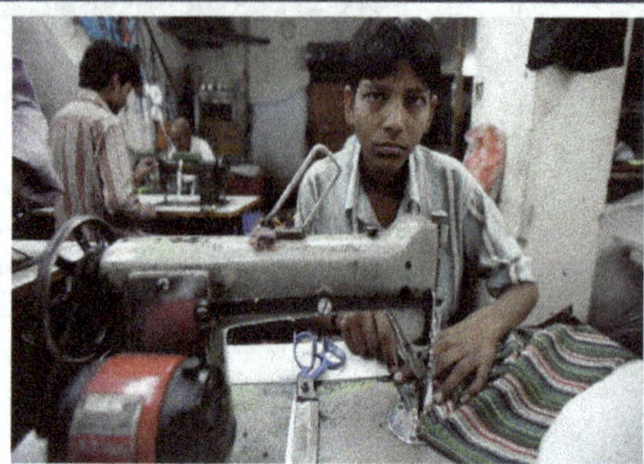

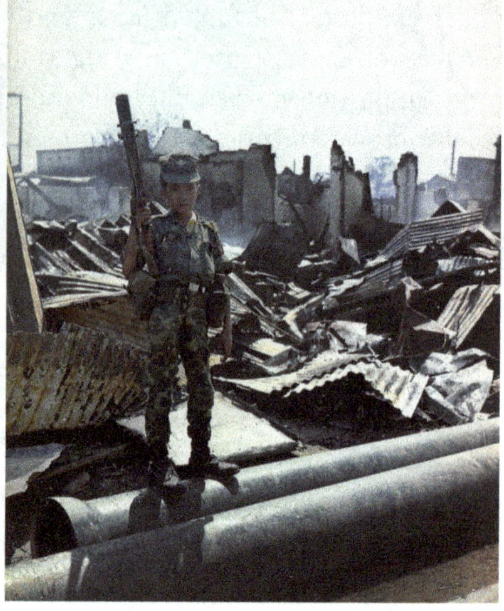

*Source*: Fig. 6.1a : Copyright © 2011 Depositphotos/paulprescott.
Fig. 6.1b: https://commons.wikimedia.org/wiki/File:Vietnam_child_soldier.jpg.

**TABLE 6-1** Worst Countries for Child Labor Worldwide (McKenna, 2012)

| Country | Child Labor |
|---|---|
| 1. Myanmar | Soldiers, agriculture, street markets |
| 2. North Korea | Labor camps, factory work, agriculture |
| 3. Somalia | Soldiers, prostitution, agriculture, mining |
| 4. Sudan | Soldiers, prostitution, agriculture |
| 5. Democratic Republic of Congo | Mining |
| 6. Zimbabwe | Mining, forestry, agriculture |
| 7. Afghanistan | Cement production, textiles, food processing, agricultural |
| 8. Burundi | Agricultural work, brick making, mining, and prostitution |
| 9. Pakistan | Production of rugs, musical instruments, sports equipment |
| 10. Ethiopia | Domestic work, agricultural work, and mining |

**FIGURE 6-2** Child labor risk worldwide (maplecroft.com). The red areas on this map represent the countries where child labor rates are at their highest.

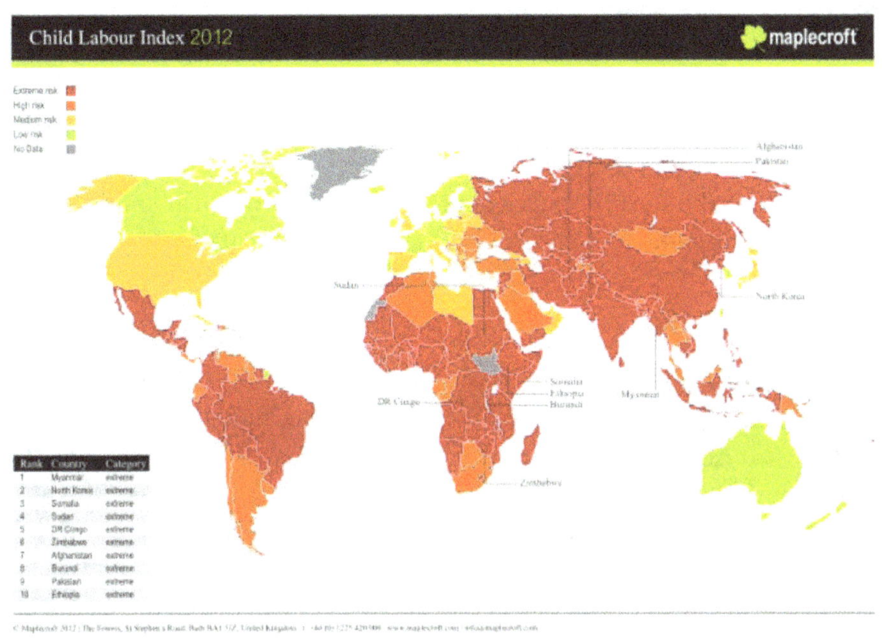


*Source*: https://reliefweb.int/map/world/world-child-labour-index-2012.

**TABLE 6-2** What's Going on in Middle Childhood? (Centers for Disease Control and Prevention, 2014)

| Age | Emotional and Social Changes | Thinking and Learning |
|---|---|---|
| 6–8 | • Greater independence from parents and family<br>• Greater understanding of their place in the world<br>• Greater focus on friendships (being liked, acceptance) and teamwork<br>• Less focus on the self, greater concern for others | • Can think generally about the future<br>• Rapid development of cognitive abilities<br>• Greater ability to describe experiences and to talk about thoughts and feelings |
| 9–11 | • Greater independence from parents and family<br>• Formation of stronger, more complex peer relationships<br>• Increasingly important to have friends, especially of the same sex<br>• More peer pressure<br>• Greater awareness of body as puberty approaches | • Increasing academic challenges and responsibilities<br>• Better able to see others' points of view<br>• Increasing attention span |

# Biological Development

**LO 6-1** **What structures and processes continue to develop in the brain during middle childhood?**

**LO 6-2** **Describe some changes in motor functioning during middle childhood.**

Since beginning this journey, I have discovered many other advantages to homeschooling, which I never expected. I love that my kids are able to follow their own interests and learn at their own pace. My oldest child is gifted, my middle child has ADHD, and my youngest is on the autism spectrum. Although we made the decision to start homeschooling before we knew these things about them, I think that teaching them at home has really been beneficial in dealing with these challenges. Homeschooling allows them each to follow an educational path that works for them. My oldest has been able to complete work at an accelerated pace. At age 13 she is currently working on high school–level geometry and Spanish. My middle child is able to do his work in short sessions with breaks in between, to help him sustain his attention. My youngest child's autism makes it difficult for him to understand abstract concepts, so math is particularly challenging for him. Homeschooling allows him to spend as much time as he needs to grasp concepts and allows me to give him the one-on-one instruction that he requires.

I also love the opportunities we have for "real-world" learning. We have learned about the ocean while standing knee-deep in the Atlantic with a marine biologist. We have studied trees and animals out in the woods at our local Audubon reservation. We've learned about our government by visiting our state house and talking to politicians. We've spent many of our days at libraries, museums, and historic sites. These experiences have allowed my kids to make real-world connections to things they read and learn about.

Every day holds different adventures for us, but typically we start our day around 7:00 a.m. with breakfast and chores. The kids then spend the morning working on their "sit-down" schoolwork. For math, my two oldest kids use independent study curriculums that they do on their own.

Anthropologists believe that middle childhood became a distinct developmental phase when we evolved into the modern humans we are today. It is comparable to the juvenile stage observed in our primate cousins (Thompson & Nelson, 2011). During this phase, children are able to feed themselves, but they cannot reproduce, and they are still under the watchful eyes of their parents. Their brain is nearly the same size it will be once the person reaches adulthood, but development within the brain will continue into early adulthood (Thompson & Nelson, 2011).

## Neurological Development and Functioning

During middle childhood, the brain's volume is roughly 95% that of an adult brain (Caviness et al., 1996). At the start of this developmental period, a child will have the greatest number of neuronal synapses, or connections between neurons, that he will have during his entire lifetime. The neurons in certain structures of the brain, including the corpus callosum, the brain structure that connects the right and left hemispheres of the brain, also undergo myelination that allows the two hemispheres to communicate with one another at a faster rate.

At the same time synaptic pruning continues throughout middle childhood and allows for more specialized processing of information in certain areas of the brain. We see this when we observe a child who has learned to more quickly solve a math problem or be able to dribble the ball with greater ease down the basketball court. Over the course of middle childhood the strengthening and solidifying of neurons and neuronal paths, known as **consolidation**, occurs. Remember, all these processes occur alongside environmental experiences, so stimulating environmental interactions continue to be crucial (Mah & Ford-Jones, 2012).

Middle childhood coincides with maturation in certain areas of the **cerebral cortex** around age 6. The cerebral cortex is the outermost layer of the brain that looks like a cauliflower. It is responsible for much of our cognition and many of our conscious processes including memory, attention and language. Development of the cerebral cortex coincides with many behavioral changes observed in middle childhood, and hormone changes are responsible for the emergence of body odor during this period. Middle childhood then ends with the onset of puberty (Campbell, 2011a, 2011b).

## Motor Development and Functioning

At the start of middle childhood, children show far more unnecessary movements when trying to perform a coordinated task such as throwing a ball. When they reach the end of middle childhood, their precision of movement while performing the same task is evident. This is due to the synaptic pruning taking place in the brain. Researchers argue

My youngest does daily lessons with help and plays math games. They also practice writing and work on any special projects they may be doing. After lunch, we often have field trips, classes, or activities with our homeschool group. They participate in various clubs and events, such as geography group, civics club, book groups, science fairs, history fairs, and various social activities such as park meet-ups and games days. All of my kids are avid readers. The oldest two read several books each week, and the youngest reads at least one per week. In between all the activity, I always make sure they have downtime to play and daydream.

Although I am satisfied with the choices we have made, and I wouldn't change a thing, homeschooling has not been without its challenges. It does require a large amount of dedication and effort, to plan outings and classes and to make sure that the kids are getting what they need. We happen to live in an area rich in resources to enhance our homeschooling experience, so that makes things a bit easier. But there have been times when it has been hard. When I had to go back to work full time after a divorce, it became difficult to keep up with homeschooling. The idea of giving up our homeschooling life wasn't really an option, as my kids really wanted to continue, and I saw how they were thriving. We managed to work it out, as I was able to work from home, but juggling full-time employment with homeschooling definitely stretched me to my limits at times. Fortunately, I have received help from fellow homeschooling families when needed, and I have the support of an amazing partner. Having a solid support system is so important.

We've always said that we would homeschool as long as the kids wanted to keep doing it. If they ever ask to go to school, we'll put them in school. But as of now, they all plan to continue until college, which is just fine with me.

Think about what you would do in this situation after reading the chapter, and then decide the following:

- If you were Jenney, what factors would you weigh most in making the decision to homeschool?
- If you were Jenney, how would you enhance your child's homeschool experiences and activities?
- If you were Jenney, how would you assess your child's performance at home?
- If you were a teacher or administrator, how would you advise Jenney on her decision to homeschool?
- If you were a teacher or administrator, in what ways could you support Jenney's efforts to homeschool?
- If you were a neighbor of Jenney's, in what ways could you support her decision to homeschool?

this is why increased physical activity during elementary school years can impact motor skills across the life span and instill lifelong habits of increased physical activity, rather than sedentary lifestyles. This is important now that we know children in the United States, in particular, are part of an obesity epidemic, with the childhood obesity rates increasing from 7% in 1980 to 18% in 2012. Physical activity helps hone motor skills and provides a stimulating environment that also promotes synaptic pruning (Mah & Ford-Jones, 2012). Later on in this chapter we will learn more about how physical activity promotes cognitive and psychological development and instills a positive sense of self, and we will go into aspects of diet and physical activity in greater detail in the next chapter.

# Psychological Development

**LO 6-3** **What kinds of thinking and reasoning do children exhibit during this age?**

**LO 6-4** **What are some characteristics of children with ADHD?**

Thinking, learning, and intelligence come to the forefront during middle childhood as many children enter the world of formal schooling. Do you remember what you were like at this age? What kinds of things were you interested in? What were your school and classroom experiences like? The child is making tremendous strides across many social domains throughout this period, in the way she views the world, how she interacts with others, and her ability to self-regulate by exhibiting greater attention and self-control.

## Cognitive Development and Learning

During this period there is an increase in independent decision making and behavioral and emotional inhibitory processes. Children develop better executive functioning skills as they show increased cognitive control over incoming external stimuli in the environment through attention and control over their internal cognitive processes such as reasoning and memory. There is better communication between the forebrain, which handles functions like planning, and the midbrain, which is responsible for a number of motor skills. So, for example, a child is able to focus on material that is being taught in the classroom and control the urge to squirm in his chair or speak out of turn while doing so. Physical activity helps promote these refinements in the brain by changing its chemical make-up and producing proteins that support myelination and consolidation to allow for certain complex memory functions, concentration, and attention. In fact, structures of the brain such as the **basal ganglia** and the hippocampus, which play a large role in memory, are actually larger in physically active children of this age (see Figure 6-3) (Mah & Ford-Jones, 2012).

FIGURE 6-3 The location of the basal ganglia and the hippocampus within the limbic system of the brain. Basal ganglia are responsible for movement, certain kinds of learning, and many routine behaviors and habits. The hippocampus plays a role in memory function.

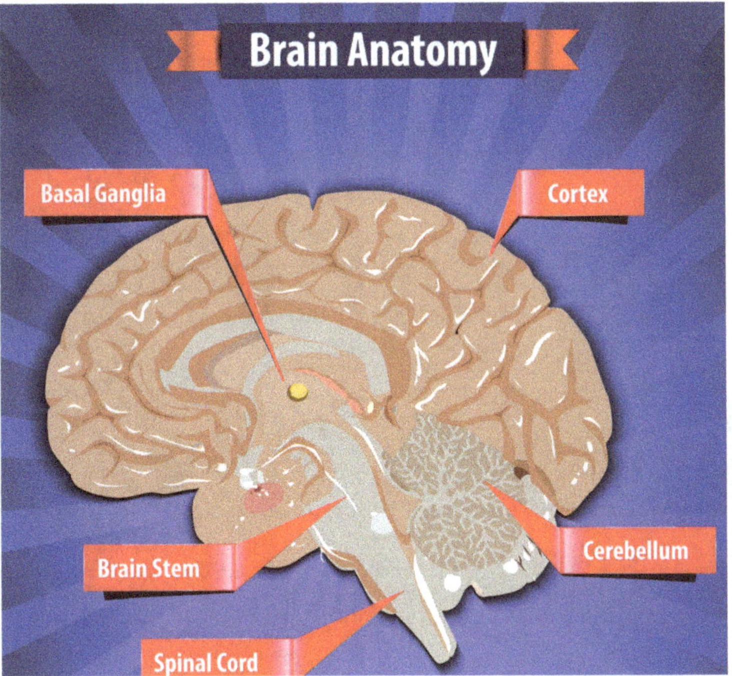




**Concrete operations.** According to Swiss psychologist Jean Piaget, **concrete operations**, known as the systems of internal mental actions that underlie logical thinking, emerge during middle childhood. At this stage, a child's thinking is still grounded in concrete experiences and concepts, rather than the abstract. Children typically use **inductive (or bottom-up) reasoning** during this stage. Inductive reasoning involves using individual observations to make generalizations about the world. For example, if a child was bit by a stranger's dog, he might think that all dogs bite. However, it is difficult for children of this age to use **deductive (or top-down) reasoning**. This means that they have difficulty applying generalizations about the world to specific events to predict their outcomes. So even if this child is taught that most dogs do not bite, it will be hard for him to believe that his neighbor's dog will not bite him.

The ability to classify objects into categories according to size or number emerges and the "operations" that were missing during the preoperational stage come together and allow the child to now mentally manipulate objects. Given this, the hallmark of middle childhood is the ability to understand concepts of conservation. Remember from the previous chapter that conservation is the realization that objects or sets of objects remain the same, even when they are moved or made to look different. Once conservation is achieved, children are able to "conserve" (keep, preserve) the original form of the object and know that it is the same, even though it has changed in shape or appearance. Figures 6-4a and 6-4b depict the conservation task for liquid.

**FIGURE 6-4A, and B** The conservation task for liquid.

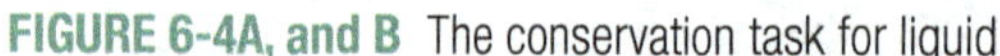

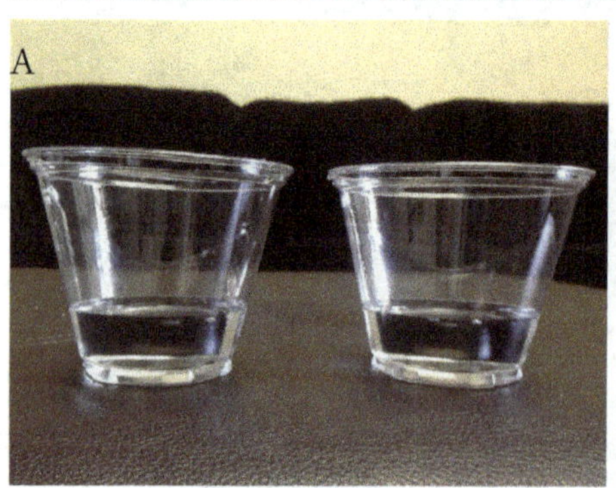


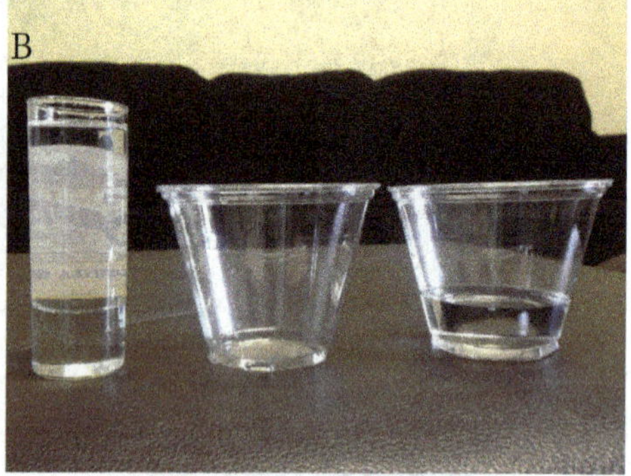


*Source*: Copyright © Waterlily16 (CC BY-SA 3.0) at https://en.wikipedia.org/wiki/File:Conservation1.jpeg. Fig. 6.4b: Copyright © Waterlily16 (CC BY-SA 3.0) at https://commons.wikimedia.org/wiki/File:Conservation2.jpeg.

## Theory Then and Now

**Theory then:** Piaget believed in the notion of **horizontal decalage**, or the gradual emergence of each conservation task in a particular order. Specifically, Piaget believed that conservation of number emerges first, followed by length, mass, and liquid and then area and weight.

**Theory now:** Many cognitive psychologists now believe that horizontal decalage actually represents increases in information processing capabilities and the automatic ways familiar mental tasks can be performed, leading to increases in working memory. This means new problems can be conceptualized in more advanced ways.

According to Piaget, children without cognitive delays, regardless of their sociocultural backgrounds, will reach the concrete operational stage if they participate in daily activities that require conservation. These activities may be practical activities of daily living or those associated with more formal and structured learning environments. However, the timing of the emergence of conservation skills may vary, particularly in developing areas of the world. This is another area in which contemporary theorists disagree with Piaget. Many believe it is problematic to state that all children develop their cognitive abilities in a stepwise and universal stage-like pattern.

**Language.** Children continue to refine their understanding and use of language throughout middle childhood, and by the end of this developmental period the average child will have a vocabulary of about 40,000 words. They begin to grasp more subtle meanings and differences, such as the way that a change in pronunciation of a word can change its meaning (for example, lead—*the past tense of to guide* versus lead—*a metal*) and that words that sound the same may have more than one meaning (for example, *cent, sent, scent*). This allows them to better understand things, such as metaphors and riddles.

**Memory.** Changes in the hippocampus contribute to advanced memory abilities in middle childhood (Ghetti & Bunge, 2012) and episodic memory improvements. This is due to changes in the organization of memories, the ability to retrieve memories, memory encoding (storage) skills, as well as memory retention and memory retrieval. Memory skills related to recognition do not depend as much on age in this stage, but as children continue to grow, they require fewer contextual cues to help them remember. For example, a child at this age will need fewer cues or prompts to remember what steps are necessary to carry out a long division problem. Some believe this is because of changes in the prefrontal cortex and greater and more specialized use of the prefrontal cortex, as well as changes in the hippocampus (Ghetti & Bunge, 2012).

Traumatic brain injuries that may occur during this period can be particularly impactful, such as a child falling off her bike and hitting her head without a helmet on. Injuries of this nature can result in impairments that do more damage to cognitive functioning at this stage of development compared with similar injuries that may occur during infancy, preschool, and later childhood stages (Crowe et al., 2012). Problems with episodic memory may arise in situations where negative childhood experiences are prominent, such as exposure to chronic stress and maltreatment, environmental toxins, as well as maternal stress. These experiences can affect both the development of the hippocampus and the prefrontal cortex. Negative childhood experiences can go hand in hand with low socioeconomic status environments, which put children at greater risk for exposure to other harmful circumstances such as malnutrition. This can put children at greater risk for compromised neurological and cognitive development. However, some of these processes can be influenced positively by parental warmth and care during early childhood. Certain kinds of early interventions, such as cognitive training, can help improve episodic memory and the structure and function of the hippocampus and prefrontal cortex. Physical activity has also been shown to promote memory performance. In studies that conduct research on animals, exercise appears to facilitate the growth of new neurons from stem cells found in the brain. Taken together we see the continued importance of the environment on neurological development and functioning and their associated cognitive processes (Ghetti & Bunge, 2012).

**Theory of mind.** Children during this stage can also distinguish their thoughts and perceptions as unique and independent of the thoughts of others. This awareness is known as **theory of mind**. They start to observe, monitor, and reflect on their own cognitive processes, a behavior known as metacognition, and they are beginning to develop internal skills that can help them become better thinkers and doers by reflecting on their own thoughts and actions.

**Attention.** During middle childhood, the ability to focus and sustain attention becomes increasingly important, especially within structured educational environments, such as classrooms. **Selective attention**, or the ability to focus on what's relevant in any given context, begins to develop, and a child's attention span typically becomes longer and more focused across middle childhood. They show increased **inhibitory processes**, ignoring irrelevant or distracting stimuli in the environment or thoughts in their heads, to focus on the task at hand. As you can imagine, these capabilities translate well into school environments and those where focused instruction is important.

**Attention deficit hyperactivity disorder (ADHD).** There are several reasons why children struggle with structured school environments, testing methods, and other contexts in which attention is important. These differences can impair an individual's cognition, making it more challenging to learn and to demonstrate one's abilities. **Attention deficit hyperactivity disorder (ADHD)** is one of the most common childhood neurobehavioral disorders. It presents largely as a learning difference that affects attention and impulse control and requires continuous management. Children with ADHD may need special instruction, tutoring, and medication to help them succeed in many academic settings (Centers for Disease Control and Prevention, 2020). The first signs of ADHD often appear in middle childhood (see Table 6-3).

Many of the behaviors listed in Table 6-3 can be considered "normal" behaviors of childhood. However, for a child with ADHD, these behaviors can be seen across a variety of situations, and they can impair their ability to function well in school, at home, and with friends. To considered symptoms of ADHD, these behaviors cannot be attributed to something else, such as a "stage" of development, a conflict at home, or another mental health issue.

The exact causes of ADHD are unknown, but researchers believe that there is a genetic component. ADHD may also be caused by environmental factors such as brain injury, a woman's prenatal alcohol and tobacco use, or premature delivery (Centers for Disease Control and Prevention, 2020). Additionally, children who are adopted from institutionalized care, such as international orphanages, show increased ADHD symptoms (Wiik et al., 2011). Contrary to some popular beliefs, there is no research that supports claims that eating too much sugar or watching too much TV causes ADHD. However, there is reason to believe that these things can make symptoms worse. Other factors, such as inconsistent discipline or lack of parental warmth, can also lead to worse symptom, whereas parental involvement can help improve symptoms (Hawes et al., 2013; Keown, 2012).

**TABLE 6-3** Symptoms of Attention Deficit Hyperactivity Disorder (Centers for Disease Control and Prevention, 2010)

| A child with ADHD might do the following: |
|---|
| • Have a hard time paying attention<br>• Daydream a lot<br>• Not seem to listen<br>• Be easily distracted from schoolwork or play<br>• Forget things<br>• Be in constant motion or unable to stay seated<br>• Squirm or fidget<br>• Talk too much<br>• Not be able to play quietly<br>• Act and speak without thinking<br>• Have trouble taking turns<br>• Interrupt others |

Parents of children who are diagnosed with ADHD should work with teachers, therapists, counselors, and doctors to determine which treatment will work best for their child. Treatment often requires a combination of medication and behavioral therapy, but is very much tailored to each individual child. Similar to its causes, success for children with ADHD depends on a number of factors. Helping a child to develop organization and planning strategies are linked to better academic outcomes with homework and grades (Langberg et al. 2013). It can take time to figure out the right form of treatment, but it is important to find ways of managing ADHD early. If not, a person can continue to struggle well into adulthood. However, many children and adults can lead very successful and fulfilling lives if they find a treatment and environments that work for them.

ADHD has three distinct types. Symptoms of the **predominantly inattentive type** include challenges with organization or follow-through. A person diagnosed with this type of ADHD may lose sight of important details or have difficulty following instructions, and they may have been diagnosed with ADD in the past. However, ADD no longer exists as a diagnosis. Someone diagnosed with the **predominantly hyperactive-impulsive type** may have difficulties controlling their behaviors for what is considered a socially appropriate amount of time. They may have difficulty sitting still or listening to directions. They may interrupt or be unable to wait their turn. Lastly, a person with the **combined type** will show symptoms of both inattentiveness and hyperactivity/impulsivity.

# What Is Intelligence?

No doubt if you are reading this book you have taken some kind of test in your lifetime thought to be a measure of your intelligence. In many cultures, we have an idea of what it means to be intelligent that is grounded in traditional psychological theories. Before we examine those theories, ask yourself a couple questions: How do I define intelligence? Is someone either an intelligent person or not? What is a good measure of one's intelligence? Does a person's intelligence depend on the particular ability you are measuring?

Contemporary psychologists think of **intelligence** as an ability that allows us to acquire knowledge, to think abstractly, to learn from experiences, to act with reasoned intention, and to adapt to the environment. Many believe intelligence is domain specific. (i.e., a person is not simply intelligent or not intelligent, and intelligence is not something that a person either has or doesn't have). We believe a person's intelligence varies depending on the situation at hand and what's being asked of them. For example, you may be highly skilled in math. Learning new math skills or formulas may have always come relatively easy for you. At the same time if someone asks you about your car's leaky oil pump and to determine exactly what the problem is and how to fix it, you may struggle because mechanics is something that has always baffled you. But your best friend, who may have always struggled in math, was the first of your friends to take apart his bike and reassemble it (so it still worked!), and he can tell you in 2 minutes what the problem is and how to fix it. Likewise, your girlfriend may be very adept at reading and responding to your emotions, but you always struggle to find the right words or understand when she is upset. Each of these things, mathematics, mechanics, and emotions, are considered different domains in which someone can demonstrate their intelligence, or lack thereof. Just because a person is "smart" in one area doesn't mean she's good in all areas. The opposite is also true. Just because a person struggles in one area, it doesn't mean that his other capabilities should be overlooked or undervalued.

**Measuring intelligence.** Assessments of intelligence usually include questions that focus on general information and abilities, such as "Today is Wednesday, two days from tomorrow will be ... ?" and "Which shape is not like the other?" that a typical person in our society should be able to answer. Once a person takes the test their scores are compared with other people of a similar age. At their core these tests are trying to measure what the typical person

### Theory Then and Now

**Theory then:** There was a belief among scientists and in popular culture that 10,000 hours or a minimum of 10 years of intense practice makes someone an expert at any given task (Ericsson et al., 1993; Gladwell, 2008).

**Theory now:** Practice only accounts for roughly one third of the differences we see individuals who are experts compared with nonexperts. Researchers say there are many factors that go into making someone an expert in any given field, including how old you were when you began, how well you learn from your mistakes, and your innate intelligence (Hambrick et al., 2014).

at a specific age should know and be able to do. The knowledge and capabilities measured in these tests reflect abilities that a person may be "born with," or those that are gained by the experience of living in a particular culture.

The results of these tests vary because the experiences of each person are different. For example, a person's particular cultural background may align with the culture in which the test is being given (see Table 6-4). This can give the test-taker an unfair advantage. Some believe that measuring intelligence cross culturally in a valid way is not possible, because intelligence is 100% dependent on a person's native cultural environment (Sternberg, 2004). If this is true, then our current tests of intelligence need to be adapted to fit the experiences of the culture where the test is taking place and the type of knowledge the person taking the test values.

Some cognitive processes that underlie intelligence may be universal, such as the ability to use different types of inductive or deductive reasoning, but intelligence does not always translate into test performance, especially in a cross-cultural context. Test-taking strategies and problem-solving abilities can also vary from culture to culture. For example, Robert Sternberg, a contemporary psychologist whose work focuses on intelligence, gives the example of Mayan children who wouldn't think of taking a test independently. In this culture, it is unusual not to collaborate on a test. This is one reason why it's important that we avoid broadly applying what we know about intelligence based on dominant cultures to people who may find themselves in the minority of a dominant culture or to those who come from a different culture altogether. This is a good example of where an intersection with culture can come into play. In fact, people who show greater cultural assimilation to a nonnative cultural context perform better on tests within that nonnative culture (Sternberg, 2004).

**TABLE 6-4** Cultural Values and Intelligence

| Cultural Values and Experiences That Affect a Person's Test Taking |
|---|
| • Attitude toward exams<br>• Comfort in the settings required for testing<br>• Motivation<br>• Rapport with test provider<br>• Competitiveness<br>• Ease of independent problem solving<br>• Attitude toward intelligence (is it innate or learned)<br>• Attitude toward education, academic standards, and studying |

*Note.* Adapted from Sternberg, R. J. (2004). Culture and Intelligence. *American Psychologist*, 59(5), 325–338.

**Theories of multiple intelligences.** Contemporary theorists such as Howard Gardner (1993) have advanced the notion that intelligence is more varied than the singular characteristic that Binet suggested and IQ tests measure. Gardner's theory of multiple intelligences proposes eight distinct areas of intelligence that a person uses individually and/or in conjunction with one another to solve problems. These eight intelligences are presented in Table 6-5. Gardner's work also suggests that of these intelligences only linguistic and logical mathematical intelligences, in other words academic intelligence, are valued and tested in today's schools. Although the tides appear to be changing in some countries and in certain U.S. schools regarding the importance of recognizing, valuing, and teaching to multiple intelligences, traditional academic achievement tests are still the gold standard in evaluating a student's and school's success.

## Theory Then and Now

**Theory then:** In the early 1900s, a French psychologist named Alfred Binet developed what is widely accepted as the first standardized intelligence test. Early versions of this test assessed aspects of attention, memory, and problem-solving abilities. Over time, Binet noted the limitations of his test, stating that it is almost impossible to reduce something such as intelligence down to one, single, all-encompassing number.

**Theory now:** Many psychologists now believe there are several domains of intelligence and numerous psychological and social skills necessary to succeed that are not captured by standardized intelligence tests.

**TABLE 6-5** Gardner's Eight Intelligences

| Intelligences | Associated Abilities |
|---|---|
| Linguistic | Analyze information and create products using oral and written language |
| Logical/mathematical | Develop equations, make calculations, and solve abstract logic and reasoning problems |
| Spatial | Recognize and manipulate both large- and small-scale spatial images |
| Musical | Produce, recall. and make sense or meaning of different sound patterns |
| Naturalist | Identify and distinguish various plants, animals, or weather formations found in nature |
| Bodily-kinesthetic | Use one's body and physical abilities in creative or problem-solving ways |
| Interpersonal | Recognize and understand other people's moods, desires, motivations, and intentions |
| Intrapersonal | Recognize and understand one's own moods, desires, motivations, and intentions |

*Note.* Adapted from *Multiple intelligences: The theory in practice*, by H. Gardner. New York: Basic Books.

Another contemporary theory is Robert Sternberg's "triarchic" theory of intelligence that describes three types of intelligence: componential, experiential, and contextual. A person may rely on one type of intelligence over another or an integration of all three. How well a person uses his knowledge to adapt to a situation often relies on knowing which type of intelligence to use and when to use it (Sternberg, 2011).

**Componential (analytic) intelligence** works with IQ tests and traditional academic problem solving similar to analogies. It relies on a combination of mental processes, including executive functioning skills, such as controlling, monitoring, and evaluating other cognitive processes. Being able to analyze problems, efficiently choose problem-solving strategies, and apply those strategies is also involved. And the ability to gain and store new knowledge, such as working memory, encoding, retrieval, and processing speed, is needed. People who rely on componential intelligence may spend more time trying to understand a problem, but once it is understood they tend to reach a solution faster. People who rely on this type of intelligence are sometimes less adept at creating unique ideas or solutions of their own.

Those who rely on **experiential (creative) intelligence** are usually good at inventing or designing new solutions to problems. They rely on insight and the ability to think and adjust creatively and effectively to new situations. Cognitively, they are better at **automated processing**, in which a task that has been done many times before can be done with little thought or extra effort. This process "frees up" mental effort, in a sense, to be able to focus on more complex aspects of a problem or task. People who possess this type of intelligence are also better at applying existing knowledge in new situations so they can focus on the important and new components. There are no known tests that exist to assess this type of intelligence.

**Contextual (practical) intelligence** relates to a person's ability to quickly assess, understand, and deal with everyday tasks and problems. It relates to all the important information fundamental to success in this world that you don't learn in a textbook or in a lecture hall. Some people call this "real-world" intelligence or "street smarts." Individuals who rely on this type of intelligence are good at getting along with others and getting out of trouble. There are certain skills that go along with this kind of intelligence, in particular those related to one's environment, which include an ability to adapt to the environment at hand, to shape the environment if changes are necessary, and to recognize the need to change environments altogether if necessary. Each of these works in a way that sets the person up for success. Personality characteristics and emotional factors, like temperament, are also an important part of contextual intelligence.

## Moral Development

The innate levels of moral development observed in early childhood are believed to continue into middle childhood. For example, in middle childhood children are focused on avoiding punishment and act in self-serving ways. However, they begin

to make moral judgments in more subtle ways as they start to understand that certain behaviors that may appear "wrong" have justifications. They also start to value the importance of forgiveness (Jambon & Smetana, 2013).

# Social Contexts and Development

**LO 6-5** **What factors can affect academic outcomes during middle childhood and beyond?**

**LO 6-6** **What are the four types of parenting styles?**

**LO 6-7** **What is peer victimization?**

Social responsibilities increase throughout middle childhood, especially if we look cross culturally. Gender segregation in terms of peer group formation occurs for many children, with boys preferring to be with other boys and girls preferring to be with other girls. At the conclusion of this developmental period, children enter adolescence and become increasingly mature, both in their thinking and in the responsibilities placed on them (Lancy & Grove, 2011). As you may know, many cultures have rites of passage and rituals that mark the end of middle childhood. Yet, as you saw at the beginning of this chapter, the unfortunate truth in many places around the world is children are placed or forced into more adult-like roles during this stage of development and their rights as children and fundamental aspects of childhood are ignored. Clearly, what is expected of children socially depends on the culture and communities in which they live. In the next section, we will focus on social aspects of middle childhood that are common in many Western and industrialized nations.

## Developing School Responsibilities

In the United States, education—whether it is through public, private, or homeschooling—is required for all children. Ages for compulsory education vary by state in the United States, with most requiring children ages 6 to 16 be enrolled in school. School is a critical social institution during middle childhood in the United States and many other cultures. It is during this time that children's developing capabilities and independence also signal an increase in responsibilities, particularly in terms of academic expectations. At the same time, children are in greater control of their own behaviors, making their own decisions, and developing their own attitudes toward school and academic achievement.

**Traditional schooling.** Traditional schooling, by far the most popular form of schooling in the United States, provides a wealth of opportunities for children to grow. **Traditional schools** are thought of as places where there are classrooms, teachers, and similar-aged peers. They provide a venue for children to master their minds, bodies, and social skills alongside their classmates. However, in the United States and elsewhere, academic knowledge and related skills are viewed as the fundamental outcomes of these school years.

Many factors contribute to the variations we see in academic outcomes for children during middle childhood. As we discussed in this chapter, one factor is how educators and researchers value and measure intelligence. A strong social and academic starting point can also impact success in elementary school. The NICHD's Study of Early Child Care and Youth Development, discussed in Chapter 4, found that higher-quality childcare earlier in childhood promotes school readiness skills that can lead to math and reading achievements. Meanwhile, television exposure during early childhood can contribute to reduced classroom engagement and math achievement, and aggression early on can lead to difficulties in math and reading during middle childhood (Hooper et al., 2010). If a child continues to have problems in school during middle childhood, she is also more likely to have difficulties into adolescence. This can impact a child's academic competence and self-esteem and lead to social problems such as withdrawal from peers (Moilanen et al., 2010).

When a child experiences a road block in their academic performance or even their social interactions, the teacher is often the first point of contact so the child can be assessed for broader difficulties. This emphasizes the teacher's role in recognizing the learning differences and academic achievements of their students. Teacher observations also provide a valuable additional assessment of child performance that goes beyond standardized testing (Speece et al., 2010).

**Variations on schooling.** In the United States, the decision to send a child to public school or private school is largely based on family preferences. Some may choose private schools for religious reasons, whereas others may feel better educational results can be yielded from private schools. The latter aspect is not necessarily true when you factor in certain characteristics that can be associated with those likely to enroll in private schools. However, there seems to be some benefits in the areas of mathematics and sciences for nonreligious private schools, in addition to more favorable retention rates, greater security and discipline, and a wider variety of specialties and activities, both in school and during extracurricular time (Figlio & Stone, 2000). As children grow older, technical and vocational schools become available, which can have certain benefits (for example, postsecondary school employment opportunities) and drawbacks (for example, risk for diminished work opportunities later on in life) (Hanushek et al., 2017).

**Homeschooling.** In the late 20th century, roughly 850,000 children in the United States were homeschooled, but now this number has grown to nearly 1.8 million children (Noel et al., 2013). Homeschooling families are also growing in diversity, as now approximately 15% of all families who homeschool are non-White/non-Hispanic. The idea of homeschooling children is also growing in popularity in Canada, the United Kingdom, Australia, Japan, and Kenya. Reasons for homeschooling vary from family to family and include concerns over the traditional school environment or dissatisfaction with academic instruction in traditional schools and a desire to provide religious or moral instruction (Noel et al., 2013).

In the United States, homeschooling is legal in all 50 states, but specific practices and policies can be different from state to state. For example, some states will allow children who are homeschooled to participate in public school activities, such as sports, whereas other states prohibit their inclusion (Home School Legal Defense Association, 2013). Some states require that homeschooled students take standardized tests along with their public school peers (Cooper & Sureau, 2007).

Critics of homeschooling often view it as an attack against traditional public schooling and view the families who participate in homeschooling as narrow-minded individuals who are trying to shelter their children. However, parents who homeschool are more likely to join community and volunteer organizations, be politically active, and contribute money to political causes (Cooper & Sureau, 2007), suggesting that these individuals are very much engaged and active in their communities and in the public sector.

Parents who homeschool rely on prepared curricula, textbooks from local schools, public libraries, technology, and instructional specialists and teachers. In addition to this, homeschool families network with other homeschooling families and may form homeschool groups in communities where there is a substantial number of homeschool families (Hanna, 2012). Children who homeschool regularly participate in extracurricular activities, such as field trips, scouting, and community sports leagues just as public and private school children do.

There is limited research on differences between children who participate in homeschooling and those enrolled in traditional schools. One study found no differences on standardized tests between children who are homeschooled and those who are not (Barwegen et al., 2004). Many colleges, including Harvard and MIT, admit homeschooled students (Cooper & Sureau, 2007).

**Out-of-school time.** In the United States, as of 2012, 75% of children enrolled in public school were involved in at least one extracurricular activity (23% in sports, 16% in clubs, 36% in both). For those enrolled in private school, 87% participated in at least one extracurricular activity. These numbers varied by certain household demographics. For example, 80% of children from two-parent homes participated in extracurricular activities, compared with 66% of children from single-parent (mother only) homes. Only 35% of children from homes where no adult completed high school participated in extracurricular activities. In terms of race/ethnicity,

50% of Hispanic children, 65% of non-Hispanic Black, and 85% of non-Hispanic White children participated in extracurricular activities. However, factors such as school and community safety impact enrollment in extracurricular activities (Howie et al., 2010).

Children who participate in extracurricular activities perform better in school, have fewer behavioral problems, and are less likely to drop out. In addition, extracurricular activities help build self-esteem and interpersonal skills such as conflict resolution (Howie et al., 2010). Some suggest extracurricular activities help explain, at least a little bit, why kids from higher socioeconomic status backgrounds have advantages with regard to noncognitive and cognitive skills (Covay & Carbonaro, 2010). The benefits of extracurricular activities hold true not only for American children, but those from other nations as well. Similar results have been found in Finland, Spain, and China (Metsäpelto & Pulkkinen, 2011; Molinuevo et al., 2010; Shiah et al., 2012).

There may be a downside to participation in extracurricular activities, too. For example, children who are involved excessively in extracurricular activities, or feel parental pressure to perform well at these activities, may feel overwhelmed and stressed. This can negatively impact the overall well-being of a child. However, parents who are supportive and encouraging with regard to extracurricular activities promote greater overall well-being in their children (Lagacé-Séguin & Case, 2008).

Structured time out of school is fast becoming the norm for many children. In the United States, many school districts also offer fee-based, extended-day programs for children. As with early childcare, the quality of these programs is important in terms of fostering a child's work habits and promoting good grades and good social skills with peers. Enrollment in a program with a staff that maintains good relationships with the children and that offers a variety of age-appropriate activities often results in good outcomes in children (Pierce et al., 2010).

Physical activity remains vital during this age, as much as it was during toddlerhood and early childhood. This is true not only for physical health, but for the development of individual and social skills as well. This can also be seen across different cultures in vastly different parts of the world. For example, one study examined play in both an urban Chicago community and in the East African nation of Angola. Both communities valued play and sports. In Chicago, play was viewed as an activity that allows children to develop seriousness, competitiveness, and individualism. In Angola, play was seen as something that fosters inclusion in groups and helps children understand and develop social roles (Guest, 2011). Recreational physical activities can boost self-esteem, which can also lead to better academic performance. Participation in sports can promote friendships and a sense of competency that can be particularly beneficial for children at risk for developing behavioral and emotional problems (Mah & Ford-Jones, 2012).

Out-of-school time that includes creative play, reading, and studying, as well as physical activities, now competes for time with various forms of media during middle childhood. It makes sense that the more time children spend engaged with media, such as television, video games, smart phones, computers, and tablets, the less time they spend playing and sleeping. These types of media can negatively impact reading, studying, and physical activity—all vital parts of childhood (Hofferth, 2009). Greater television exposure is also associated with an increased chance of being victimized by bullies, higher consumption of soft drinks and snacks, and a larger body mass index (BMI) (Pagani et al., 2010).

## Family

Although school is a major focus for parents and children during childhood, the family is still a strong factor that shapes a child's development and well-being. Family structure (for example, two parent versus single parent) and positive support from parents can influence development in a number of ways during middle childhood.

Historically, many of the comparisons researchers make related to family structure focus on single-parent family households and two-parent family households. Much of what is known about single-parent families is based on information we gather from single-parent mothers. As we know, differences in family structures in the United States and elsewhere are becoming more prominent, within both single-parent and two-parent family structures. For example, there are single-parent father families, as well as families with children who share time between mothers and fathers in joint custody agreements. Some single parents are divorced, whereas others have never been married. Further, some divorced parents remain single, whereas others remarry. Some two-parent families have two mothers; others have two fathers. Some have two grandparents raising a child, and some have a parent who spends extended periods of time away from the home.

Compared with two-parent families, single-parent families, regardless of whether they are headed by a mother or a father, often experience greater socioeconomic difficulties and face other challenges, such as a parent's work schedule that may impact parental stress, monitoring, and supervision of children's activities, as well as family cohesion. The lack of these resources, both financial and psychological, can put a child at risk for certain negative learning outcomes. In countries outside of the United States, such as Germany, children from single-mother homes are at increased risk of being overweight, having asthma, and being in poor health, in addition to an increased risk for psychological problems (Scharte & Bolte, 2013). These children experience challenges with academic achievement and show slightly more behavioral problems. These problems are often more likely to occur while the family structure is transitioning, for example, going from a two-parent home to a single-parent home (Magnuson & Berger, 2009).

**Parenting styles.** Perhaps not surprising, variations in parenting styles can influence children behaviorally, psychologically, and physiologically. Parenting styles (Baumrind, 1991) are characterized by the amount of demandingness and control and acceptance and responsiveness, resulting in **authoritative**, **authoritarian**, **permissive**, and **neglectful parenting styles**, presented in Table 6-6.

**TABLE 6-6** Parenting Styles

| | Low Acceptance and Responsiveness | High Acceptance and Responsiveness |
|---|---|---|
| Low demandingness and control | Neglectful | Permissive |
| High demandingness and control | Authoritarian | Authoritative |

In Ireland, authoritative parenting, compared with permissive parenting, is linked to higher scores on reading and math for children. This may be due to greater parental monitoring and the ways that authoritative parenting can promote a more positive self-concept in children (Murray, 2012). In Canada, authoritarian parenting is linked to increased risk for childhood obesity (Kakinami et al., 2014). This may be due to chronic family stress that can contribute to the likelihood of a parent utilizing an authoritarian parenting style, especially if socioeconomic factors are part of the equation. Family stress can also be a result of authoritarian parenting. As we've discussed in previous chapters, this type of stress can impact allostatic load and disrupt metabolic functioning, thus leading to obesity.

There are other aspects of a family's structure and functioning that can impact a person during middle childhood. For example, boys whose fathers work longer hours are more likely to act out (Johnson et al., 2013). Changes to the family structure, socioeconomic factors, family size, and parental mental illness can also lead to more aggressive behaviors in children in general (Pagani et al., 2010). When it comes to aggression, there appears to be a bidirectional relation between the parent and child as harsh parental discipline at earlier ages leads to aggressive behaviors in children at later ages, which in turn leads to more parental discipline, and then to even more child aggression. This represents what developmental psychologist call the **transactional model of human development** (see Figure 6-5) (Sameroff & MacKenzie, 2003). This model shows how the individual and the environment are constantly interacting with one another to influence development.

FIGURE 6-5 An example of transactional model of human development (Sameroff & MacKenzie, 2003).

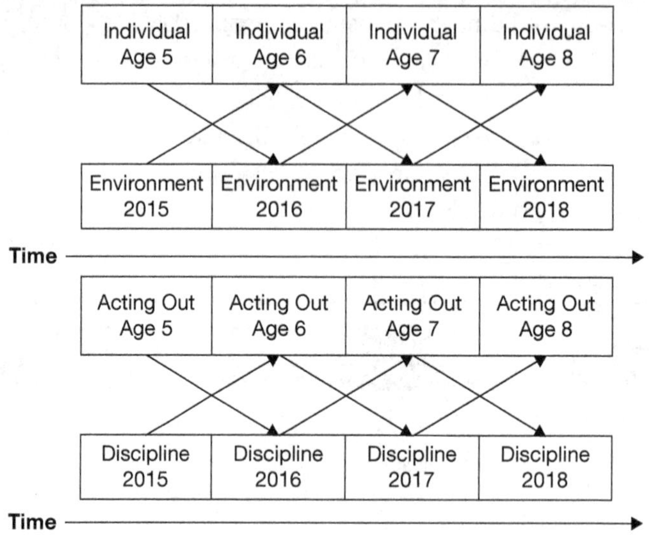

| Individual Age 5 | Individual Age 6 | Individual Age 7 | Individual Age 8 |
|---|---|---|---|
| Environment 2015 | Environment 2016 | Environment 2017 | Environment 2018 |

Time →

| Acting Out Age 5 | Acting Out Age 6 | Acting Out Age 7 | Acting Out Age 8 |
|---|---|---|---|
| Discipline 2015 | Discipline 2016 | Discipline 2017 | Discipline 2018 |

Time →

*Source*: Cynthia R. Davis

On the other hand, family support can be critical in stopping a chain of events like this and in buffering a child who is exposed to school- or community-level violence. In these cases, family support can help lessen the impact of these environmental factors and help reduce negative mental health symptoms such as anxiety (Kennedy et al., 2009).

# Developing Friendships

During middle childhood, friendships typically focus on a child's identification with other children who are of the same gender. Within friendship groups, a social hierarchy takes place, where there are leaders, those who are second in command, and so forth. Academic achievement can sometimes be a strong predictor of status within a peer group; those who are higher achievers climb higher up the social ladder within any given group. A child's achievement level can also lead to greater peer acceptance, which can in turn boost the achievement level of the child's friends. On the other hand, peer rejection predicts worse academic achievement throughout this developmental period and on into early adolescence (Brendgen et al., 2010). Peer rejection is also linked to greater aggression in children, which, in turn, predicts greater peer rejection (Lansford et al., 2010).

**Bullying.** Bullying, or what is sometimes referred to as "peer victimization" has become a central focus of considerable research during middle childhood. At some point, almost all children are on the receiving end of peer victimization at least once during childhood, whereas roughly 10% of children are chronically bullied by their peer(s) (Storch & Ledley, 2005). Bullying and **peer victimization** can take the form of direct bullying through teasing or physical aggression, or through less direct, but no less hurtful behaviors, such as gossiping or group exclusion. Peer victimization, which can be prominent during middle childhood, typically decreases as a child makes his way through adolescence, when it may also take on different forms, which we will discuss in later chapters. Nevertheless, the long-term impact of peer victimization can still be felt across childhood and beyond. Several longitudinal studies have shown that being on the receiving end of peer victimization is strongly linked with depression and anxiety symptoms (Schwartz et al., 2014). There is also evidence that bullying itself is linked to acting out and, over time, to criminal offending outcomes in adulthood (Fergusson et al., 2013). Research shows, however, that if teachers take a more disapproving stance toward bullying in the classroom, then instances of bullying go down (Saarento et al., 2013).

## Socioeconomic Status and Environmental Resources

As in other developmental periods, parental socioeconomic status, including parental education level, household income, and financial resources, remains a strong predictor of a child's well-being across multiple areas, including physical health, mental health, social functioning, and school/academic functioning (Nuru-Jeter et al., 2010). However, regardless of a child's socioeconomic status, contextual assets that are strong predictors of a child's overall well-being include the availability of and connections to peers and supportive adults in the family, school, or neighborhood; academic self-concept and positive school climate; general health, nutrition, and sleep; and constructive use of out-of-school time. The more assets a child has, the greater his well-being (Guhn et al., 2012).

Whether it is by providing material resources or by fostering a more enriching environment in other ways, any investment in a child's environment remains crucial to development during this stage. By stimulating the child's mind and body, she is set up for success not only at the observable behavioral level, but at the neurobiological level as well.

# CHAPTER 7 Preadolescence

A post to my social media account recently asked, "Parents of tweens ... what are your kids into these days?" This is some of what parents had to say: "Taylor Swift ... Minecraft ... iPad games in general." "Sports and deciding if he wants to be a rapper or an architect when he grows up." "Instagram, snapchat, friends, dancing all the time." "The Thundermans, Austin & Ally, Drake & Josh." "Violent video games that he doesn't own and isn't allowed to play."

Does this sound familiar? Some of it may not, because the children in this age range (10 to 12 years old) and throughout adolescence are very in tune with trends, especially those related to music, clothing, television shows, and video games, which are constantly changing. Keeping up with trends reflects the preadolescent's strong motivation to "fit in" and is much more prevalent at this developmental stage than in previous stages. Fitting in will becoming increasingly important for the child across adolescence.

If someone had asked what you were into during your "tween" years, you may have said *Harry Potter* or *iCarly*. Some interests during the tween years remain the same from generation to generation, such as riding a bike or playing a game of truth or dare with friends. Activities and friendships will always be on a list of what preadolescent children are into. Along with these interests comes the urge to have or do something that is forbidden by those in authority, namely parents and other caregivers.

As friendships and social acceptance become increasingly important during this period, it is typical for children to show a greater capacity and desire for independence from their families. The preadolescent child is also undergoing some pretty incredible neurological changes, and some will start to show physiological changes, as the conclusion of this developmental stage coincides with the onset of puberty.

# Biological Development

**LO 7-1** **Describe some of the typical changes that take place in the bodies and brains of preadolescents.**

**LO 7-2** **What are the dietary needs of preadolescents?**

We often notice growth changes in height and body shape during this stage, and both development and change are taking place in the brains of preadolescent children. Preadolescents are also becoming more skilled at mastering their bodies and certain motor skills than ever before.

### What Would You Do?
### Joe's Story

Parenting a tween is difficult. I just reluctantly got her an iPhone, and a lot of it had to do with the fact that all her friends have iPhones. She had an old phone that she never really used. I wanted her to use it for sleepovers and stuff, but she wouldn't. My wife and I were convinced she was embarrassed by it because 90% of her friends have iPhones. I'm sure she didn't use it because she's the one kid in the circle who didn't have the iPhone. Then there was a pair of sneakers that she needed. Like really needed. She gave us a whole list of reasons why she needed them. "I'll wear them for hip hop dance class." "I'll wear them pretty much every day." I think it's one of those things where the circle of friends acts like a magnet dictating whatever is in or whatever that circle is into is what you want to do. I get it. Because being in that circle is a hell of a lot better than being out of the circle. What drove her to need those sneakers is that other kids in school needed them, too.

Dance means a lot to her. She's always said it gives her the opportunity her express herself. She was a tiny little kid when we signed her up for classes. It wasn't like she was naturally gifted at it, but she was naturally in love with it. Now, her typical weekly dance schedule is extremely busy. I think she's at the studio at least 3 days a week, and she just asked to sign up for a fourth different kind of dance. It's her thing, and there's nothing that's even close. It's amazing from seeing her first dance in a chicken outfit to see her up there doing ballet now. I do worry sometimes that she picked something that is such a major focus. It shows because none of her friends from our town are in her dance classes, so you know this is something she's really serious about and invested in if she's willing to give up time with her school friends. It's good, though, because she has two different sets of friends, ones from school and ones from dance. I think at this age it's important to experience a lot and try new things, but she doesn't really try new things because dance takes up so much time. She does do that to a certain extent by trying different dances and being on a travel team that challenges her. It's a big contributor to her self-esteem. It shows her that if you work at something, you actually see the improvement. I also think doing dance and meeting new kids must help her gain confidence in talking to new people. Her future, her goals, all involve dance. In terms of whether they're realistic goals, I don't know. I'm sure they'll change. I just say if you like it, keep doing it.

It's not easy for my wife to manage the different activities, especially now that our younger daughter is playing lacrosse, too. I coach my younger daughter's team and their practices are different nights of the week, so we have to divide up our time because our schedules never line up. My wife has hooked up with another dance parent from a neighboring town and they trade pick-ups and dropoffs, which makes it a little easier. I don't know if my wife tries to schedule the different classes and practices so they're on the same nights, but it's a lot of traveling back and forth. My daughter is not necessarily overscheduled compared to many of her friends. She has a lot of dance, but her friends play all sorts of sports, so I think that's what it is for a lot of kids. Their schedules are just full. I think back to when I was a kid, and I don't think that I had nearly as many activities. I was doing baseball, but when you're a kid you don't look at it as a schedule. You just think this is what I do. Even so, it seems like there's less spontaneous stuff, like pick-up stick ball or basketball. And when kids these days are not doing a scheduled activity they want to be in front of the TV or on their phones. When I was a kid and you wanted to talk to your friends, you had to get out of your house and go down to theirs.

Still, she's a great kid. Really. She's the greatest kid on the planet. In terms of maturity, she's pretty on par for her age. She does really well in school, and she's well liked. My guess is that she's one of the more popular girls in school, only because of the tremendous number of friends she has. She has a friendship group with about five other girls that she considers a pretty tight group. They're all good kids and they really get along. She's going to summer camp with all of them next week, and she plays lacrosse right now because these five best friends do it. I bet if all of them said, "I don't want to play lacrosse anymore," she'd say "I don't want to do that either." This is one of the reasons we know dance is so important to her. She does it because she loves to do it. And if three of her friends said, "We're not going to dance next year," she'd still be in dance class.

One her friends put glue in her hair the other day, and there have been times when someone has done something they shouldn't do, so I tell her to stick up for herself and don't try to be a friend to everyone. She tries to please a lot of people and it's something that I reiterate with her. Don't let people walk all over you because you think they won't be your friends. But she and her friends are of the age where they don't want to do anything to hurt the friendship, because having five friends is better than having four friends. I say to her, when you're older you're going to find that the number of friends is not what you strive for, but I'm sure that for a lot of girls her age quantity of friends is a big thing. I try to tell her that if you can have one friend who likes you and respects you, that one friend is better than 10 friends.

## Neurological Development and Functioning

The volume of **grey matter** in the brain peaks as the brain continues to grow during preadolescence. Grey matter includes the parts of the brain that contain the neurons responsible for much of how we view the world, our behaviors, as well as memory and emotions. Grey matter is found in the cerebral cortex and in other structures of the brain. In the frontal lobes of the cerebral cortex, grey matter peaks slightly earlier for females (11.0 years) than for males (12.1 years), whereas temporal lobe grey matter peaks later (16.2 years for females and 16.7 years for males) (Tanaka et al., 2012). Parietal lobe grey matter peaks around 10 years for females and 12 years for males (Gogtay et al., 2004).

Grey matter volume then begins to decline into adolescence. The volume of both the amygdalae and the hippocampus also peaks during preadolescence, occurring about a year and half earlier for females than for males. The gradual peak of these brain structures suggests that preadolescence is a critical period for neurological development (Uematsu et al., 2012).

## Physiological Development and Functioning

Growth is slow at the start of preadolescence but can speed up toward the end of the preteen years. During this time the early stages of **puberty** begin to show as the body becomes more adult-like in size and function, and sexual reproduction becomes possible. In preadolescence, boys and girls may begin to develop pubic hair and hair under their arms.

For females, breasts begin to develop, and they may experience **menarche** during this stage, which is the start of menstruation. For males, the penis and testicles grow, and they experience more frequent erections and become capable of ejaculating. Hands, feet, arms, and legs grow faster than other parts of the preteen male body, hence the common use of the word "gangly" to describe some boys this age. Soon they will experience their voice beginning to crack as it deepens.

By now, the child is growing roughly 2 inches in height and gaining 6.5 pounds in weight every year. Muscle mass also increases. Keep in mind, though, that these numbers represent averages for all children. I'm sure you remember when growing up that some children are at the bottom end of the range, growing more slowly, whereas others may shoot up in terms of height and weight. Some children can also experience a period of rapid growth over the course of a few months, followed by a slow period, such as a small kid who returns from summer break twice his size. And although physical activity can promote bone strength and density for preadolescents, there is no evidence to suggest that physical activity stimulates growth.

## Motor Development and Functioning

A preadolescent's motor abilities continue to become more refined during this age. However, in some areas they still lack **automacy**, or the ability to carry out a single action requiring several detailed steps, such as shooting a basketball. Complex actions still require significant thought and cannot be carried out as easily or automatically as they can later on in young adulthood (Ruitenberg et al., 2013). Still, a preadolescent child can make great strides

All the families of these girls were out together not too long ago, and the girls made a pact that this was the group and they were the besties. So, she has these good friends, and will they be best friends in high school? I don't know. Within that group, her "best friend" can switch from month to month. And in a month if that friend slept over at someone else's house, then those two would be the besties. She's sensitive, though. There's times when a friend has done something intentionally or unintentionally that upsets her, and I can see how it affects her versus her just rolling with it. I think that's partly because she cares what other people think about her. Still, her group of friends seem good. I don't really think it's like "You're my friend so I can say I have five friends." Some of them will go to her dance events, even though it's a couple towns away, or she'll go to their stuff, so they seem like a good group of kids who want to be supportive of one another.

She says she's never getting married, but boys are definitely a thing for her. Some of her friends have started going on dates with boys and one of her friends has a boyfriend. Recently at a family wedding, she was dressed up with a bracelet on that said "love dance." She told me a boy gave it to her. She thought that I would be upset that she got it from a boy and so she waited to tell me. She looked at me in a way, wondering if I was upset, sort of testing the waters on whether I'd be mad. I said, "That's nice that he gave it to you. You love to dance and it's a nice gesture." Other things are changing, too. I definitely can't walk into her bathroom anymore, and I think she likes that I give her privacy. I've heard stories from friends about their daughters who are older and I feel like I've got a few more years until she's sexually active. I can't tell you whether she's had the HPV vaccination because I know that's a thing now. You'd have to ask my wife. But I would want her to get it.

I know some other parents with kids her age definitely trust them at home, but my wife and I think she's probably about a year or two away from her being alone with her younger sister. I'm definitely overprotective. She has other responsibilities around the house, though. She's started to take the garbage out. She's been vacuuming. She puts dishes away. She doesn't cook. She gets her own breakfast, but she doesn't use the stove. She'll make stuff in the toaster, but she's never done stuff on the stove top. In terms of outside the house, we live in a bit more rural area, so if she wanted to walk to a friend's house, she'd need to go on a busy road. It's not just that. In my mind every single person is someone to be wary of. Right or wrong that's the mode of thinking I have. We have let her walk with friends to and from places in our downtown area, but if she wanted to walk from home to downtown for a couple hours with her friends I probably wouldn't let her do that. I grew up in a city, so when I was a kid I could walk four blocks to a friend's house. Sometimes I wonder if it would be different if she was a boy. I don't know. A friend has a son and he feels like there's less fear surrounding a boy walking down the street, where you think a girl is a lot more susceptible to "bad guys."

There's a long list of worries. Their health by far. I don't want her to worry about what she eats. I just want both my kids to be happy and to pursue their dreams. I worry about her self-disclosing things when she's on Instagram and those sites, and the number of friends she has on there is staggering. We have talked to her about chatting and remind her if there's someone you don't know, you never disclose anything about yourself. Sometimes there's no way around her disclosing things to her friends or boys, but it's the strangers I really worry about. The people you don't know. I'm worried about her sending inappropriate pictures, all that stuff. It's different from my tween years because when I was that age, we were into being outside all the time. My friends and I would think about playing stickball and relievio tag in the streets. Still, I'm sure I dealt with the same things she is, without even knowing I was dealing with it, whether it's fashion or trying to look cool or be cool or fit in.

Think about what you would do in this situation after reading the chapter, and then decide the following:

- If you were Joe, would you worry about your daughter's focus on dance?
- If you were Joe, would you be concerned over the influence of his daughter's friends?
- If you were Joe, would you place similar restrictions on independence and put forth similar responsibilities?
- If you were Joe's daughter, would you feel overscheduled?
- If you were a pediatrician, would you recommend the HPV vaccination?

over what they could and could not do during middle childhood. Unlike a typical 6-year-old, a 10-year-old can catch a fly ball, build a model airplane, or knit a scarf (Stricker, 2014).

**FIGURE 7-1** Performing a "changement" in ballet can be performed with a certain level of automacy for the trained dancer in young adulthood, but for many preadolescents in ballet classes, this move still requires considerable thought and effortful motor coordination.

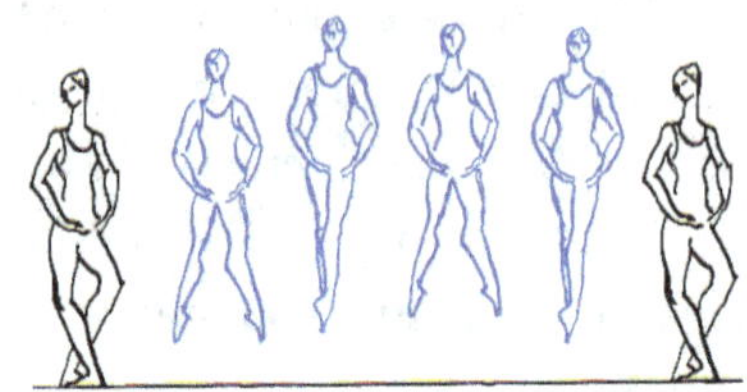

*Source*: https://commons.wikimedia.org/wiki/File:Entrechat_six.jpg.

## Diet, Physical Activity, and Well-Being

In the preadolescent stage, children need more healthy calories and protein than adults do to promote development in all areas, especially during periods of rapid growth. Many parents and caregivers are concerned about the fluctuating eating habits of their children, which may coincide with their child's slow versus rapid periods of growth. However, pediatricians are confident that nutritional needs are being met as long as a child gains between 4 and 7 pounds each year and she eats a variety of healthy food (Stricker, 2014).

**Body dissatisfaction and disordered eating.** Even during preadolescence, as many as 40% of children restrict calories and more than 60% exercise in attempts to maintain or lose weight (Eaton et al., 2010). Body dissatisfaction may emerge during this period for some children and can occur in children of all body types. In other words, it is not just limited to children who are overweight or obese, or to those children who are of normal weight but consider themselves overweight. For many preadolescent girls, an ideal figure is an extremely slender one that is more slender than girls actually are, and more slender than they perceive themselves to be. This can sometimes lead to disordered eating.

**Disordered eating** includes problems with food and/or body image, and a number of abnormal eating behaviors. Symptoms are similar to those of anorexia (restricting calorie intake) or bulimia (purging after eating a large amount of food). Children's thoughts and perceptions related to disordered eating can start earlier than previously thought, and disordered eating is more prevalent among preadolescent girls than previously believed (Evans et al., 2013). Research suggests more than 10% of girls this age binge eat, whereas almost 7% of girls purge food by vomiting (Combs et al., 2011). The thin ideal many children and adults possess can lead to body dissatisfaction, health risk behaviors such as disordered eating, and serious health problems, as well as negative mood and decreased self-esteem (Hawkins et al., 2004).

**Obesity.** Overeating may also be a concern for some parents. According to the Centers for Disease Control and Prevention (CDC, 2018), being overweight means "having excess body weight for a particular height from fat, muscle, bone, water, or a combination of these factors," whereas obesity means "having excess body fat" specifically. Both are due to "caloric imbalance" or consuming too many calories and expending too few calories. Since the 1970s, rates of childhood obesity have tripled. Now roughly 20% of children in the United States are overweight or obese (Centers for Disease Control and Prevention, 2018).

Obesity should be taken very seriously. It puts a child at risk for developing chronic diseases such as type 2 diabetes and cardiovascular disease during childhood and into adulthood. Because of the increases we have seen in recent years in childhood obesity, some think for the first time ever children of the up-and-coming generation may actually live shorter and less healthy lives than their parents (Kamijo et al., 2012).

**The human papillomavirus (HPV).** Preadolescence is also the time when the CDC recommends that parents and caregivers consider giving children the **human papillomavirus (HPV)** vaccination. They recommend children as early as 9 years old (and up to age 26) be vaccinated. HPV is the most common of all sexually transmitted infections, known as STIs, and the CDC reports that almost all of sexually active adults will have HPV at some point in their lives. HPV can be transmitted not only through sexual intercourse, but through intimate touching or sharing sexual objects.

There are many different types or strains of HPV. Some strains have no signs or symptoms, some can cause genital warts, and others can lead to certain types of slow-growing cancers. This is why the CDC believes that early vaccinations are important. Still, parents and caregivers may be reluctant to have their children vaccinated. In the United States, only 48% of females and as few as 2% of males have been vaccinated. Factors such as race, religion, knowledge about HPV, and encouragement from a partner contribute to vaccination rates. The CDC recommends that physicians discuss HPV vaccinations alongside the administration of other vaccines such as hepatitis B (Thomas et al., 2013).

# Psychological Development

**LO 7-3** **What are some important aspects of cognition that develop during preadolescence?**

**LO 7-4** **What are some factors related to low self-esteem during preadolescence?**

**LO 7-5** **Describe the typical types of friendships children make during preadolescence.**

**LO 7-6** **Describe the reasons why shy children do not engage in social interactions.**

As with middle childhood, Freud considered preadolescence as a sort of "holding pattern" stage and believed there was not much going on developmentally. As psychology and allied fields have progressed and become more sophisticated in their observational methods and theories, we recognize that this most certainly is not the case. In fact, there is a lot of development and change happening during this period. For example, preadolescents begin to abandon many fantasy-based notions from previous stages, such as fearing monsters under the bed, and move toward more reality-based thoughts and ideas. Instinctually, most preadolescents make progress in emotional and cognitive maturity, having better abilities to regulate emotions such as frustration or hurt feelings.

## Cognitive Development

Children during preadolescence show increasingly higher-level thought processes, problem-solving skills, and goal-directed behaviors. There is greater use of logic, and preteens and early adolescents are on the cusp of developing more expansive abstract thinking while making the move away from more strict, black-and-white thinking. They can solve more complex math and science problems, and they have better memory skills, attention abilities, and inhibitory skills.

However, the automacy that is limited in motor skills is also underdeveloped in certain areas of cognitive functioning, as well, such as number and word processing (Ruitenberg et al., 2013). But both their bodies and their minds are improving in ways that make things such as playing sports or solving certain math problems much easier. Preadolescents are developing the ability to plan ahead, to think on their feet, and to act on those movements and ideas more automatically through processes related to automacy. All of this coincides with improvements in executive functioning so that multiple stimuli, such as different pieces of a math problem and the rules to solving it, are easier to manage. The brain can also utilize selective attention better by paying attention to what is relevant and ignoring what is not to process information more efficiently (Stricker, 2014).

Preadolescents do well in certain areas of **self-regulation**, those cognitive, behavioral, and emotional skills related to monitoring one's thoughts and actions, such as control and impulsivity, but they can still struggle in other areas. The executive functioning skills that are closely linked with self-regulation are growing in their capacity but are still limited. Factors in the environment, such as neglectful, rejecting, or harsh parenting, as well as other stressful life events, are related to self-regulation skills. Preadolescents who show better self-regulation skills are less likely to exhibit internalizing problems such as depression or anxiety and externalizing problems such as acting out. They also show better coping skills, in addition to greater social competence and overall well-being (King et al., 2013; Zalewski et al., 2011).

At the start of preadolescence, children's cognitive systems for perspective taking are also underdeveloped. However, as they make their way through this developmental period, perspective-taking abilities advance, and they become more adept at reading others' mental states based on nonverbal cues. More refined perspective-taking abilities begin to emerge in subsequent adolescent stages as formal operational thought develops (Choudhury et al., 2006; Rusnáková & Rektor, 2012).

## Developing Competence

Children this age continue to develop their independence and autonomy, not only in terms of their physical space, but also in terms of what they think for themselves, what they know they are good at, and what they can do that makes them unique. Given this autonomy, there is usually an increase in risk-taking behaviors that will eventually peak during adolescence. Risk taking can occur in many typical behaviors at this age, such as riding a bike, and have been linked to aspects of cognition. **Inhibitory control**, which is the act of keeping irrelevant stimuli in check such as external distractions from the environment (a car's horn honking) or internal distractions from thoughts ("What is Dad making for dinner tonight?"), is one of these cognitive processes. Inhibitory control can guard against risk-taking behaviors in these scenarios by helping the child to stay focused on the task at hand.

Perhaps not surprisingly, factors such as aggression can also lead to more risk-taking behaviors (Stevens et al., 2013). Inhibitory control is thought to occur largely in the **prefrontal cortex**, which is still developing during this period and will continue to do so into a person's 20s. The prefrontal cortex is part of the cerebral cortex located at the very front of the frontal lobe. Researchers believe the prefrontal cortex is responsible for processing information on goals, such as "I better get home for dinner." Inhibitory control works alongside these goal-directed thoughts. The prefrontal cortex can enhance signals in the brain related to that goal, causing greater focus, and it can send signals to other parts of the brain to stop processing other information that is not related to the goal (Munakata et al., 2011).

## Self-Esteem

Preadolescents display a more heightened sense of self-identity and develop greater self-concern for how they dress, what and whom they like and dislike, and what they can and cannot do relative to their close friends and other peers. This self-identity is the basis for **self-esteem**, or one's general positive attitude about the self. Up until the adolescent period, self-esteem is relatively high.

In adolescence, and especially for girls, self-esteem begins to decline. It then gradually increases across adulthood, but experiences another decline in old age. These shifts in self-esteem are true regardless of other characteristics such as socioeconomic status, ethnicity, and other cultural factors. And increases and decreases in self-esteem are relative. For example, someone with high self-esteem going into adolescence will only experience a slight decrease, but will still seem like someone with relatively high self-esteem to most people. Similarly, for someone with extremely low self-esteem in adolescence, the increase in adulthood will likely be small, so they might still exhibit lower levels of self-esteem compared with their peers (Robins et al., 2002).

As we discussed earlier, aspects of dieting and body image can be important for children at this age, and especially with regard to their self-esteem. Much research has been done on childhood obesity and self-esteem, and not surprisingly the areas of self-esteem hardest hit by obesity include physical competence, appearance, and social functioning (Griffiths et al., 2010). Boys who are obese show slightly lower levels of self-esteem, but obese White and Hispanic girls show the lowest levels of self-esteem compared with their peers who are not obese (Strauss, 2000). This does not mean girls of other races and ethnicities are invulnerable. African American girls who are obese and experience more teasing tend to have lower levels of self-esteem and higher levels of depression (Porter et al., 2013).

During this age, obese children whose self-esteem continues to decline tend to be more sad, lonely, and nervous, and they eventually become more likely to engage in health risk behaviors, such as smoking cigarettes and drinking alcohol (Strauss, 2000). Aspects of family relationships are also associated with self-esteem. For example, children who show disorganized attachment patterns associated with abusive or neglectful parenting during preschool tend to have lower self-esteem as preadolescents, in addition to higher levels of anxiety and depression (Lecompte et al., 2014). Peers are also powerful players in preadolescent self-esteem. Peer approval can lead to increases whereas disapproval can lead to decreases in self-esteem (Thomaes et al., 2010).

**FIGURE 7-2** Up until the adolescent period, self-esteem is relatively high.

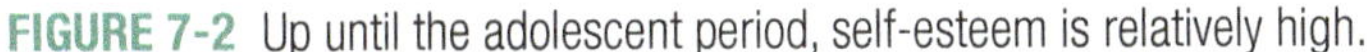

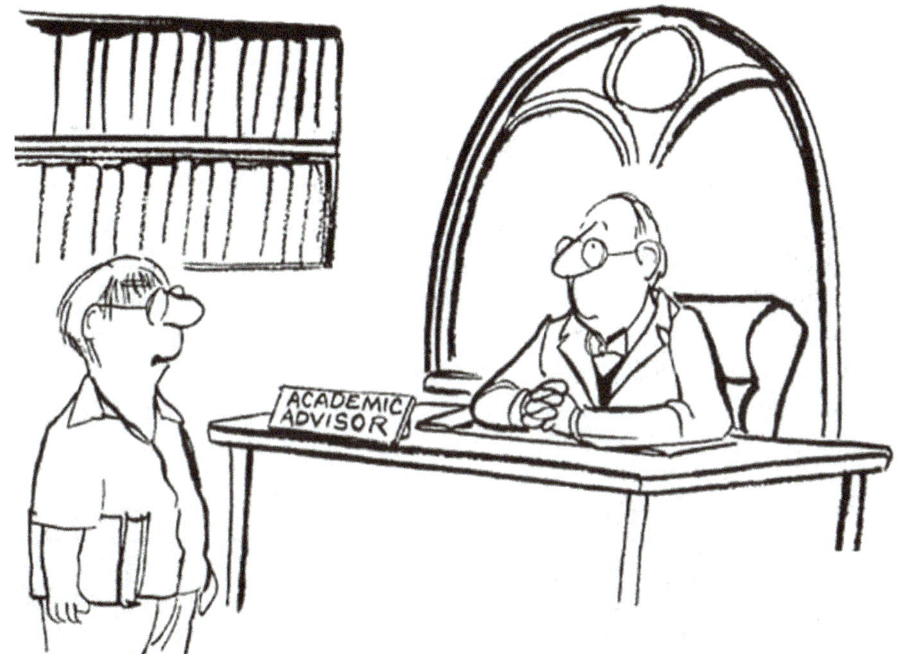


"I've decided to forego trigonometry and make myself eligible for the NBA draft.

*Source*: Copyright © 2013 Depositphotos/andrewgenn.

# Social Contexts and Development

**LO 7-7** **What are some concerns related to preadolescents' use of social media?**

**LO 7-8** **What are some of the factors that can impact a parent or caregiver's willingness to leave a child home alone during preadolescence?**

Parents and family remain important to preadolescents, but parents and children spend less and less time together across childhood and into adolescence. In place of parents and family members, friends become a substantial focus during later stages of childhood and throughout adolescence. During this time friendships and friendship groups become more complex. Friends serve as models for what is acceptable and what is not, as well as a basis for judging one's self, even if it is through the eyes of others. A lot of time is spent with friends or in extracurricular activities at this age.

For some, however, being outside the home can be unsafe. Think about children living in high-poverty urban neighborhoods who may not feel safe enough to play on the street, especially when neighborhood violence is high. The same holds true for children in war-torn areas of the world. Children who live in high-risk neighborhoods are also less likely to participate in after-school programs and activities. This can be attributable to several factors, including fewer resources available in these neighborhoods, less community engagement and cooperation, as well as a lack of trust among neighborhood members. Families can make a difference though. For children in high-risk neighborhoods, only 18% of children who come from low-risk families do not participate in any after-school activities, compared with 49% of children from high-risk families (Moore & Kahn, 2008).

**FIGURE 7-3** Involvement in activity outside the home can be dangerous for some children.

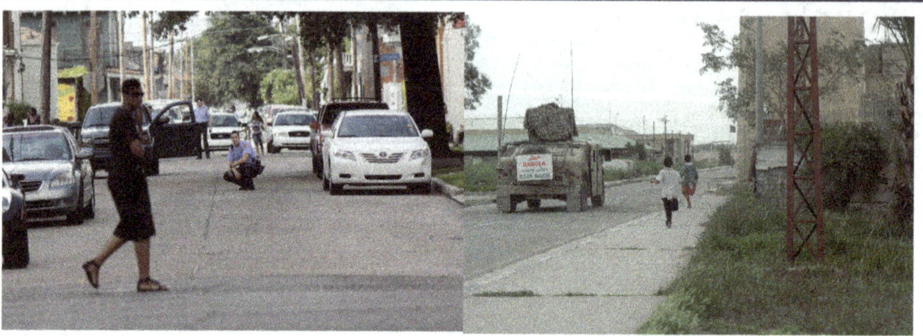

*Source*: Copyright © Derek Bridges (CC BY 2.0) at https://www.flickr.com/photos/derek_b/5027402768.
Fig. 7.3b: : https://commons.wikimedia.org/wiki/File:Task_Force_Vigilant_Works_to_Make_Baghdad_Streets_Safer_DVIDS38429.jpg.

## Peer Groups and Peer Interaction

Children at this age typically spend time with their closest friends in small friendship groups. These small groups or pairs are usually comprised of age mates who spend a considerable amount of time together and who are engaged in similar activities. Within these groups, "best friend" relationships can sometimes be a child's first experience with social conflict situations. For example, a fight may arise about who is best friends with whom, and much more. Still, even if there is conflict among a pair or small group, larger friendship groups tend to remain relatively stable in terms of their members. Hierarchies and rules exist within these groups, and the preadolescent aims to be similar to the group in terms of the social norms and behaviors the group adopts. Some of these behaviors and norms may reflect positive aspects, such as academic achievement and motivation, whereas other behaviors and norms may put the child at risk or be dangerous in and of themselves, such as depressive thoughts and self-harm (Brechwald & Prinstein, 2011).

Children at this age become like their peers because their peers serve as models for social behavior. Most preadolescents have a strong desire to be similar to their peers to "fit in." Friendship groups within the child's larger social network may also transmit important social cues and information, such as how to behave in public. For example, "Should I let my mom give me a kiss goodbye in front of my friends or is that a no-no?" Popular peer role models and even enemies can influence a child's behaviors, attitudes, and emotions (Brechwald & Prinstein, 2011).

**Shyness.** What about those children who do not connect with a larger group, or who may only have one or two friends, or who struggle with aspects of peer interaction and group socialization? These characteristics, similar to most other characteristics and behaviors, can range from mild to extreme. We often consider many of these children shy, and we define **shyness** as discomfort and self-consciousness in unfamiliar or new social settings. Shyness is certainly not unusual, given between 25 and 42% of people are shy (Spooner et al., 2005). It is a relatively stable trait across the life span. So if you are shy in childhood, chances are good you will also be somewhat shy in preadolescence, and into adulthood.

Some children who appear shy may have perfectly good social skills but simply prefer to be alone, and may be viewed very positively by their peers for this behavior. Others who are shy may desire peer interaction but do not possess the social skills or confidence to engage in social interactions. In turn, these children avoid social settings, such as after-school events and parties. Shyness at a more extreme level, and especially in cases where there is a lack of social skills, is linked to social withdrawal, social anxiety, and symptoms of depression across the life span (Coplan & Weeks, 2010; Eggum et al., 2012; Goodwin et al., 2004).

## Virtual Worlds and Social Media

Using social media is one of the most popular activities among preteens and adolescents, and it is increasingly more common for tweens to have personal profiles on social network sites such as Facebook and Instagram even though both websites state in their *terms of use* that users must be at least 13 years old to sign up. Websites and applications, or "apps," are platforms for social interaction, self-expression, entertainment, and information gathering. There are of course benefits and drawbacks to the use of social media. In a positive sense tweens using social media can enhance communication and social connections among their peers, and even promote certain technical computer skills and literacy for their own development (O'Keeffe & Clarke-Pearson, 2011). These social outlets for children are not without their drawbacks though, including cyberbullying and online predators. Time spent engaging with social media also detracts from time devoted to other important parts of a preadolescent's life. Remember, children at this age also lack appropriately developed self-regulation skills to monitor how much time they spend using social media as well as who they are interacting with on these websites. Academics, physical activity, and sleep help to keep a child healthy at this age and should not be replaced with hours of online recreation.

Another drawback to allowing children to participate in social media is their level of self-disclosure. Younger children are more likely to self-disclose personal or sensitive information than older children. Young children's self-disclosure and inappropriate sharing can occur for a number of reasons, including peer pressure or a desire to portray themselves in a particular light. Even the way a website is designed, asking for information on telephone numbers or home addresses, can lead children to disclose more than they should over the web. Self-disclosure of the preadolescent's thoughts, actions, and characteristics on social media sites and in virtual worlds increases during this age and can often serve as a "rehearsal stage" for making the same disclosures in the real world (Valkenburg et al., 2011). However, those who tend to value privacy "in real life" tend to share less on these sites (De Souza & Dick, 2009).

Self-disclosure may make a child vulnerable to ridicule by peers, especially if they disapprove of the personal or sensitive information, and more dangerously may expose a child to online predators, which can lead to far worse consequences. Sexual offenses that are initiated online represent a small but important proportion of sex crimes in the United States. And many victims are already at-risk youth who may have been previously abused or have problems at home or in school (Wolak et al., 2013).

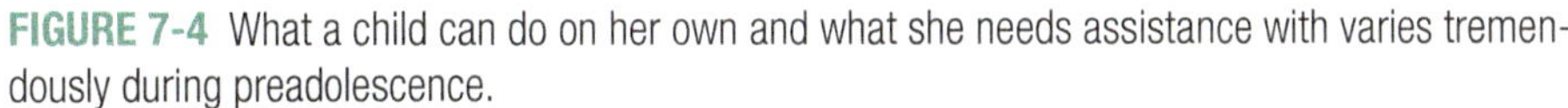

**FIGURE 7-4** What a child can do on her own and what she needs assistance with varies tremendously during preadolescence.

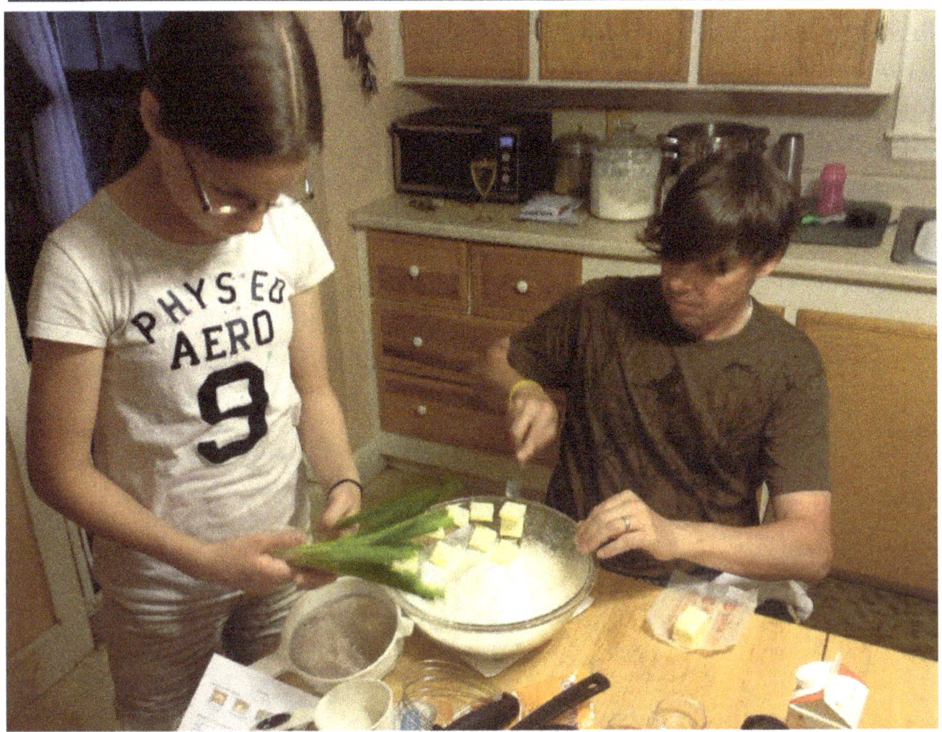


*Source*: Cynthia R. Davis

# Family

Within the family dynamic, preadolescents have greater household responsibilities than when they were younger. Household responsibilities, such as cooking or cleaning, involve a child in the types of chores they have seen their parents doing up until this point. In this respect, a child may begin to feel a sense of community, contribution, and self-worth when they do chores around the house.

Some parents may even feel comfortable leaving children of this age home alone, or allow them to babysit younger siblings at home or other young children outside the home. Of course these decisions are based on a number of factors, including the child's maturity level and logistics such as the length of time they will be alone, the time of day, whether there are other adults nearby, and rules for when the child is on their own, for example, no turning on the stove or no going outside. In addition, the parent's level of comfort or anxiety plays a huge role in determining what the child is permitted to do.

As their independence and abilities grow, it is not uncommon for children of this age to be more challenging toward their parents and caregivers. However, despite these developing capabilities, children are still very much reliant on their parents for things such as their physical care and certainly for their emotional well-being. Children of this age may be vulnerable to family shifts such as divorce in different ways than younger children, as they may become part of parental conflicts, be forced to choose a side, or be called on for instrumental (helping with household tasks, supervising younger siblings) or emotional support by a single parent.

# CHAPTER 8 Adolescence

It may surprise you that the term "teenager" first appeared in print in the magazine *Popular Science* in 1941. Adolescence as a formally recognized developmental period is a relatively new trend in many societies. It was not recognized as a part of childhood until the mid-19th century with the introduction of compulsory education and child labor laws and the juvenile justice system in the United States. Since then age limits for certain rights and responsibilities such as driving, smoking cigarettes, voting, enlistment in the Armed Services, and marriage have also been established. Adolescence as a developmental period prolongs one's entrance to adulthood because of these societal factors.

A host of developmental markers exist during adolescence. **Developmental markers** can act as identifiers for other people in terms of the adolescent's developmental status (physical, psychological, and behavioral) and expectations that can be placed on her. These markers are related to physical changes that have taken

### What Would You Do? Glen's Story

Looking back into my early adolescence, I'm not sure whether to hate myself or to be thankful for the life lessons I was taught. Being in a military family I had a very strict upbringing, with my parents controlling everything from my friends to my haircut. Getting older I was allowed more freedom, and I used it to the fullest extent. I was always trying to sneak things past my parents, whether it was hiding a stash of Halloween candy under my bed or playing Pokémon on my Gameboy under the blankets until midnight. I always thought that I knew best and the benefits always outweighed the risks.

One of the best decisions I ever made was when I was 13 years old, deciding to go to a technical high school instead of my failing town high school. My town's high school had an enormous dropout rate, and I wasn't a very popular child, so I didn't have many friends there. By going to a new school I was getting a fresh start at a much more successful high school where I would also learn a trade. I would also be getting a fresh social start, which was something I was very excited about as a young teenager, and I ended up making several friends from the next town over. We had a good time hanging out. They had a lot more freedom to do what they wanted so I spent most of my time over at their houses.

Multiple family members have had serious medical issues from tobacco use, mostly smoking. However, even after seeing this I still chose to ignore it all and start at first experimenting, then regularly using tobacco in all forms my freshman year of high school. I thought I was doing it because I liked it, and I really believed that I did; thinking back though I think the most appealing part of it was that I was defying my parents' wishes. I finished freshman year without too much conflict with my parents and went off to Boy Scout camp like every summer previous to that. However, that year one of my fellow scouts introduced me to smoking pot, one of the few things I actually regret doing during my life. During the time I smoked pot I cared for little else other than smoking it and getting money to buy more pot. I offered to do extra chores any chance I got to pay for it, and when there was nothing else for me to do I even stole money to keep my habit going.

As this was happening my grades started slipping quite badly; I had never really applied myself in school, but at this point I had just stopped caring all together. It was at this time my parents started getting suspicious, but I thought I was the smarter one, so I kept on my downward spiral thinking nothing of it. My parents were never exposed to

place, cognitive abilities that are developing, and skill enhancement. Cultural practices or rituals also serve as markers as we progress through life and may be closely tied to cultural beliefs, such as first communions and confirmations, bar and bat mitzvahs, quinceañeras, and sweet sixteen birthdays. Alongside these markers are social milestones, for example being able to go into town without an adult, getting a driver's license or staying out past midnight (Crockett, 1997). There are also markers related to clothing, interests, and activities, such as music or sports, as well as information sharing, both in terms of how the information is shared (a note passed in class versus a post on Instagram) and what information is shared (being candid about private or serious matters such as a family's financial concerns). These markers differ from family to family, from culture to culture, and from generation to generation.

Most pubertal change takes place during early adolescence, or in the United States what we consider the middle school or junior high school years. During late adolescence, or the latter half of the second decade of life, career interests may emerge, as does a greater interest in dating and romantic relationships and fundamental aspects of identity exploration. Adolescence as a whole is very much a transitional period. Children are trying to master a new "adult" body while maintaining a continuing and stable sense of self and managing changes in expectations and social norms. New and differing risks and vulnerabilities also emerge. School dropout, pregnancy, and substance abuse are worries of many teenagers, parents, and caregivers, and there are numerous social programs targeted at preventing these things. Still, these potential pitfalls must be managed while promoting appropriate exploratory behaviors for the adolescent as he figures out who he is and what he is capable of.

# Biological Development

**LO 8-1** **What is the brain's role in risk-taking behaviors?**

**LO 8-2** **What are some factors that influence the onset of puberty?**

**LO 8-3** **Why is sleep important during adolescence?**

Tremendous biological changes related to pubertal processes are already underway at the start of the adolescent period. There is an interplay between continued development within the brain, physical growth, and hormonal changes that result in a new body, new capabilities, and new ways of thinking.

## Brain Development

The pruning, or elimination, of synapses continues to occur during adolescence that leads to a reduction in grey matter (discussed in the previous chapter). As this happens the pathways that remain become consolidated or strengthened. For example, if an adolescent is inclined toward academics, those areas of the brain will become strengthened. If she is more interested in television and video games, those pathways in the brain will become strengthened as the other areas are pruned away. The speed of information flow also increases due to continued myelination of the axon of the neuron, which leads to increases in information processing capabilities.

Many of these processes continue not only over the course of adolescence, but into subsequent developmental periods. The prefrontal

any of this during their lives so they were oblivious as to what was happening to me at first. Eventually I got caught; it was inevitable given how careless I was being with the whole situation. I packed a bowl that morning for when I got home and thought nothing of it. I thought I was slick. However, when I got home my dad asked me to go for a drive with him and after a couple of minutes in the car he pulled out the bowl and confronted me about it. He asked me why I was doing it, and I couldn't give him an answer. "I'm just doing it because I want to" is what I told him over and over again. I didn't care that it was illegal. I just wanted to do it.

After that whole encounter I was grounded for 6 months and wasn't allowed to go out and see my friends outside of school the whole time. It was during this time I tried to fix my failing grades and met someone who would affect me for the rest of my life. I was sitting around on Facebook one day and got a friend request from a girl from the next town over where my friends lived. I was 15 and it was a girl, so I naturally accepted it and began talking to her, beginning my longest and most mentally scarring relationship I've ever had. After the first couple times meeting her we began dating and everything seemed pretty normal. She was about a year younger than me, but we had a lot in common and I was content with our relationship. She didn't have the best home life, and I did what I thought was appropriate at the time to try to keep her happy. It got to the point where when I wasn't at school, I was on the phone with her just to keep her happy. I would look at the call logs and some of them would be more than 6 hours long of just talking to her. I would sit in my room completely ignoring my family talking to her. My friends I made the previous year didn't see me for months because once I wasn't grounded anymore, I spent every bit of free time I could either talking to her on the phone or at her house.

About a year into the relationship I started to miss seeing my friends outside of school, so I tried to balance the two of them in my life, and my girlfriend was not pleased. She was used to having all of my attention and wasn't going to settle for anything less. I remember her being passive aggressive the first couple times I was with them, nothing too drastic, but it didn't stay that way for long. She started a whole thing about being able to talk to ghosts and my gullible, then 16-year-old self never thought she would lie to me, so I believed every word of it. I would be stressed to no end with her attention grabbing. She would go through phases of it, whether it was pretending to be haunted, being suicidal, or the one that affected me the most, being pregnant.

We started having sex about 8 months into the relationship; being a 16-year-old kid I was petrified. This was my first time doing anything of the sort, and like any normal teenager I was terrified of getting her pregnant, which I guess shows some maturity because I knew there was some sort of risk that was definitely a realistic outcome. We were always safe when it came to sex, never doing anything risky, but when she told me she thought she was pregnant I believed her. That didn't seem like anything anyone would ever lie about. She sent me a picture of a positive pregnancy test a few days later. I aged about 10 years in the weeks following, constantly thinking about ways I could afford to raise this baby at 16 years old. I even started thinking of different ways I could get full custody of the child because at that point I realized I no longer wanted to be with this girl and didn't want my child growing up in an environment with her in it. We even agreed on a name, Sophia.

What I did next was one of the hardest things I've ever had to do in my life, tell my mother I got a girl pregnant and was expecting a child. One night I decided to sit my mom down and tell her everything, and I talked for what felt like hours explaining everything and telling her about all of the symptoms my girlfriend was experiencing. After I was done my mother had a simple response for me. She wasn't pregnant. My mother was a nurse and had me and my two sisters and knew everything about a pregnancy, and my girlfriend's symptoms were not even close. That was like my whole world had flipped upside down again. I went from accepting that I was having a child at the age of 16 and even going as far as to name the child, to being guaranteed that the child was a lie. I went to my girlfriend and told her that it was over, that I didn't care what she had to say, and that was that.

I was very skeptical about dating for the rest of high school; I would date girls but try not to get overly attached, to avoid the emotional roller coaster that one relationship gave me over the year it lasted. However, near the end of high school I made one of the most important decisions of my life, to serve my country and join the Army National Guard. My father was in the military and it never really seemed like an appealing choice to me. However, as I matured and realized college was approaching and someone needed to pay the bill, I started looking around. One of my friends went to a recruiter and told me all about it. He heard our state had a full tuition and fee waiver for National Guard members, which was the perfect solution to my issue. I went to go see the recruiter and about a month later I was sworn into the National Guard. I left for basic training a month after my high school graduation. Basic training was a huge challenge, but it sharpened my discipline and

cortex continues to develop and is responsible for many higher-level processes in the brain, such as executive functioning. Pruning and myelination lead to better impulse control skills that are used more consistently over the course of adolescence (Luna & Sweeney, 2004). **Emotional maturity**, or the ability to interpret and regulate one's emotions, develops well into adulthood (Benes, 1998) and becomes more sophisticated as the adolescent brain becomes better at integrating cognitive information with affective information. This leads to several aspects of social cognition, which we will discuss later in this chapter. Cognitive skills, socioemotional skills, and associated areas of the brain can develop at different paces during adolescence, and some speculate this is why we see increases in risk-taking behaviors (Dahl, 2001; Steinberg, 2007). Adolescents may be better at physical and cognitive tasks, but they can lack aspects of emotional maturity and social experience to fully understand potential outcomes or consequences.

During puberty, hormone changes impact the amygdalae, which are responsible for processing emotional information and for our more primitive fight-or-flight responses to threats in the environment. This leads to more "bottom-up" or emotion-based ways of thinking and reasoning rather than "top-down" or logic-based thought. Many aspects of our thinking are initially considered bottom-up and based on quick, emotional responses to cues in the environment. As we develop, thinking becomes more top-down and is governed by aspects of executive functioning rather than quick, gut reactions to what's going on in the environment. Stressful and emotional conditions stimulate the amygdala for rapid and instinctive behavioral responses that lead to more emotional thinking. These emotional responses can limit aspects of cognitive functioning such as logical thinking and executive control, especially during adolescence when structures of the brain are sensitive to rises in sex hormones because of pubertal changes (Romeo, 2003).

changed me into the productive member of society I am today, ready to serve our country at a moment's notice.

Think about what you would do in this situation after reading the chapter, and then decide the following:

- If you were Glen's father, how would you have approached the marijuana smoking?
- If you were Glen's mother, how would you have reacted to the news of the pregnancy?
- If you were Glen's teacher, how could you have identified something was wrong?
- If you were Glen, would you have made a different decision about joining the National Guard?

## Hormones

The phrase "raging hormones" is often used when describing adolescents' thoughts, emotions, and behaviors. Hormones are chemical messengers produced by glands and tissues that send messages to cells all over the body. They also regulate physiological and behavioral activities including metabolism, sleep, stress, growth, and reproduction. There are approximately 50 known hormones circulating through the body. The hypothalamus, which plays a major role in regulating basic drives such as eating, thirst, and sex, regulates the pituitary gland and begins to produce greater amounts of adrenal stress hormones, growth hormones, and sex hormones during adolescence.

### Myths and Misconceptions

Teenagers are full of raging hormones that cause them to be moody and make bad choices. **Myth**

Hormones contribute only modestly to adolescent mood and male risk-taking behaviors. **Fact**

Gonadal hormones contribute to roughly 4% of the variation in things such as negative affect among adolescents, whereas social factors contribute between 8 to 18% of the variation (Brooks-Gunn & Warren, 1989).

**Sex hormones and puberty.** The organization of sex hormones according to male or female occurs pre- and perinatally, whereas the activation of sex hormones occurs during puberty. The activation of sex hormones and adrenal hormones affect the physical appearance of the body, the brain, and behavior. The hypothalamus releases gonadotropin-releasing hormone, which causes the pituitary gland to release follicle-stimulating hormone and luteinizing hormone, which signal the start of sexual development in both young males and females. In females, these hormones act on the ovaries. The ovaries are responsible for ovulation and produce specialized hormones such as estrogen and progesterone. Estrogen is responsible for most of the changes in a female's body during puberty. In males, these hormones act on the testicles (testes). The testes produce sperm and specialized hormones such as testosterone, which is responsible for most of the changes to a male's body.

Pubertal processes and physical changes during adolescence lead to the ability to reproduce, the establishment of a more adult-like appearance, and the development of secondary sex characteristics such as pubic hair, enlarged breasts for females, and the appearance of facial hair and the emergence of an Adam's apple in males. Adolescents start to develop more adult-like physical capabilities. These changes can bring about a new body image and a new sense of self. As we've discussed, there can be considerable variation in the timing and sequence of physiological changes from person to person, and the same is true for puberty.

**Pubertal timing.** Factors that affect the onset of puberty include genetics and environmental influences such as nutrition, infectious diseases, chronic diseases, pollution, and exposure to certain insecticides. A long-term trend exists with regard to the onset of puberty. In the United States and other countries, the onset of puberty has occurred earlier and earlier over the past century. Children are growing faster and taller and sooner. However, some say this trend has leveled off in recent years. We must also keep in mind there are biological limitations in terms of just how early puberty can start (Boaz & Almquist, 1999).

**FIGURE 8-1** Secular trend in the decrease in age of menarche in Western European and North American girls (Boaz & Almquist, 1999).

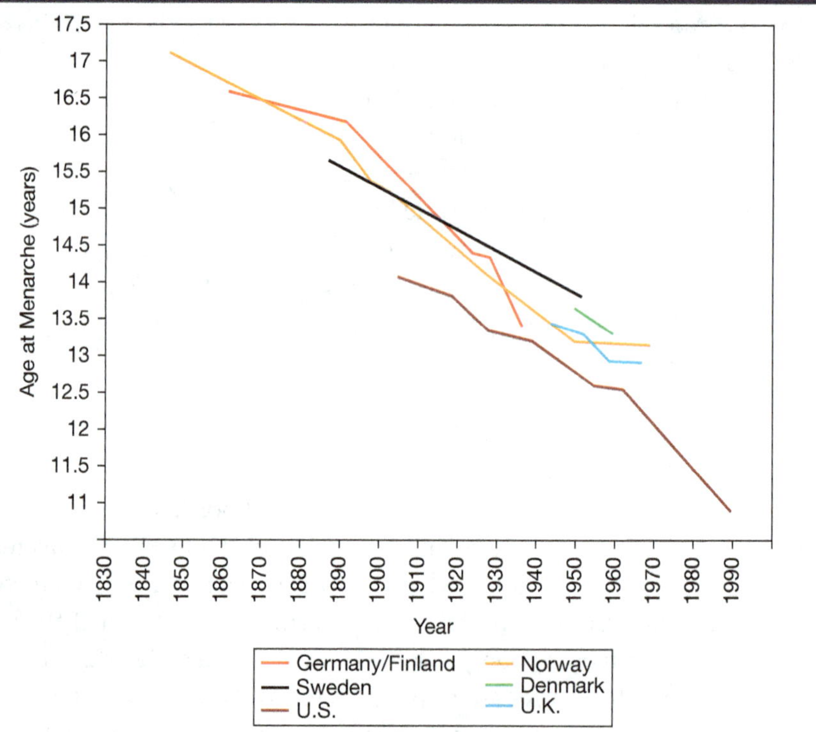


Fig. 8.1: https://commons.wikimedia.org/wiki/File:Acceleration1.jpg.

Whether an adolescent experiences puberty at an earlier age or a later age seems to have an impact on psychological and social functioning. Early maturing females are more likely to show internalizing symptoms such as depression, as well as psychosomatic symptoms (physical symptoms based on psychological factors like stress), including stomach pain, headaches, and sleep disturbances. Self-esteem levels tend to be lower for early maturing females. On average, they report greater body dissatisfaction and are more likely to engage in disordered eating behaviors. Academic functioning (for example, achievement, subject-matter interest, truancy) is also problematic for early maturing females compared with on-time or later maturing females. They are more likely to engage in substance use and early sexual activity and show more delinquent behaviors. Research suggests that later maturing females tend to be less popular, have higher grades, and are more likely to abstain from substance use (Mendle et al., 2007).

Early maturing males are more likely to show externalizing behaviors such as aggression, risk-taking behaviors, delinquency, association with deviant peers, and substance use and abuse. They are more likely to be threatened with or victims of violent assault that may be a result of engaging in more delinquent behaviors. Early maturing males are also more likely to engage in early sexual activity and are less likely to use contraception. Late maturing males are also at an increased risk for certain problem behaviors such as substance use (Mendle & Ferrero, 2012).

Social factors such as friendship groups, supportive parenting, and parental monitoring (which we will discuss in more detail later on in the chapter) can either reduce or increase the likelihood of problematic outcomes for early or late maturing males and females.

## The Need for Sleep

The biological changes during adolescence can affect a teenager's **circadian clock**, the internal, daily biological clock that influences many functions, including waking, eating, and sleeping. The timing of our circadian clock shifts later during adolescence and makes it more difficult to fall asleep at normal hours. As you may know, it's difficult to go to sleep earlier than the body wants to, because the brain is still promoting wakefulness. Because it naturally takes longer to fall asleep, adolescents are inclined to wake up later. These changes in our daily rhythms affect not only the human species during adolescence, but other mammals during similar developmental periods (Kelley et al., 2015).

What do established school schedules in the United States and other countries mean for adolescents and sleep? For one, they can lead to unrecoverable sleep loss on a regular basis during a very important stage of biological development. Not only do school times require

### Myths and Misconceptions

"Adolescents are tired, irritable and uncooperative because they choose to stay up too late, or are difficult to wake in the morning because they are lazy" (Kelley et al., 2015). **Misconception**

"If they simply went to sleep earlier, it would improve their concentration" (Kelley et al., 2015). **Fact**

It's ideal for adolescents to get 9 hours of sleep, fall asleep later, and set the alarm for later.

adolescents to wake or be woken up earlier than they should for optimal health and development, adolescents' schedules and workloads often limit the time available for sleeping, and less than 6 hours of sleep a night can have potentially harmful effects on the adolescent (Kelley et al., 2015). Older adolescents appear to be affected the most. They experience the greatest difference between their biological clocks and the typical social clocks we maintain in many cultures. They also show the greatest difference between the amount of sleep they get on school nights compared with what they get on weekends, and "sleeping in" on Saturday doesn't make up for sleep time lost throughout the week (Kelley et al., 2015).

Think about it this way, a 7:00 a.m. school start time for older adolescents is like having a 4:30 a.m. school start time for a teacher in his 50s. Table 8-1 presents a schedule of what biological wake times that are synchronized with school start times might look like.

**TABLE 8-1** What Synchronized Wake and School Start Times Might Look Like

| Age | Biological Wake Time | Synchronized School Start Time |
|---|---|---|
| 10 | ~ 6:30 a.m. | ~ 8:30 a.m.–9:00 a.m. |
| 16 | ~ 8:00 a.m. | ~ 10:00 a.m.–10:30 a.m. |
| 18 | ~ 9:00 a.m. | ~ 11:00 a.m.–11:30 a.m. |

Most studies that have examined later school start times used times before 9:00 a.m., which may still be too early for adolescents, but even those adjustments showed benefits for adolescents (Kelley et al., 2015). Keep in mind, too, there may be important trade-offs with later start times. Can you think of things that might be affected if school start times were later?

## Nutrition and Diet

It is recommended that adolescents eat anywhere from 2½ to 6½ cups of fruits and vegetables daily, along with 6 to 7 ounces of whole grains. Calcium is a necessary component of an adolescent's diet because of the significant increase in skeletal growth they experience during this time. It is recommended that adolescents intake 1,300 milligrams of calcium daily. Milk, cheese, ice cream, and frozen yogurt are common sources of calcium for teenagers. Sweeteners and added sugars account for roughly 20% of adolescents' total caloric intake, and they eat more than the recommended daily allowances for fat and sodium (Story & Stang, 2005). According to the CDC, most young people in the United States don't meet the recommended daily servings presented in Table 8-2.

TABLE 8-2 Recommended Daily Allowances for Adolescents (Gidding et al., 2005; Story & Stang, 2005)

| | Females | Males |
|---|---|---|
| Calories* | 1,800/day | 2,200/day |
| Proteins | 46 grams/day | 52 grams/day |
| Carbohydrates | 130 grams/day | |
| Fats | 25–35% of daily caloric intake | |
| Added sugars** | <10% of daily caloric intake | |
| Sodium | <2,300 milligram/day | |

*Increased physical activity (moderately or very physically active) requires more calorie consumption per day

**Added sugars are those that come from "snack" foods, sugar-sweetened beverages, and desserts

Look at the Table 8-2 and consider this: A fast-food meal with a cheeseburger, large french fries, and a medium, 12-ounce soda has 1,250 calories, 49 grams of fat, and 1,500 milligrams of sodium. This doesn't leave much room for additional calories to be spread across two other meals. A 15-year-old, 110-pound adolescent would have to jog for 30 minutes or walk for 3 miles to burn off 250 calories (the typical calorie content of a 20-ounce soda) (Bleich et al., 2014).

Diet has an impact on adolescents beyond physical health. For example, eating a healthy breakfast can promote aspects of cognitive functioning and memory as well as better mood, and adolescents who eat a healthy breakfast are less likely to be absent from school (Taras, 2005).

# Psychological Development

**LO 8-4** **What cognitive skills emerge during the formal operations stage?**

**LO 8-5** **How does identity development occur?**

**LO 8-6** **Why are aspects of child and adult mental health different?**

The transitions that occur over the course of adolescence lead to new ways of thinking about ourselves, others, and the world. Adolescents are also discovering who they are and what they are capable of. Some challenges can occur along the way as risk-taking behaviors are not uncommon, and hormone changes can bring about complex emotions.

## Cognitive Development

An adolescent's intellect is on par with adults, but there are differences in how adolescents and adults carry out mental tasks. Adolescents and adults differentially engage parts of the brain during tests that require calculation and impulse control, as well as parts of the brain that react to emotional content. Increases in our cognitive capabilities are a result of both physiological changes in the brain and experience.

**Information processing.** The development of information processing systems is a product of increases in both our cognitive capacity (how much we can handle) and our speed of processing (how fast we can handle it) and the efficiency with which we can process information (how well we can handle it). Specific areas that show improvements across adolescence include working memory, executive functioning, selective attention, response inhibition (the ability to stop ourselves from doing something), and response speed accuracy (how quickly we can do something correctly the first time). As information processing develops, memory and problem-solving performance also improve. It's not only how much and how quickly information is processed, but how it's thought about or considered as well. Knowledge, or what we know, becomes organized with increasing complexity. We don't simply accumulate knowledge. There are qualitative differences between someone who's a novice or new at a task and someone who's an expert in terms of how knowledge is organized. If we compare novices and experts on a certain subject their verbal responses and pictorial representations differ in describing or explaining concepts, principles, behaviors, and functions with more integrated elements (Hmelo-Silver & Pfeffer, 2004). Adolescents are becoming more knowledgeable on a day-to-day basis across multiple domains.

**Formal operations.** According to Piaget, most adolescents reach the formal operations stage (roughly from age 12 through adulthood). During this stage, **abstract thought** emerges and thinking moves from what is concrete and tangible, existing in the here and now, toward hypotheticals and what is possible. Physical objects become abstractions, and these concepts can be manipulated through thinking, without the need of actually doing, using **abstract reasoning**. Ideas, not just objects, can be compared and classified. An adolescent's understanding of the world and problem-solving abilities are no longer limited to actual concrete experiences. Thinking about the future becomes prominent. Logical thought is based in **hypothetico-deductive reasoning**, so a more methodical and scientific approach to problem solving is used. Hypotheses can be made about how to solve problems rather than relying on trial and error. For example, if a 15-year-old fails a test, she can think about all the factors that play a role in someone passing or failing, such as whether she paid attention in class, what were the quality of her notes, how intensively she studied, how long she studied, how much sleep she got the night before, and so on. She can then mentally compare each of these with her own behavior and decide which course of action makes most sense. She does not need to try each of the possibilities before deciding on a possible solution for the next test. **Metacognition**, the ability to think about one's thinking, to understand and self-evaluate how we learn and what we know, grows stronger. The well-known quote within the field of adolescent cognitive research describes the act of metacognition well, "I began thinking about why I was thinking what I was. Then I began thinking about why I was thinking about why I was thinking about what I was" (Santrock, 2015, p. XX).

**Social cognition. Social cognitive theory** focuses on interactions among the environment, the person, and their behaviors. According to this theory, many behaviors are not simply a response to a stimulus in the environment, as other theories contend. A person's inner processes help him interpret his experiences and the environment in which they occur, thus affecting how he behaves (Bandura, 1989). For example, the chances of a teenager being loud at the dinner table and his understanding of its consequences may be different if he's at home or out at a restaurant and depend also on whether his parents are strict or lenient.

**FIGURE 8-2** Interactions among the environment, the person and their behaviors.

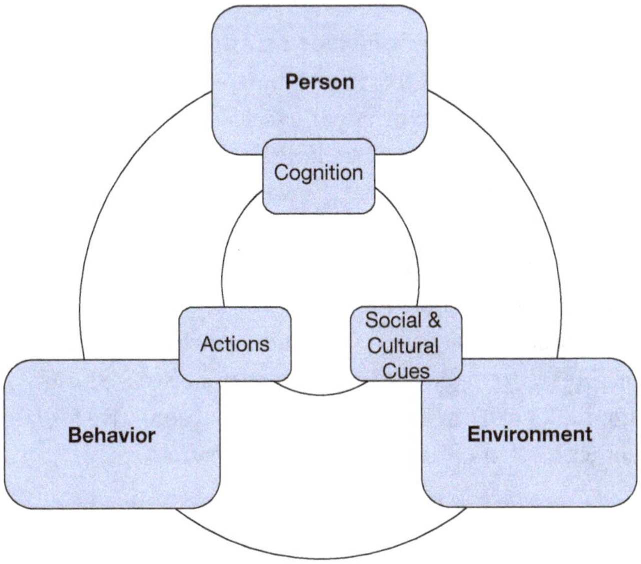

*Source*: Cynthia R. Davis

The inner processes a person uses in social cognition include aspects of cognition, such as attention or retention, as well as characteristics such as motivation and features of intelligence. Social cognition incorporates social or **observational learning**, or ways we learn by observing the behaviors of others and the consequences of those behaviors. Observational learning occurs through **modeling**, or those instances when we imitate or choose not to imitate others' behaviors, as well as **vicarious learning** when we learn ourselves based on what happens to others through observing and understanding consequences, namely rewards and punishments (Bandura, 2002). All these things lead to our perception, judgment, and memory of environmental cues and ultimately influence our behaviors. However, learning also does not necessitate a change in behavior. We can learn that something is the wrong thing to do, but still do it ourselves.

Self-regulation, introduced in the previous chapter, is also important to social cognition. Remember, self-regulation refers to the inner processes we use to control thoughts, emotions, and behaviors. Many of our regulatory processes (self-regulation, emotion regulation) come from external sources in early childhood, for example, from a parent or a caregiver who helps a child think through or plan out their actions or who controls impulses or urges that may be inappropriate for a given situation in addition to upsets the child may feel. As the child grows, these regulatory functions become increasingly internal, so they are able to self-regulate and maintain inner control. These are certainly expectations we hold for adolescents, to be planful, to act appropriately, and to control their own emotions. Self-demands, self-motivation, self-direction, and self-evaluation also play important roles in self-regulation for adolescents.

Other social cognitive functions include **forethought activity**, or the ways we think about the future, how we put it into perspective, set goals, and anticipate what might happen under certain circumstances. **Self-reflecting capabilities** contribute toward our behaviors and include thoughts such as "How might I do?" "How am I doing?" "How well did I do?" As we do this we evaluate our capabilities and performance, as well as moral considerations of what should be done. These evaluations affect our thoughts, feelings, or behaviors (Ford & Lerner, 1992). **Self-efficacy** relates to our beliefs, positive or negative, in our ability to learn or perform a task. It governs whether we view things in our environment as opportunities to engage with or threats to avoid, or somewhere in between, based on our understanding and confidence in our abilities. Other social cognitive functions can affect how we interact with others. Table 8-3 lists just a few.

**TABLE 8-3** Examples of Social Cognition That Impact Our Interactions With Others

| Social Cognition | Definition | Example |
|---|---|---|
| Joint attention | Maintaining attention on something within the environment with another individual | Following a teacher's lesson in class |
| Perspective taking | Spontaneously adopting the psychological point of view of others | Understanding the differing opinion of a classmate during a group discussion |
| Empathy | Experiencing feelings of sympathy and compassion for unfortunate others | Crying because a best friend's parents are getting divorced |

Adolescents differ from adults in the extent to which social expectations, social pressure, and peer modeling, all contributors to social cognition, affect their behaviors (Muuss, 1988). If we want to alter the behavior of an adolescent, we may use certain social-cognitive interventions that address how accurately adolescents perceive the intentions and behaviors of others. These methods help an adolescent identify situations or emotions that have been problematic in the past and think of ways they could have responded differently. One may also work with the adolescent to predict outcomes of each of these alternatives.

**Adolescent egocentrism.** Adolescent egocentrism is a feature of adolescent thinking, conceptualized by child psychologist David Elkind, that coincides with adolescents' developing cognitive abilities to think about hypothetical situations, consider their own thoughts, and focus on what others may be thinking. In an adolescent's mind, much of this is related to the adolescent's own behaviors as well as their outward appearance. Elkind argues that adolescents often fail to differentiate their thoughts from others,' and because of this, they believe their own behaviors and appearance are on the minds of others, as well. Elkind describes an **imaginary audience** that the adolescent plays to with all eyes on them. This audience can be either critical or adoring. Accordingly, an adolescent may become embarrassed or obsess over minor things. For example, they may feel self-conscious walking to the front of the class to write on the board because they're worried about their new haircut or whether their handwriting is neat enough, and they believe everyone else is concerned with those things, too. Along with the imaginary audience, a **personal fable** develops. Because adolescents think others are fascinated by them, they also think they must be unique in some way. This differs from characteristics such as high self-esteem, because adolescents can believe they are unique, even if they are not particularly good. Elkind (1967) believes the personal fable can be linked to adolescent risk-taking behaviors, because if adolescents are special or different from others, then regular rules don't apply and nothing bad can happen to them. There is research challenging the notion that egocentrism of this nature is limited to adolescence, as it can be viewed across the life span (Frankenberger, 2000). Also, there is support for the notion that girls are more likely to experience thoughts and behaviors in line with an imaginary audience, whereas boys are more likely to experience those related to a personal fable (Goossens et al., 2002; Schonert-Reichl, 1994). Elkind believes that adolescent egocentrism is a natural progression of development that can lead to a greater awareness of the self and one's identity, both considered important developmental tasks of adolescence.

## Identity Development

Adolescence is a time for developing one's **identity**, consolidating roles, relationships, talents, abilities, or failings into a whole that is connected with

### Theory Then and Now

**Theory then:** Until recent decades, developing occupational interests and deciding on a career path was a hallmark of adolescence and identity development (Erikson, 1968).

**Theory now:** Many aspects of identity development continue into what theorists have termed "emerging adulthood," a relatively new developmental phase that will be covered in the next chapter (Arnett, 2000).

the expectations of society. The adolescent is figuring out who he is, what he believes, and how he wants to behave. There can be a new focus on occupational interests at this age, as some decide whether college or work is the right path. Sexual intimacy that adolescents may experience is believed to be the precursor to developing the ability to achieve true, mutual intimacy with another person. Developmental theorist Erik Erikson, who did considerable work on identity development, believed that one cannot achieve true intimacy during this stage unless he has first developed a solid identity (Erikson, 1968). Erikson felt that this is why so many adolescent love relationships fail.

**Identity development status.** Psychologist James Marcia expanded on Erikson's work in identity development to describe where individuals may be as they seek to establish an identity. Marcia described four statuses of identity development, each marked by some combination of exploration, or the seeking out and experimenting with alternative life paths and beliefs, and commitment, or the choice of one among alternatives that have been explored (see Table 8-4). These paths and explorations can lead to beliefs, behaviors, interests, or involvement in certain social groups. Once a person has committed to an aspect of their identity, it is typically abandoned only with great consideration and/or reluctance (Marcia, 1980). These four statuses are *identity diffusion*, *foreclosure*, *moratorium*, and *identity achievement*.

**TABLE 8-4** Marcia's Identity Statuses According to Exploration and Commitment

| | No Commitment | Commitment |
|---|---|---|
| No Exploration | Identity diffusion | Foreclosure |
| Exploration | Moratorium | Identity achievement |

**Identity diffusion** describes those who may have done relatively little exploring and who still have made no commitment to a particular identity or path. These individuals may be characterized as more socially remote, apathetic, or isolated. Alternatively, they may be viewed as carefree and nonchalant, showing little concern over areas in which we would expect to see some identity development occur. Between these two types of identity-diffused individuals, lack of exploration may be for totally different reasons, whether it's not really wanting to engage with opportunities for exploration, or not really caring about them in the first place.

**Foreclosure** status includes individuals who have made a commitment to some aspect of their identity without undergoing any exploration. They can sometime be characterized as inflexible, self-righteous, or authoritarian but also as goal-directed, neat, clean, or well organized. They may like to be told what to do or set high, rigid goals for themselves. The may come from families with close ties, subscribe to family values, and often follow parental choices.

**Moratorium** is a state of total exploration with little or no commitment. However, this doesn't mean the person will not make a commitment at some point. Many adolescents find themselves within the moratorium status. These individuals may be defined as struggling, intense, even somewhat anxious. However, part of their exploration includes being actively engaged in working through relationships and personal dilemmas. They may find themselves going back and forth between rebellion and conformity as they explore different paths. They can also be personally engaging because they are so lively and involved in exploring themselves and the world.

**Identity achievement** characterizes those who have explored and then made a commitment to a particular identity or life path. They may seem settled and exhibit a solid self-assuredness. They can clearly articulate their choices as well as their reasons for making them and are resistant to manipulation.

FIGURE 8-3 Can you think of areas in which personal or social identity exploration can take place? Consider these among others.

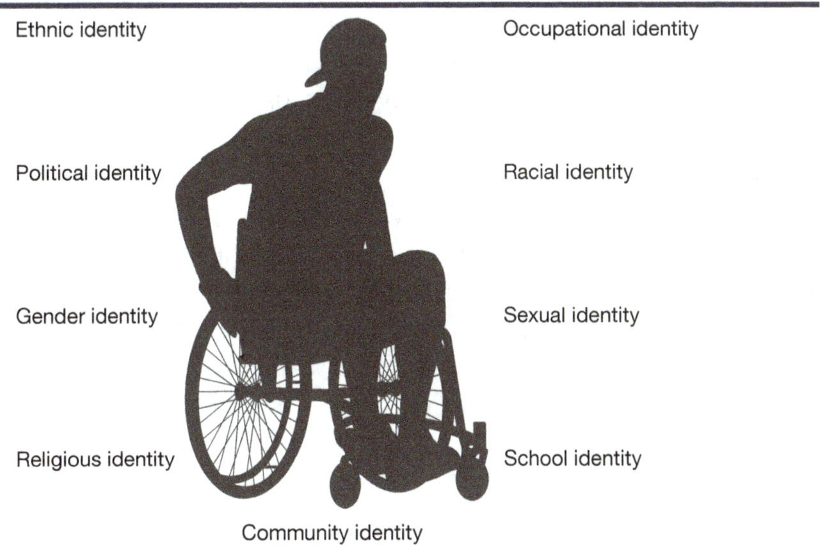


*Source*: Copyright © 2013 Depositphotos/k3studija.

As you can imagine, role models can play an important part in identity development, exploration, and commitment. Identification with a role model may begin in early adolescence as more idealizing. For example, a 13-year-old who wants to be a football player because Tom Brady is the greatest of all time may be basing this on an idealized view of what it means to be successful. As the adolescent grows older, he may view other figures who play an important part in his day-to-day life as successful, such as teachers, coaches, mentors, and family members, and choose to emulate those figures instead. The adolescent also tends to move away from wanting to be "just like" a role model toward being able to differentiate positive and negative characteristics of that person. For example, a coach may have a tremendous impact on the way a 17-year-old wants to interact with younger generations, but the coach may struggle in other areas of his life that the 17-year-old chooses to avoid (Marcia & Archer, 1993).

## Risk-Taking Behaviors

Part of identity exploration for adolescents will likely include risk-taking behaviors. Many things can lead an adolescent toward risk-taking behaviors, such as alcohol or drug use and unsafe sex, to name a few. Risk-taking behaviors are often associated with risk contexts such as living in a high-risk neighborhood or in a high-risk family situation. However, some risk-taking behaviors are considered typical during this developmental period. People take calculated and noncalculated risks all the time. However, adolescents are more inclined toward risk-taking behaviors for several reasons, including development and change occurring within brain regions, brain structures, and brain functioning associated with socioemotional functioning such as reward seeking, especially when peers are present. As we grow and develop greater cognitive control and better self-regulation abilities, risk-taking behaviors tend to decline (Steinberg, 2008).

Taking risks can be costly or beneficial. Often times the benefits of a particular risk add up before the costs do, for example, condom use. One factor that contributes to the perception of costs and benefits related to risk-taking behaviors is peer presence. As we know, peers become more important across childhood, and that is particularly true for adolescents. In situations when and where risk taking may occur, peers can influence how an adolescent views potential costs or benefits. Even if they know the costs are high and the benefits are low, teens are still more likely to take a risk when a peer is present. Additionally, if the reward of a risk-taking behavior is immediate (as opposed to more long term), adolescents are more likely to engage in the risk if a peer is present than when they are alone (Smith et al., 2014).

There is also an association between when a child begins to exhibit risk-taking behaviors and how likely they are to maintain those behaviors, as well as the extent and severity of risk associated with the behavior (Hanna et al., 2001; Kendler et al., 2013). For example, an adolescent who starts smoking cigarettes at age 13 is more likely to continue smoking cigarettes throughout their lifetime. An adolescent who starts smoking marijuana at age 14 is more likely to try a variety of other drugs, with increasingly dangerous effects and addictive properties.

As we've mentioned, some associate risk-taking and other problematic behaviors with certain risk contexts, such as lower socioeconomic status backgrounds.

However, in reality adolescents from high socioeconomic status backgrounds, who grow up in environments that can provide a great many opportunities, experience psychosocial risks as well. Adolescents from both high and low socioeconomic status backgrounds are more similar to one another than they are different in terms of adjustment and socialization. And adolescents from high socioeconomic status backgrounds can have problems with substance abuse, anxiety, and depression, just as those from low socioeconomic status backgrounds can. Some believe that two factors are at work in the case of adolescents from affluent backgrounds. First, excessive pressure to achieve can put added stress on an adolescent, and second, isolation from parents, be it actual isolation in cases where the parent is simply not around or emotional isolation when an adolescent does not receive the emotional support they need (Luthar & Latendresse, 2005).

## Adolescent Mental Health

The National Alliance on Mental Health (2016) reports that approximately one in five adolescents are diagnosed with a serious mental illness and 50% of lifetime mental illness cases begin by age 14. Recent statistics show 11% of adolescents have a mood disorder, 8% have an anxiety-related disorder, and 10% have a behavior or conduct disorder. Among this group, 37% drop out of school and 70% of those in the juvenile justice system have a mental illness. In 2014, suicide was the second leading cause of death among 10- to 24-year-olds at 17.4% of all deaths (Heron, 2016). Mental health during adolescence is certainly something we need to be aware of.

There are distinct differences between child mental health and adult mental health related to their underlying causes and processes. In adolescence, certain brain structures related to the processing of emotion-based content are fully online while others are not, which can influence the emotionality of adolescents and how they interpret information from their environments. Consider, too, potential hormonal influences and sleep disruptions that may exacerbate faulty cognition, increased emotionality, and mental health symptoms. The symptoms of mental health disorders and how we make diagnoses are also different between adolescents and adults, as are some commonly used treatments.

We must be careful to separate symptoms of mental health disorders from more normative or expected mental health issues. Remember, during adolescence, there is greater concern over things like body image, looks, and clothes. Adolescents tend to focus on themselves and can go back and forth between setting high expectations for themselves and having a significant lack of confidence. More moodiness is not uncommon, and they tend to express less affection toward parents as they develop a greater interest in and are more influenced by their peer groups. They may sometimes seem rude or short-tempered, which can be concerning for someone on the receiving end. They may also feel increased stress from more challenging school work. Furthermore, aspects of identity development, as well as family and peer relationships, may contribute to mental health symptoms adolescents may exhibit.

# Social Contexts and Development

**LO 8-7** **How do parents and caregivers stay involved in the lives of adolescents?**

**LO 8-8** **What are some benefits and drawbacks of social media use?**

Autonomy and independence become increasingly important as the adolescent navigates the world around him. Social settings beyond the family and the home are important and influential places where identity development can occur. Engagement with school and peers can lead to both positive and negative experiences and feelings about the self.

## Parents and Families

Given the varying contexts in which adolescents spend their time, parents and custodial caregivers are competing for time and influence with peers, siblings, other adult relatives, and close adults, teachers, coaches, religious leaders, gang members, bosses, and coworkers. However, parents continue to exert influence over their adolescent children, despite teenagers' ever-increasing autonomy. Parents may have less direct supervision and monitoring of adolescents' behaviors, activities, and time, but supervision and monitoring are important in terms of a parent or caregiver's awareness of activities and friends, and monitoring of environments when the parent or caregiver is unable to directly supervise, for example calling, texting, monitoring online behaviors, being familiar with peers or adults such as teachers, coaches, or other parents. Parents who are more proactive to begin with tend to exhibit higher levels of monitoring behaviors (Pettit et al., 2001). Parental supervision and monitoring in adolescence can have an impact on academics, peer choice, health behaviors, and risk-taking behaviors, such as delinquency and teen pregnancy (Abar et al., 2015; Criss et al., 2015; Miller, 2002; Pettit et al., 2001). Adolescents whose parents show greater involvement are also less likely to engage in bullying behaviors (Wang et al., 2009). Furthermore, adolescents whose parents have more authoritative parenting styles are less likely to drink heavily, compared with those whose parents were more permissive or neglectful (Hoffmann & Bahr, 2014).

In describing ways parents show love, adolescents in Western societies typically include themes of warmth and support, whereas in Eastern cultures, guidance and advice are common themes. Across a variety of cultures, caring, support, and encouragement, as well as being given things, especially if it is something special, are viewed as parental expressions of love by adolescents (McNeely & Barber, 2010).

**Siblings.** The average number of siblings in a home was 1.51 in 2010, with 80% of children and adolescents living with at least one sibling (one sibling = 40%; two siblings = 25%; three or more siblings = 15%). These rates differed across racial/ethnic groups. The average number of siblings was 1.41 for Asian families, 1.49 for White families, 1.64 for African American families, and 1.68 for Hispanic families, and more than 10% of homes included step- or adoptive siblings (King et al., 2010).

Many things shape sibling relationships, from the personal characteristics and behaviors of the siblings to cultural norms and expectations. Siblings influence one another through direct interaction, whether positive or negative, via support or conflict, or indirectly through impacts on other family members or through opportunities for vicarious learning. Parents' relationships with each another impact sibling relationships, especially if parents are more hostile or the parental relationship is high in conflict. Parents' relationships with their children can also impact siblings' relationships with each other in two different ways. There can be "spillover effects," in which we see negative parent-child relationships leading to negative sibling relationships, or "compensatory processes," in which negative parent-child relationships can lead to more positive sibling relationships, perhaps through forming close sibling relationships. Research is inconsistent with regard to sibling relationships across different family constellations (married, single-parent, divorced, or remarried families). In some circumstances, relationships may be more positive and in others more negative depending which aspect of the relationship is being measured, for example, conflict or closeness. In divorced families, there seem to be more emotionally intense relationships that have both positive qualities and negative qualities (McHale et al., 2012).

Achievements of older siblings can influence younger siblings both positively and negatively. And sibling relationships can place a child at further risk, particularly if one of the siblings is modeling risk-taking or negative behaviors, or be protective in risk contexts and compensate for negative circumstances, for example, by acting as a caregiver for siblings. Recent research also shows that among some of the poorest families in the United States, older, adolescent siblings (especially boys) sacrifice their nutritional needs by going without food for the benefit of their younger siblings (Moffitt & Ribar, 2016). Caregiving among siblings has practical benefits for the entire family and can instill a sense of responsibility, agency, and competence in older siblings. However, if demands become too overwhelming, caregiving can result in frustration, anger, and lowered self-esteem (Hetherington, 1989).

## Peer Relationships

Peers are people of approximately the same age with whom we share some similarities, and many theorists including Piaget, Erikson, and Bandura believed peers are integral to cognitive, social, and emotional development by serving as models and providing feedback for our own behaviors. They give us opportunities to learn and demonstrate cooperation, reciprocity, perspective taking, and empathy. Adolescent peer relationships can become more intimate as they increasingly turn to their close friends to help with personal problems and to be companions as they explore aspects of their environment and avenues for identity development. A reciprocated best friend relationship can be particularly protective, especially for adolescents who are bullied or victimized by their peers (Fitzpatrick & Bussey, 2014). Peers and friends also pose a risk to adolescents in certain circumstances. Perhaps not surprisingly, adolescents are more likely to start drinking if their friends drink, and if an adolescent drinks, they are more likely to seek out other friends who drink (Leung et al., 2014). In fact, being friends with a substance-using peer is one of the strongest predictors of substance use for adolescents. Yet there are many factors that can influence whether an adolescent whose friends are substance users will become a substance user himself, including the nature of the friendship, parental monitoring, personality characteristics, and tendencies toward sensation-seeking behaviors (Marschall-Lévesque et al., 2014).

**Romantic relationships and sexual experiences.** Romantic relationships in adolescence are normative experiences, and sexual experiences are often explored. In many Western countries, most adolescents report having had at least one romantic relationship, and in the United States more than half report engaging in sexual intercourse by the age of 18 (van de Bongardt et al., 2015). These romantic relationships and sexual experiences are influenced by many factors, including traits such as self-esteem, as well as other relationships with parents and other peers. This is not surprising, given what we know about the importance of early attachments with caregivers in creating internal working models of how we view ourselves and others in relationships. Our preferences and behaviors in romantic relationships during these years can influence the romantic relationships we have in during adulthood. Peer relationships also seem to set the stage for future romantic relationships, as high-quality peer relationships during adolescence are associated with high-quality romantic relationships in adulthood (Yu et al., 2014). However, adolescent romantic relationships that result in early marriage are associated with greater marital dissatisfaction and higher rates of divorce (Whisman et al., 2014). This, coupled with rates of sexually transmitted infections and unwanted pregnancies among adolescents leads some to consider romantic relationships and sexual experiences at this age potential risk-taking behaviors.

Yet recent research has explored strategies that promote relational and sexual health among adolescents and has started to move away from viewing romantic relationships and sexual experiences during adolescence from a strictly risk-based framework (Connolly et al., 2014; van de Bongardt et al., 2015).

**Sociometric status.** Imagine back to your high school days. Now think about some of the people you liked the most and those you liked the least. Think about your class or your grade or your school. Were there students who were generally well liked or disliked by everyone or who were more influential than others? These opinions are related to a person's **sociometric status**, or the degree to which children are liked or disliked by a peer group. A person's sociometric status can be based on many factors, including their personality, social behaviors, attractiveness, and athletic abilities, as well as the sociometric statuses of their friends. Table 8-5 shows the descriptions of the established sociometric categories: popular, rejected, neglected, and controversial. In early studies using these categories, a child's classification was generally stable from sixth grade through ninth grade (Coie & Dodge, 1983).

**TABLE 8-5** Characteristics of Sociometric Status Categories

| Sociometric Status | Liked Most | Liked Least | Social Preference | Social Impact |
|---|---|---|---|---|
| Popular | ↑ | ↓ | ↑ | |
| Controversial | ↑ | ↑ | | ↑ |
| Rejected | ↓ | ↑ | ↓ | |
| Neglected | ↓ | ↓ | | ↓ |
| Average | | | ↔ | |

↑ rated high by peers on this characteristic
↓ rated low by peers on this characteristic
↔ rated average by peers for on characteristic

Those in the popular category are rated by their peers as high in cooperation and leadership but low in disruptive behaviors, fighting, and help seeking, and are more likely to be viewed as good students. Controversial children are rated high in disruptive behaviors, fighting, help seeking, and leadership; low in terms of shyness; and average with regard to cooperation. They are also less preferred students according to teacher ratings. Neglected children tend to be viewed favorably by teachers and show higher levels of school motivation. Rejected children, on the other hand, seem to be opposite and are rated high in disruptive and help-seeking behaviors and fighting, rated low in cooperation and leadership; and tend to be rated less favorably by teachers. Rejected children have been further categorized into submissive-rejected children and aggressive-rejected children.

Submissive-rejected children are more like average children in terms of academics and social behaviors. Aggressive-rejected children have more problematic academic and social profiles. Yet not all aggressive children and rejected by their peers. This is true especially when we look at the characteristics of controversial children (Coie et al., 1982; Wentzel & Asher, 1995). Some research suggests that sociometric classifications are also associated with quality of friendships in early adulthood, as well as other outcomes in adulthood such as education level, employment, and mental health symptoms (Almquist & Brännström, 2014; Lansford et al., 2014).

**Bullying in adolescence.** Aggression, hostility, and bullying are not atypical in adolescence, and those who are low in peer acceptance or high in peer rejection are not the only victims. Bullying can take on different forms and involve acts of direct aggression (physical or verbal) and indirect aggression (social group exclusion and rumor spreading). Although victims of indirect aggression can be wide-ranging, children who are low in peer acceptance are more likely to be the victims of direct aggression. Adolescents who *engage* in more direct forms of aggression and bullying also tend to have emotion regulation and conduct problems, low peer acceptance, and high peer rejection. Those who engage in more indirect forms of aggression and bullying tend to have more internalizing problems such as poor mood or low self-esteem.

Aggressive and bullying behaviors can also vary by gender. When it comes to bullying, boys are more likely to engage in physical or verbal bullying, whereas girls are only somewhat more likely to engage in relational bullying through behaviors such as exclusion from the social group or rumor spreading (Card et al., 2008; Wang et al., 2009). There are several theories regarding why girls engage in more relational aggression, including the tendency for girls to have lower physical strength, making physical aggression less impactful, and smaller friendship circles, making relational aggression more impactful, as well as social norms related to adolescent women's sexual reputations, making rumor spreading more impactful on the individual being targeted (Card et al., 2008).

Peer aggression and victimization can lead to many challenges during adolescence and into adulthood. Both victims and bullies are at an increased risk for anxiety, depression, suicidal ideation (thoughts), and suicide attempts in young adulthood (Copeland et al., 2013; Klomek et al., 2010).

## School Engagement and Connectedness

**School engagement**, or the ways youth are behaviorally involved and emotionally identify with their school, is a consistent predictor of adolescents' well-being. Those who are more engaged in school programs and academics have better grades and fewer depressive symptoms and exhibit fewer risk-taking behaviors, including delinquency and substance use. School engagement may have a lasting impact on a person, too, as those who are disengaged are more likely to be unemployed, exhibit delinquent behaviors, and engage in substance abuse even into young adulthood (Henry et al., 2012; Li et al., 2016; Wang & Fredricks, 2014). There appears to be a reciprocal relation between school engagement and academic achievement. In other words, school engagement predicts how well a student does in school, but how well a student does in school also predicts how engaged they feel with their school (Chase et al., 2014). Students' perception of the school environment affects their motivation to achieve, which influences how they engage with the school on behavioral, emotional, and cognitive dimensions (Wang & Eccles, 2013). Perception of the school environment is related to **school connectedness**. School connectedness is "the belief held by students that adults and peers in their school care about their learning as well as about them as individuals" (Centers for Disease Control and Prevention, 2013f). School connectedness is also associated with better academic functioning, including attendance, performance, and high school completion, as well as fewer risk-taking behaviors such as disruptive behaviors and aggression, delinquency, sexual initiation, emotional distress, and suicidality (Centers for Disease Control and Prevention, 2013f).

## Social Media and New Technologies

New technologies and social media provide a new stage on which normal aspects of adolescent development, be they cognitive, emotional, or social, can be played out (Barth, 2015). As has been the trend for a number of decades, mass media are important parts of adolescents' day-to-day lives. What teenagers learn on television, in movies, and online dictates what's important and what's not, what's cool and what's not, what they should be doing and what they should not. For earlier generations, it was Elvis Presley and the Beatles on evening television, moving to the generations who grew up on the *MTV Top 20 Video Countdown* and *Total Request Live*, to MySpace, to Facebook, to Instagram, and Snapchat.

When it comes to various forms of media and technology, girls are more likely to use social media, whereas boys are more likely to play video games. Still, for today's youth, being "online" appears to be the predominant medium of choice. According to a report from the Pew Research Center, in 2015, 92% of teens report going online daily, with 24% saying they are online "almost constantly" and only 12% saying they go online once a day. At that time, more than half of all teens had access to a tablet, with 87% having a desktop or laptop. This is perhaps not surprising given the requirements for computing technology in many middle and high schools these days. Gone are the handwritten assignments, with computer use now during and outside school time a necessity. Still, smart phones are the most common way teens go online. There appear to be differences across racial and ethnic groups, at least in the United States, in terms of who has smart phones and how often they use them. African Americans are most likely to have a smart phone (85%) compared with White and Hispanic teens (71%), whereas 34% of African Americans are online "almost constantly" and 32% of Hispanic teens are online "almost constantly" compared with 19% of White teens who are online "almost constantly" (Lenhart, 2015).

Adolescents use their phones to go online and to communicate with their peers. The average teen sends and receives 30 text messages per day. Some (35%) have also used their phones to cheat on exams, but less than half of adolescents surveyed thought texting answers to others was a form of cheating.

A majority of teachers (63%) think media can help students find information quickly and efficiently, but a smaller number (34%) think entertainment media can help students multitask effectively. However, if a teacher is comfortable with new media and technologies they are more likely to perceive benefits of various forms of media and its impact on students' creativity (Common Sense Media, 2012). Other research on the benefits of media use and new technologies is contradictory. On the one hand, texting and online messaging can carry over into face-to-face situations but on the other hand it may improve teens' social skills and interaction behaviors (Barth, 2015).

Social media sites such as Facebook can make a lonely adolescent feel worse, even if they believe the site is a source of support and connection. In terms of health, some have linked the recent rise in the childhood obesity rate to long hours spent in front of computers as opposed to being physically active (Barth, 2015). A recent review of research on online technologies, including usage other than social media, found both benefits (increased self-esteem and social capital, perceived social support, safe identity experimentation, and increased opportunity for self-disclosure) and costs (increased exposure to harm, social isolation, depression, and cyberbullying) to online technology use, but no clear effects of social media on adolescent well-being (Best et al., 2014). There are clear risks involved in certain online technologies. In a study of abused and nonabused girls of ages 14 to 17, 40% reported experiencing online sexual advances and 26% met someone "in real life" they first met online (Noll et al., 2009). In 2000, 95% of internet-initiated sex crimes were statutory rape (Wolak et al., 2008).

**Media violence.** Many wonder whether engaging with violent content through media causes violent behaviors. Research suggests it increases the likelihood of engaging in violent behaviors later on in life, and being more aggressive and growing up in environments where violence is prevalent further increases the likelihood. Still, there are many more factors that affect the likelihood of someone committing violent acts. Given this, engaging with violent media is considered a risk factor for violent behavior, rather than the cause of violent behavior (Common Sense Media 2013).

# CHAPTER 9 Young Adulthood

In keeping with the biopsychosocial perspective we've highlighted throughout childhood and adolescence, we see that physical changes in adulthood work in tandem with psychological and social factors, including well-being, socioeconomic status, aspects of racial and ethnic backgrounds as well as sex and gender. Think about the ways women in Western culture may be socialized to care about their appearance in different ways that men are. Some women may experience negative feelings of self-worth as youthful "beauty" changes across adulthood. Similarly, women may be more likely to take measures to maintain their appearance, such as altering their diets and exercise habits, which may have additional benefits on health and wellness.

## What Would You Do? Jarrod's Story

My story begins when I was 31 years old. I was a healthy and active person, had a nice apartment, was the marketing and design director for a thriving company, was dating a terrific woman, was driving the car I always wanted, and was preparing to go back to school to earn an MBA. I was healthy and living my life as if it would go on like that forever.

But over a period of several months, I had some strange health changes. I had some very bad migraine headaches; a dizzy spell in a restaurant that left me on the floor unconscious for several minutes; incremental weight gain, and small skin rashes and sores in my armpits coming and going. I wrote it all off to stress and the fact that my roommate had recently obtained a cat (to which I was allergic). My energy level plummeted. After work, I hit the couch and couldn't do much more than rest for the entire evening. In addition to extra rest and sleep, I was taking an increasing number of herbal remedies, vitamins, and energy boosters. None of those remedies helped me either. I can't explain how strange I felt and couldn't put my finger on what was wrong. I felt like I was becoming a hypochondriac.

Several months after I first started feeling different, I went in to see my doctor, who told me to remove the cat immediately and return for a long overdue regular check-up, which I scheduled for a few weeks later. By the time I got to that check-up, I was having trouble breathing at night, and the skin rashes were more frequent. My doctor tested me for the AIDS virus, scheduled an appointment with an immunologist, and told me to take Benadryl to keep the symptoms at bay. I ended up eating those like candy! The immunologist found nothing unusual except an abnormally high allergy to cat dander; I moved out my apartment and away from the cat. But the "allergy" symptoms persisted, and I began to feel worse. And the doctors sent me home with no follow-up appointment or plan.

Finally, when I developed a severe pain in my lower abdomen that would not go away with ibuprofen, I was referred to a surgeon, who listed about a dozen things that might be wrong with me. Nobody ever mentioned the word cancer and I was completely ignorant that it was a possibility. When I went for a second opinion at one of the top hospitals in Boston, the surgeon looked at my X-rays and CT scan results for 30 seconds and said, "You have a mass in your abdomen the size of my fist." He gave me another list of what that mass could mean and mentioned cat scratch fever. Again, at this point I still never thought about cancer and no one had uttered the word. But by then, I could not

# Biological Functioning

**LO 9-1 Explain how cancer develops and identify ways we can prevent certain types of cancer.**

**LO 9-2 Describe some of the body's physical changes that begin to take place during young adulthood.**

**LO 9-3 Identify the major bodily systems and briefly describe their functions.**

Certain age-related changes can be prevented or slowed to promote successful aging regardless of whether you're a young adult or older. Physical activity of course can help in some cases, but adopting healthy habits are also important. If you started smoking in early age, quitting can have immediate impacts.

Chronic illnesses in adulthood affect quality of life. Some illnesses and symptoms have minimal impacts whereas others can affect many facets of everyday life, including the ability to move, the experience of pain and anxiety, and the inability to think clearly or to complete simple mental tasks. It is important to clearly differentiate major and chronic illnesses from normal aging processes, even in early adulthood. Health is more than the absence of illness or disability. According to the World Health Organization (1948) health is a state of complete physical, mental, and social well-being.

## Physical Changes

**Skin.** Our skin is the largest organ in the body. Age-related changes to the skin can be visible in the early 20s for some and continue across adulthood. What influences the rate of skin aging? Genetics and factors such as skin type can certainly play a part. For example, certain people with fair skin show more rapid effects of aging than those with darker skin. Lifestyle habits, such as sun exposure, are also tremendously important and cause age changes known as photoaging (Coelho et al., 2009). Other harmful lifestyle habits can interact with sun exposure, cigarette smoke in particular (Burke & Wei, 2009).

The use of sunscreen is perhaps the most important protective lifestyle habit that can minimize skin aging due to sun exposure. It's not possible to avoid the sun's rays completely, nor would we want to avoid the sun altogether, as sun exposure promotes vitamin D production in the body. However, it is extremely important for people to use sunscreen with a sun protection factor (SPF) of at least 15 that blocks two types of ultra violet (UV) light (UVA and UVB) to protect against the harmful effects of sun-exposure on the body. Most health-conscious people know sunscreen is important. However, they may not use it appropriately to prevent sun damage (Wang & Dusza, 2009). Others may know about its importance but not care. Younger adults in particular still tan excessively, either outdoors or in a tanning salon, despite growing evidence regarding its dangers.

There are numerous products that take advantage of people's desire to look younger, and this is not a new trend. Pig fat was a popular moisturizer in the 18th century, and at the time there were strawberry and gin facial washes. We've come quite a long way since then indeed, with newer products that utilize advances in the biology of aging combined with the improved microdelivery systems of such ingredients as collagen and tretinoin (the active ingredient in retinol) (Tucker-Samaras et al., 2009). The addition of alpha-hydroxy acid agents to a basic moisturizer can stimulate cell growth and renewal to offset sun damage. Regardless of its touted antiaging effects, the best type of moisturizer combines such active ingredients with SPF-15 and UVA/UVB protection. Used regularly, these types of moisturizers can help counteract the fragility, sensitivity, and dryness of the exposed areas of skin (Yamamoto et al., Me 2006).

stand up straight, had pain in my lower back and neck, my arms were sore, I had trouble breathing at night and sleeping, and I had rashes and hives coming and going all the time. I had digestive trouble, couldn't make love, couldn't exercise, and I had very little energy.

The biopsy proved what I knew already—something was very wrong with me. I was right! But I did not have cat scratch fever, or a hernia, or diverticulitis. I had a progressive cancer in my lymphatic system that would need radiation and chemotherapy treatment immediately. It was tough news to hear, but I felt relieved that I was not crazy and that I finally knew what I was up against, and I planned to fight. My hope is that with more awareness—from patients *and* the medical community—we can identify cancer symptoms earlier and get young adults to go the doctor regularly, "just because" it can save your life.

Think about what you would do in this situation after reading the chapter, and then decide the following:

- If you were Jarrod, how would you interpret your symptoms? Which would both you the most and lead you to seek medical advice?
- If you were Jarrod, how would you react to such a cancer diagnosis?
- If you were Jarrod's doctor, would you have done anything differently after the initial cat allergy diagnosis? If so, how?
- If you were part of Jarrod's health care team, how would react to the initial misdiagnosis?

**Body build.** Being "grown up" often implies that you are done growing and your body has reached its adult form. Yet throughout adulthood, the body can continuously change in size and shape so that by the time many people reach their 50s and 60s, their bodies have only a passing resemblance to their physique in early adulthood. The body's lean tissue, or fat-free mass (FFM), decreases. Changes in body composition over adulthood are reflected in the body mass index (BMI). The BMI is calculated by dividing weight (in kilograms) by height (in meters squared). According to the Centers for Disease Control (CDC, 2010b), a BMI between 18.5 and 25 is considered normal weight. However, there are racial differences in BMI ranges for normal weight. For example, the range for normal weight in Asians is lower, whereas the range for Blacks is higher (Heymsfield et al., 2016). Also, think about it this way, people who are the same height and the same weight can certainly have different proportions of fat and muscle. If we look to BMI as an indicator of other health problems, such as metabolic syndrome, these are factors that must be taken into consideration. To calculate BMI, divide your weight (in kilograms) by the square of your height (in meters) ($kg/m^2$). The overall pattern of body weight in adulthood shows an upside-down U-shaped trend by age. Most people experience an increase in their weight from their 20s until their mid-50s, after which they tend to lose those added pounds.

**Mobility.** Our bones, muscles, tendons, and ligaments, essentially everything that allows us to move around in the world, from big movements such as heavy lifting and running to small precise movements such as threading a needle, undergo age-related changes that compromise their ability to function effectively. Muscle strength, as measured by maximum force, peaks, in young adulthood, but you may hear someone refer to a professional ball player as "being on the wrong side of 30." That's because there is progressive age-related loss of muscle mass across adulthood. Coinciding with this is a loss of strength, a process known as **sarcopenia**. The number and size of muscle fibers decrease, especially the fast-twitch muscle fibers that you use in speed and strength.

Bone is living tissue that continuously reconstructs itself through the process of **bone remodeling**. Old cells are destroyed and replaced by new cells. Fortunately, most people aren't significantly affected by bone loss until they are in their 50s or 60s. We can ward off this bone loss by exercising, not smoking, and maintaining a healthy BMI (Wilsgaard et al., 2009). Resistance training with weights in particular, eating high amounts of dietary protein, increasing calcium intake prior to menopause, and taking vitamin D can also help minimize bone loss (Dawson-Hughes & Bischoff-Ferrari, 2007; Devine et al., 2005; Tolomio et al., 2008). Getting enough magnesium, found in foods such as bananas, certain types of nuts, and potatoes, as well as carotenoids found in carrots, squash, and apricots, are also important (Ryder et al., 2005; Sahni et al., 2009). Beyond individual factors, aspects of the environment also play a role in maintaining bone health. People who live in climates with sharp demarcations between the seasons appear to be more likely to suffer from earlier onset of bone loss; for example, people living in Norway have among the highest rates of bone fracture of anyone in the world (Forsmo et al., 2005).

Most people won't report feeling "creaky" until their 40s, but the joints already undergo significant changes even before skeletal maturity is reached in late adolescence. These changes occur throughout adulthood and seem to impact women more than men (Ding et al., 2007). Even in young adulthood, the articular cartilage that protects the joints begins to degenerate, and as a result, our bones can start to suffer. The fibers in the joint capsule become less pliable, reducing flexibility even further. Unlike muscles, joints do not benefit from constant use, and stress and repeated use can cause joints to wear out faster. As this occurs, and joints become less flexible and more painful, people find it harder to move affected areas of the body. In fact, more than half of the adults in the United States report that they experience chronic joint pain or movement restriction (Leveille, 2004). However, certain precautions can be taken to reduce the effects of aging on joint mobility, such as setting up your computer workstation posture properly and wearing proper shoes (Dufour et al., 2009).

## Vital Bodily Functions

The cardiovascular, respiratory, urinary, and digestive systems house the major organs of the body that keep us alive. General estimates put age-related changes to these vital systems at 0.5% per year, but some put these rates as high as 1% (Ades & Toth, 2005; Bortz, 2005). Declines seem to be nonlinear; in other words, these changes occur faster in later adulthood, depending on the person's fitness level. Physical activity is one of the best strategies you can follow to try to prolong these changes from occurring.

**Cardiovascular system.** The cardiovascular system includes the heart, the **arteries** that circulate blood throughout the body away from the heart, and the **veins** that bring the blood back to the heart. In adulthood, the most significant changes to this system involve the heart muscle itself and the arteries. The **left ventricle** is the chamber in the heart that pumps the oxygenated blood out to the arteries and is largely responsible for the efficiency of the entire cardiovascular system. Over time, the walls of the left ventricle lose their ability to contract adequately to provide an efficient distribution of blood through the arteries, due to the aging of the muscle as well as changes in the arteries. The arteries accommodate less blood flow that, in turn, further stresses the left ventricle (Nikitin et al., 2006; Otsuki et al., 2006). The arteries accommodate less blood flow because fats circulating throughout the blood eventually form hard deposits inside the arterials walls known as **plaque**, consisting of cholesterol, cellular waste products, calcium, and fibrin (a clotting material in the blood).

Cardiovascular efficiency is indexed by aerobic capacity, the maximum amount of oxygen that can be delivered through the blood, and cardiac output, the amount of blood that the heart pumps per minute (Whitbourne & Whitbourne, 2012). Both cardiovascular efficiency and cardiac output decline as much as 10% per decade from age 25 and older. However, the rate of decline may be half that in physically fit individuals. Exercise helps maximize the heart's functioning and counteract heart problems that have already occurred such as **arteriosclerosis**, or the hardening of the arteries caused by plaque build-up and aging. In one training study, a simple program of daily walking for 12 weeks was sufficient to have beneficial effects (Teichtahl et al., 2009).

**Respiratory system.** The respiratory system brings oxygen to the body and moves carbon dioxide out. This occurs as we breathe. The diaphragm muscle and the muscles of the chest wall allow breathing to occur. The exchange of gasses takes place in small air sacs in the lungs known as alveoli. Oxygen moves from these sacs into the blood and carbon dioxide moves from the blood into alveoli.

**Urinary system.** The urinary system includes the kidneys, bladder, ureters, and urethra. The kidneys are composed of nephrons. Nephrons serve many functions: They regulate water, salts, and electrolytes, among other things, and cleanse the blood of waste that is combined in the bladder with excess water from the blood and is eliminated as urine through the urethra.

**Digestive system.** The digestive system includes the tongue, salivary glands, gastrointestinal tract, pancreas, liver, and gallbladder. Each of these helps break down food into smaller components so it can be digested and absorbed into the body. Waste is excreted as feces through the rectum and anus.

**Endocrine system.** The endocrine system is comprised of a large and diverse set of glands that regulates the actions of many of the body's organ systems. As we discussed in previous chapters, hormones are chemical messengers of the endocrine system produced by glands and tissues that send messages to cells all over the body. We've discussed hormones as they relate to pregnancy, labor and delivery, stress and allostatic load, as well as puberty. However, there are many age-related changes to the endocrine system and its hormones across adulthood. Endocrine glands themselves may release more or less of a particular hormone. Organs may also respond differently to stimulation from the hormones. And as we've discussed, the endocrine system is highly sensitive to levels of stress as well as physical illness, which can further disturb whatever changes would normally occur due to aging.

**Immune system.** The immune system regulates the body's ability to fight off stress, infection, and other threats to well-being and health. It is also closely linked to the nervous system and, consequently, to behaviors, thoughts, and emotions (Lupien et al., 2009).

## Lifestyle and Health

There are several factors related to one's lifestyle that can contribute to the onset of many chronic diseases in adulthood. Chronic diseases are those with a long duration and include cancer, chronic obstructive pulmonary disease, diabetes, or Alzheimer's disease. We differentiate chronic diseases from noncommunicable diseases. Noncommunicable diseases are those that do not stem from any type of viral or infectious agent. These may include certain chronic diseases, but may also include those diseases that are shorter in duration and may bring on sudden death, such as stroke. Taken together, noncommunicable diseases account for 40 million deaths worldwide each year (World Health Organization, 2017f), with nearly three-quarters occurring in low- and middle-income areas of the world and more likely to affect people younger than 70. Although there are certainly genetic and environmental factors that play a role in the onset of chronic and noncommunicable diseases, factors such as a sedentary lifestyle, smoking, alcohol use, and unhealthy diets are all risk factors that can be modified by the individual to some extent to promote health and well-being.

**FIGURE 9-1** Risk factors for noncommunicable disease.

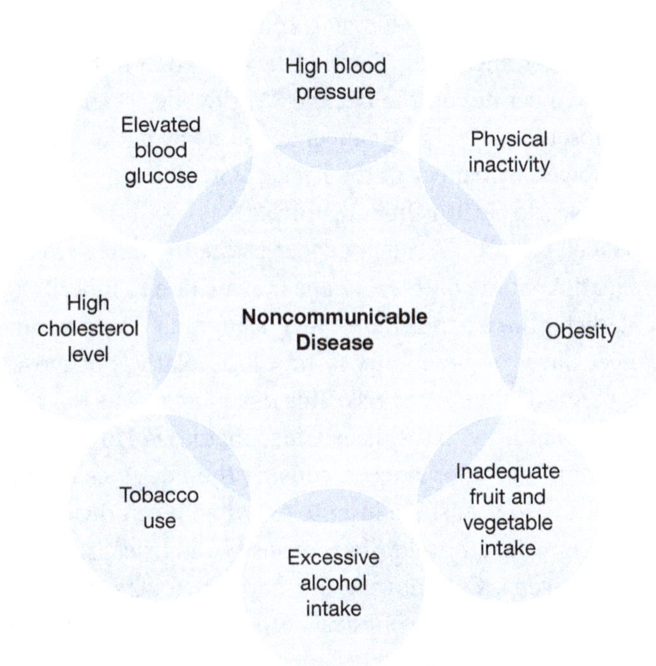


*Source*: Cynthia R. Davis

**Smoking.** In 2014, China ranked first worldwide in terms of the number of cigarettes smoked per person per year, with one in three cigarettes smoked in the world being smoked in China (World Health Organization, 2017h). According to the CDC (2020), in 2015, roughly 36.5 million (15%) American adults smoked, with higher rates among adults with lower levels of education living below the poverty line. The rates of current smokers decrease across age groups of adults, from 17% among adults aged 45 to 64 to a low of 8% among those age 65 and older. It is very possible that the smoking rates decrease not only because older adults are less likely to smoke but also because the nonsmokers are more likely to survive (Whitbourne & Whitbourne, 2012).

**Cancer.** Cancer is a generic term that includes a group of more than 100 diseases and is characterized by abnormal cell growth. Cancers may be isolated to areas of the body but can spread to other areas over the course of the disease history. Cancers can cause tumors. Malignant tumors have the potential to invade other areas of the body, whereas benign tumors do not. Each type of cancer has its own symptoms, including detectable lumps, abnormal bleeding, prolonged cough, or unexpected weight loss, as well as its own characteristics, treatment options, and overall effect on a person's life and health.

In the United States, the incidence rate for new cancers is roughly 4.6 new cases per 1,000 people annually (National Cancer Institute, 2020). These rates are highest for prostate (in men only), breast (female), and lung cancer. Black men are most likely to die from cancer and Asian/Pacific Islander women the least, and overall mortality rates for cancer are on the decline. Worldwide, 14 million new cases of cancer were diagnosed in 2012. Lung cancer accounts by far for the highest cancer mortality rate, followed by cancer of the liver, colorectal cancer, stomach cancer, and breast cancer (World Health Organization, 2018).

The abnormal cell growth we see in cancer is due to damage in the genes that control cell replication. Some of this damage may be due to inherited genetic mutations, particularly for breast and colon cancers. Roughly 5% of women diagnosed with breast cancer have the hereditary form. Close relatives of those with breast and colorectal cancers are at greater risk. This risk increases as the number of people in their extended family with the disease also increases. However, most cancers develop when random mutations occur, causing the body's cells to malfunction. Mutations may be due to a mistake in mitosis, when a cell divides to create two new cells. Cancers may also develop in response to injuries from environmental agents called carcinogens. Carcinogens are harmful toxins in the environment that can lead to cancer, including physical carcinogens (e.g., radiation), chemical carcinogens (e.g., asbestos), or biological carcinogens (e.g., Epstein—Barr virus). Cancer generally becomes more common as we age, mainly because aging is associated with greater cumulative exposure to carcinogens in the environment. In other words, over her lifetime, a typical 25-year-old has been exposed to far fewer carcinogens than a person who is 75.

Skin cancer is the most common form of cancer in adults and is directly linked to ultraviolet (UV) radiation exposure. This includes exposure from the sun and other artificial sources of UV radiation. In the United States, melanoma is most common in Utah, a state where a high proportion of the population has fair skin and lives in elevated areas, where sunlight can be reflected by ice, snow, and water. Sunlamps and tanning booths, which emit artificial UV radiation, can cause skin cancer despite the claims and beliefs about their safety. People who use tanning beds before the age of 30 increase their risk of developing skin cancer by 75%. Even so, people use tanning beds despite knowing the associated risks (Farley et al., 2015).

Cigarette smoking is often considered more dangerous than UV exposure because the forms of cancer related to cigarette smoking are far more lethal than most skin cancers (17% for lung cancer and 92% for melanoma). People who smoke are not only at risk for developing lung cancer, but they also place themselves at risk for developing cancers of the mouth, throat, esophagus, larynx, bladder, kidney, cervix, pancreas, and stomach. Exposure to cigarette smoke ("secondhand smoke") presents just as great a risk, if not greater, for developing lung cancer. Lung cancer risk lowers as soon as a person quits smoking. Furthermore, current smokers who develop lung cancer and subsequently stop smoking are less likely to get a second lung cancer compared with those who continue to smoke (Chung et al., 2015).

# Psychological Functioning

**LO 9-4** **Identify and briefly describe the types of processing we use for attentional tasks.**

**LO 9-5** **Compare different beliefs on whether intelligence changes across adulthood.**

**LO 9-6** **Summarize how the "big five" theory of personality organizes traits.**

We'll consider aspects of cognition, memory, and personality as we begin to look at psychological functioning across adulthood. Typically, in young adulthood aspects of cognition, such as reaction time and attention, as well as memory, function well. We see certain aspects of our personality manifest in core characteristics, including an individual's openness to experience, conscientiousness, extraversion/introversion, agreeableness, and neuroticism, traits psychologists have labeled the "big five."

# Cognitive Perspective

We know aging affects many areas of cognition, including attention, memory, intelligence, problem solving, and the use of language, leading to important changes in many people's ability to carry out their everyday activities. Processing speed, the amount of time it takes for an individual to analyze incoming information from the senses, formulate decisions, and then prepare a response on the basis of that analysis, is one of the most widely studied subjects across the field of cognition and aging. Researchers believe that psychomotor speed reflects the integrity of the central nervous system (Madden, 2001).

**Reaction time.** The basic measure of processing speed is reaction time. To measure reaction time, researchers ask their participants to complete an action such as pushing a computer key when the screen flashes a particular stimulus, known as a target. Stimuli that do not fit the criteria for the target are called distractors. A simple reaction time task may ask participants to make a response by pushing the key as soon as they see the target, such as a red circle appearing on the screen in front of them. In choice reaction time tasks, participants must make one response for one stimulus and another response for a different stimulus. For example, they would push the "F" button for a red circle and the "J" button for a blue circle.

Researchers know with certainty that reactions become higher (i.e., the person will be slower) as we age. The question is, by how much and under what circumstances do they increase? The documented changes in reaction time with age in adulthood are typically a matter of several hundreds of milliseconds, not enough to be particularly noticeable in everyday life, but enough to be significant under the scrutiny of the laboratory researcher.

**Attention.** As we've discussed in previous chapters, attention involves the ability to focus or concentrate on a portion of experience while ignoring other features of that experience, to be able to shift that focus as demanded by the situation, and to be able to coordinate information from multiple sources. Once your attention is focused on a piece of information, you are then able to perform further cognitive operations, such as those needed for memory or problem solving.

For the most part, studies on attentional tasks suggest that people become less efficient in the use of attentional processes as they get older. Certain attentional tasks rely on **parallel processing**, meaning that you can scan the whole environment at once, just looking for the one feature that matches that key feature you're looking for. It's as if you were at a home basketball game and wanted to spot your friend, a fan of the visiting team, in the large crowd. If all the home fans were wearing the school colors (e.g., maroon), your friend's light blue shirt would easily jump out at you. Younger and older adults perform at similarly high levels in simple visual search tasks, finding the targets quickly and accurately (Whiting et al., 2005).

A more time-consuming attentional task is **serial processing** because each stimulus must be examined in sequence to determine whether it has all the qualities of the target. The larger the number of stimuli to scan, the longer the participant will take to decide whether the target is present or not. In the case of your friend at the basketball game, should the visiting team's shirts also be maroon, it would take you much longer to find your friend's face among the fans, especially in a large arena.

If you have difficulty concentrating or focusing attention for long periods of time, you are certainly aware of how frustrating it can be to miss important information or details when you divert your mental resources away from the task. The attentional deficits associated with the normal aging process can lead to difficulties, particularly when individuals have to make complex decisions within a short period of time.

## Memory

We've described memory in previous chapters and will talk more in this and coming chapters about how memory changes across adulthood.

**Working memory.** Working memory temporarily keeps information available and active in consciousness. You use working memory when you try to learn new information or recall information you learned previously. Working memory and attention are closely linked, as controlled attention is required to juggle multiple thought processes, including working memory.

The **default network** is also important for working memory. It is a circuit linking structures of the brain active when the brain is processing internal stimuli, for example when we're daydreaming or thinking about others or the self, all those things we could possible think about when not focused on a specific task. The default network includes the hippocampus, parts of the prefrontal cortex, the parietal lobe, the temporal lobe, and part of the cingulate cortex involved in visualization. When working memory is activated, the default network becomes deactivated and other brain structures come "online" (Buckner et al., 2008). In other words, the default network acts like the parts of a computer that are active when your computer is in "sleep mode." When you need to focus on remembering information being presented to you, the sleep mode function of your brain turns off.

**Long-term memory.** Long-term memory is the repository of information held for a period of time, ranging from several minutes to a lifetime (Whitbourne & Whitbourne, 2012). It includes information about the recent past, such as remembering where you put your car keys a half-hour ago, to information from many years ago, such as what happened on your first day of kindergarten. People often confuse long-term memory with **remote memory**. Long-term memory includes your memories for what happened an hour or a day ago. Remote memory is a person's long-term memories for experiences or learning that took place years or decades ago. Long-term memory processes include encoding, storage, and retrieval. We encode information when we first learn it, keep it in long-term storage, and retrieve it when we need to use it on a subsequent occasion.

As we get older, we seem to experience a **reminiscence bump** of very clear memories for the ages of adolescence through young adulthood, especially for happy memories (Gluck & Bluck, 2007; Rubin et al., 1998). It's possible that memories are preserved so strongly in part because they are central to identity (McLean, 2008).

## Higher-Order Cognitive Functions

Researchers are certainly interested in higher-level cognitive functions that help us perform cognitive tasks necessary for adaptation and functioning that are also the basis for our ability to analyze, reason, and communicate with others (Salthouse, 2012). These functions play a major role in areas such as health, occupational performance, and relationships. Information on thinking and learning in adulthood can shed light on the potential we all have for lifelong learning. In recent years, many adults have found themselves retooling their knowledge and skills as they move to new positions in the rapidly changing labor market. Determining the factors that contribute to the effective teaching, training, and learning strategies can help people find and keep their jobs. An understanding of these cognitive functions can inform how we diagnose and treat cognitive disorders that can develop in middle and later adulthood.

**Executive functioning and its measurement.** As we've discussed, executive functioning involves higher-order cognitive skills needed to make decisions, plan, and allocate mental resources to a task at hand. An individual's executive functioning draws on working memory, selective attention, mental flexibility, and the ability to plan and inhibit distracting information (Miyake et al., 2000).

Examining how aging affects executive functioning is important because it is central to so many skills older adults need to care for themselves. Even a task such as driving, which depends heavily on speed, has a strong executive functioning component. Your executive functions will help determine the route to take to your destination, alternate between information coming from the road and your vehicle's dashboard, and make any changes along the way. Studies on executive functioning and aging increasingly focus on interventions that can protect and maximize these important skills.

**Intelligence in adulthood.** Intelligence can serve as a personal attribute that forms part of the sense of self. People seem to be aware of whether they are "smart" or "not as bright," a self-attribution that they may hold for years (Leonardelli et al., 2003). If you're one of these people who thinks of themselves as "smart," you likely value the products of the mind, such as the ability to solve tough crossword puzzles or score well in certain types of games against your friends. You may also be more vigilant for changes in intelligence associated with aging compared with those who take pride in their physical strength or dexterity. For some people, these changes may be more imagined than real, particularly as people age and relate to popular or common images that portray older adults declining in their mental abilities. Yet this may be a tough change in one's abilities to acknowledge when the declines are real.

In addition to theories presented in earlier, there is the fluid-crystallized theory, which divides intelligence into fluid reasoning, or the individual's innate ability to carry out higher-level cognitive operations, and crystallized intelligence, now referred to as comprehension knowledge, which represents the acquisition of specific skills and information people gain as the result of their exposure to the language, knowledge, and conventions of their culture (Cattell, 1963, 1971; Horn & Cattell, 1966).

Building on fluid-crystallized theory, the "extended" fluid-crystallized theory of Gardner proposes eight other broad factors that incorporate cognitive skills such as memory, speed, sensory processing, reading, writing, and mathematical knowledge. Remember his theory proposed that intelligence includes traditional abilities (logical/mathematical, verbal, visual/spatial) as well as others not usually tapped in intelligence tests (naturalistic, interpersonal, intrapersonal, musical, bodily "kinesthetic," or athleticism). Multiple intelligences theory, discussed in earlier chapters, has not served as much of a testing ground for studies on intelligence in adulthood. We might hope future researchers explore these alternate and important forms of ability that clearly impact many areas of functioning throughout the adult years.

The most comprehensive study of adult intelligence was originally conducted by K. Warner Schaie. Begun in the 1950s, what is now known as the Seattle Longitudinal Study (SLS) has produced extensive information about people's intellectual skills as they age. In addition to providing a picture of how age alters intelligence, the SLS also has provided important evidence about how cohort and time of measurement influence patterns of performance on basic intellectual abilities. Additionally, more recent offshoots of the SLS have explored the relationship of intelligence to personality, lifestyle, and the activity of various brain structures as well as patterns of intellectual development across generations.

Adult age effects on intelligence have practical and theoretical implications. For practical reasons, it may be important to understand relative strengths and weaknesses of younger versus older workers, as there appear to be differences in the styles these age groups use in decision making, a feature of cognition that can work hand in hand with intelligence.

### Theory Then and Now

**Theory then:** Age differences in intelligence across adulthood followed the classic aging pattern of an inverted U-shape, with a peak in early adulthood followed by steady decline (Botwinick, 1977).

**Theory now:** There is either no decline or a decline that does not become apparent until very late in life.

# Personality

What's your **personality** like? I'm sure three or four or more characteristics that reflect how you think about life or behave will come to mind. Are you outgoing or shy? Are you always outgoing? Are you outgoing in certain situations but not others? Psychologists view personality in many ways, and there is no one consistent meaning that all psychologists use to define it. Instead, psychologists who study personality often approach its definition from a particular theoretical vantage point.

**Psychodynamic perspective.** Sigmund Freud was one of the first psychologists to study personality. He's credited with "discovering" the unconscious, and his work indeed placed importance on hidden motives and feelings within the mind. His approach, called the psychodynamic perspective, emphasizes the ways unconscious motives and impulses are expressed through people's personalities and behaviors.

Current theories of development and personality based on the psychodynamic perspective still emphasize Freudian ideas, such as the importance of early development and the ways in which people cope with such emotions such as fear, anxiety, and love. However, the methods used to study these phenomena are far different from traditional Freudian approaches.

Although he left a rich body of work that later theorists would subsequently revise and reshape, Freud believed one's personality does not change after early childhood. In fact, according to Freud, many of the major tasks of personality development are completed by the time the child turns 5 years old. Some changes continue to occur through adolescence, but by early adulthood the individual's psychological development is essentially over and their personality is set in stone. Consequently, some traditional Freudian psychologists felt that therapy is of little value to individuals over the age of 50, because their characteristics and behaviors were so fixed they could not be radically changed.

Contemporary followers of traditional Freudian theory still emphasize early development but do not view adult personality as based on a deterministic system, where early events determine what we will become and where there is no room for change. Today, Freudian theory is divided into three main branches.

**Ego psychology.** According to Freudian theory, the mind is made up of three structures called the **id**, the **ego**, and the **superego**. If you took an introductory psychology course you may recall the id refers to the individual's biological instincts and drives, which include the need for food, sex, and water. Freud believed the id also had a death instinct, and the need to hurt, kill, and exert power over others. The superego on the other hand acts as our conscience and our moral guide that attempts to control the id's irrational instincts by providing an image of goodness to which the individual can aspire (the ideal self). The ego controls rational thought. It negotiates a way for people to meet their biological needs (based in the id) without putting themselves at risk of violating society's expectations or falling short of their ideals (based in the superego). Other theorists propose the ego is the central part of the mind that helps people find a balance between expressing their inner selves and finding ways to adapt to the world's demands.

Unlike Freud, Erikson, who also viewed development and functioning from a psychodynamic perspective, believe development occurred across the life span, from childhood through adulthood and into old age. His psychosocial model proposes that the ego matures throughout life as the individual faces particular psychological and social forces. He defined a series of eight psychosocial crises (see Figure 9-3) that individuals face in stages across the life span and believed development occurs as we make our way through the push and pull of each. A crisis is described on a spectrum between favorable outcomes (such as attaining a sense of identity) and unfavorable outcomes (such as identity confusion). Most people aren't all the way at one end of the spectrum or the other, but fall somewhere in between leaning toward one end or the other.

**FIGURE 9-2** According to Freud, aspects of personality are like an iceberg, with the ego and parts of the superego outwardly visible or expressed. All three parts also exist in the unconscious, or below the surface.

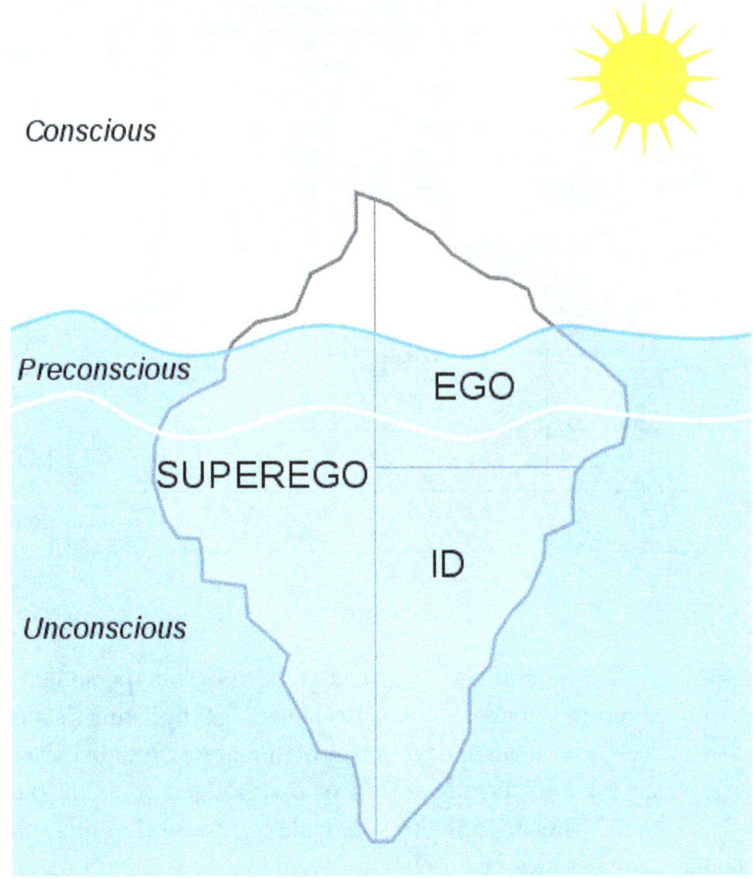


*Source*: https://commons.wikimedia.org/wiki/File:Structural-Iceberg.svg.

Once a stage is navigated, Erikson proposed that the individual moves on to the next crisis following the epigenetic principle; in other words, each crisis unfolds in a predetermined order. Recall our discussion about Erikson's view on why adolescent love relationships often fail. If a person leans toward a more unfavorable outcome during a crisis, it is unlikely he'll end up toward the favorable end when navigating subsequent crises. Although the theory proposes that particular issues are most likely to arise at particular ages (for example, identity development during adolescence and the development of intimacy during young adulthood), earlier issues may arise at a later point in life, and later stages may move to the forefront in earlier periods if conditions require the individual to confront those issues (for example, a teen mom may face crises related to parenthood and generativity that we envision happening later on in early adulthood and midlife). Research based on Erikson's theory includes studies that cover a single stage and those that incorporate all or most of the stages. Of all eight stages, identity and generativity receive the greatest attention, particularly among researchers whose work covers adolescence, emerging adulthood, and midlife.

**FIGURE 9-3** Erikson's stages.

Erikson's stages of personality development

| 1 | 2 | 3 | 4 | 5 | 6 | 7 | 8 | **Approx. age** |
|---|---|---|---|---|---|---|---|---|
| Basic trust vs. mistrust | | | | | | | | Infant |
| | Autonomy vs. shame, doubt | | | | | | | Toddler |
| | | Initiative vs. guilt | | | | | | Preschooler |
| | | | Industry vs. inferiority | | | | | School-age |
| | | | | Identity vs. role confusion | | | | Adolescent |
| | | | | | Intimacy vs. isolation | | | Young adult |
| | | | | | | Generativity vs. stagnation | | Midlife adult |
| | | | | | | | Ego integrity vs. despair | Older adult |

*Source*: Susan Whitbourne

**Trait approaches.** Remember we asked you what your personality is like. When you think about this question, you most likely begin by listing a set of a characteristics or qualities that seem to fit your way of thinking or your behaviors. These characteristics may take the form of adjectives such as "generous," or "patient," or "quiet," or "unfriendly." Trait theories of personality propose that adjectives such as these capture the essence of a person's psychological make-up based on the concept of the **trait**, which is a stable, enduring disposition that persists over time.

Trait theory in personality contends that the organization of the personal dispositions, or traits, guide a person's behavior. Trait theory is increasingly viewed in terms of genetic theories of personality that suggest the enduring nature of personality traits over time reflect the fact that they are at least partially inherited (Bouchard, 2004). One of the most generally accepted trait theories is based on Costa and McCrae's proposal of five major dimensions to personality. The five-factor model (FFM) (sometimes called the "big five") is intended to capture the essential characteristics of personality in a set of five broad traits or dispositions. The five traits in the FFM are openness to experience (or "openness"), conscientiousness, extraversion, agreeableness, and neuroticism (you can remember these as spelling "OCEAN" or "CANOE") and they're measured by the Neuroticism-Extraversion-Openness Personality Inventory–Revised (NEO-PI-R), a questionnaire containing 240 items related to these traits (Costa & McCrae, 1992). Each trait name closely fits its meaning in everyday conversation—people high in neuroticism tend to worry a great deal, those who are extraverted are outgoing and sociable, being open to experience means you are willing to entertain new ideas, having high agreeableness means you get along well with others, and being conscientious means you attend to detail and tend not to procrastinate.

**FIGURE 9-4** Key characteristics of the five-factor model of personality.

| **Neuroticism** | **Extraversion** | **Openness to experience** |
|---|---|---|
| Anxiety | Warmth | Fantasy |
| Angry hostility | Gregariousness | Aesthetics |
| Depression | Assertiveness | Feelings |
| Self-consciousness | Activity | Actions |
| Impulsiveness | Positive emotions | Ideas |
| Vulnerability | | Values |
| **Agreeableness** | **Conscientiousness** | |
| Trust | Competence | |
| Straightforwardness | Order | **Note** |
| Altruism | Dutifulness | |
| Compliance | Achievement striving | The five factors spell out |
| Modesty | Self-discipline | OCEAN and CANOE. |
| Tendermindedness | Deliberation | |

*Source*: Susan Whitbourne

Each of the five traits has six subscales or "facets." To characterize an individual completely requires knowing how that person rates on each of the 30 total facets. Where you stand within the six facets of a particular trait can make a difference in how your personality reflects in your behavior. For example, within the extraversion trait, people can be either high or low in the facet of warmth and high or low on the facet of gregariousness. Being high on both typically means you genuinely like to be around people and relate easily to others. Being low on warmth but high on gregariousness typically means you seek out being with others but people find it hard to get to know you very well.

It may come as no surprise that certain personality traits are associated with early life experiences. For example, young adults high in openness often report a higher number of stressful life events in childhood and show less physiological reactivity to laboratory stressors, such as discussing a recent highly stressful event (Williams et al., 2009).

Personality traits, even in young adulthood, such as high levels of hostility, may pose a risk factor not only for heart disease but also for the development of depression during the ensuing years. Higher hostility in the college years has also been associated with riskier health-related behaviors, including smoking and drinking. Increases in hostility also predict obesity, failure to exercise, high-fat diets, social isolation, poor health, and, for women, lower income (Siegler et al., 2003).

Clearly, personality factors are integral aspects of the biopsychosocial model of development in adulthood. Traits and behavior patterns that have their origins in inherited predispositions or in early life experiences influence the health of the individual through a variety of direct and indirect pathways. However, although personality traits may be an integral part of "who" you are, they can modulate and change over adulthood (Staudinger & Kunzmann, 2005) and even influence some of the most basic components of your ability to remain healthy.

**Cognitive perspective.** The cognitive perspective on personality believes people are driven by the desire to predict and control their experiences. Emerging from this perspective are cognitive self-theories that suggest people regard events in their lives from the standpoint of how relevant these events are to their sense of self. These theories emphasize the ways people interpret their experiences and understand themselves over time. An important principle of the cognitive perspective is the idea that people do not always view themselves realistically. In part, this is because people strive to maintain a sense of self that is consistent (Baumeister, 1996, 1997). In other words, most people prefer to see themselves as stable and predictable (even if they are not). Another basic tendency is for people to view their abilities and personal qualities in a positive light (Baumeister et al., 2001). Cognitive perspective theories also place emphasis on **coping**, the thoughts and behaviors people use to manage stress.

We've asked you a few times now, "What's your personality like?" Going hand in hand with these characteristics is our view of the self, or **self-schema**, that guides the choice and pursuit of future endeavors (Markus & Nurius, 1986). This is part of the **possible selves** model that literally means just that: What are you now, and what could you be in the future? These types of thoughts motivate you to act in certain ways so that you achieve your "hoped-for" possible self and become the person you want to be. These self-conceptions shift as you develop throughout adulthood, and some people can remain hopeful of change well into their later years (Smith & Freund, 2002). Increasingly important as you make your way through adulthood is your health-related possible self, meaning your hope that you will remain in good shape and free of disease (Hooker & Kaus, 1994). A dreaded possible self is the opposite of the hoped-for possible self, in other words who *don't* you want to become? With regard to health, most people would rather not become ill and so they will take action to avoid that outcome.

Positive feelings of life satisfaction are theorized to emerge from the extent that someone is successful at becoming the hoped-for possible self and not the dreaded possible self. People think of themselves and view their lives negatively when they are unable to realize a hoped-for possible self or avoid the dreaded possible self (Whitbourne & Whitbourne, 2012). For instance, you probably feel better when your grades confirm your possible self as a good student and study harder to avoid the dreaded self of a person who fails out of college.

However, people can protect themselves from negative self-evaluations, for example by revising the possible self to avoid future disappointment and frustration if experiences suggest that the possible self may be unattainable. You may realize that you will not be a straight A student if your grades include a mix of A's and B's (or lower grades), so you revise your possible self accordingly. You will likely feel better about yourself in the long run if you make these revisions, even if you continue to strive for good grades.

**Identity.** A person's possible self is certainly linked to her identity. Think back to our discussion on James Marcia and his identity status model presented in the previous chapter. It can be useful to understand the identity formation process during adolescence and young adulthood. However, it is less clear how it can be applied to adults in midlife and beyond. If we followed this model, you could fall into "identity achieved" classification if you went through a period of exploration during your early teens and college years and decided on some part of your identity that fit at the time. For example, let's say you competed in motocross racing on weekends and traveled extensively for trainings and competitions. Part of your identity is a motocross racer. In 20 years, would it still be appropriate or possible for you to retain that same set of commitments despite the many opportunities for exploration and change that present themselves? Technically, you would be identity achieved, but if you never questioned your identity as a motocross racer since that initial exploration during adolescence, should someone who occasionally revisits these types of identity commitments be considered differently?

The **identity process model** examines adult development in terms of **identity accommodation**, **identity assimilation**, and **balance** and allows us to describe an adult's position on issues relevant to the self at any point in life. In this model, people who retain their adolescent commitments without questioning or challenging them are not identity achieved but instead considered high on identity assimilation. Those who make changes to the self are high on identity accommodation. Balance refers to individuals who maintain a sense of self but make changes when necessary (Sneed & Whitbourne, 2003).

# Social Contexts and Functioning

Young adulthood is a time when we become fully independent individuals. Long-term intimate relationships develop and often lead to marriage and are for some preceded by a period of cohabitation. Families are formed with the arrival of children. Friendship ties continue to develop. Career choices become solidified for many, whereas others may take longer to make their way along a career path.

**LO 9-7** **Argue why you believe cohabitation is beneficial or detrimental to the success of long-term intimate relationships.**

**LO 9-8** **Evaluate your own vocational interests, whether they coincide with aspects of your personality and whether you're affected by a calling.**

## Relationships in Adulthood

Your relationships with others are essential to your existence throughout life. From your intimate partners to your family, friends, and the broader community, your social connections are a crucial part of who you are and how you feel on a day-to-day basis. It is difficult to capture the central qualities and complexities of these many relationships, and it is perhaps even more challenging to study the way these relationships interact with developmental processes within the individual over time. Yet researchers must be able to translate that intuitive sense of the importance of relationships into quantifiable terms that demonstrate the nature and impact of social processes in adulthood.

Changes in the broader society of the country and world heavily impact the nature of individual relationships. You can see from even brief glances at news stories in the media that patterns of marriage and family life change significantly with each passing year. In the United States at least, fewer people marry today, and those who do are waiting longer than previous generations. Family compositions are continually changing as people leave and reenter new long-term relationships, often involving their children and extended families as well. In this section, we examine these changing family patterns and try to provide an understanding of what theorists say about the qualities of close relationships and how they interact with the to serve as the foundation of the entire family hierarchy that is passed along from generation to generation. You hear about the death of marriage as an institution, yet interest in marriage itself never seems to wane in the popular imagination, the media, and professional literature. The decision to marry involves a legal, social, and, some might say, moral commitment in which two people promise to spend the rest of their lives together. Furthermore, as states in the United States arrive at positions on the legality of gay marriage, with even the Supreme Court weighing in on the issue in spring 2015, it seems clear that marriage is still a very relevant social institution.

Even as the definition of marriage continues to evolve, the statistics on its success rate prove to be as discouraging as ever for those who contemplate legalizing their own relationship with a partner. Given the current divorce statistics, you know that many people are not able to maintain the hopeful promises they make to each other in their wedding vows. What factors contribute to a successful marital relationship and what might lead to its demise? Social scientists are nowhere near finding answers to these questions, but, as we will see shortly, there are a plethora of theories.

Poets, philosophers, playwrights, and novelists, among others, have attempted for centuries to identify the elusive qualities of "love." Although they have not been around for as long, psychologists and sociologists have also contributed their share of theories to account for why people develop close, loving relationships and what factors account for their maintenance or dissolution over time.

Throughout the changes of marriage, divorce, remarriage, and widowhood, most adults actively strive to maintain gratifying interactions with others on a day-to-day basis. Furthermore, for many adults, the feeling of being part of a close relationship or network of relationships is the most salient aspect of identity (Whitbourne, 1986). Whether this relationship is called "marriage," "family," "friendship," or "partnership" is not as important as the feeling that one is valued by others and has something to offer to improve the lives of other people.

As relationships in the real world seem to become more complicated, so do the theories, and there is now greater recognition of the multiple variations possible when adults form close relationships. The emotional factors involved in long-term relationships are also gaining greater attention, as it is realized that some characteristics of human interactions transcend specific age- or gender-based boundaries.

In adulthood, people structure the nature and range of their relationships to maximize gains and minimize risks according to **socioemotional selectivity theory** (Charles & Carstensen, 2010). According to this theory, people look for different rewards from their interactions with others as they age. Socioemotional selective theory describes two types of functions served by interpersonal relationships: informational and emotional. Relationships that serve an informational function provide you with important knowledge that you would not otherwise have. For example, when you started your first job, you may have sought out and got to know people who seemed to know the most about how to work the printer, who manages time cards, how to interpret the boss's latest request, and where to find a cheap but good lunch. Maybe you friended them on Facebook or followed them on Instagram, but these friends served an informational function in your life. The other function of relationships is emotional. Relationships that serve an emotional function contribute to your sense of well-being. In your friendships that serve an emotional function, you seek to find people who help you feel good about yourself and your life. These are the people you turn to when you're feeling lonely, depressed, or stressed in hopes that they will make you feel better.

Socioemotional selectivity theory proposes that as we grow older we become more focused on the emotional functions of relationships and less interested in the informational functions. We want to spend time with the people who make us feel good. Similarly, the desire to maximize emotional rewards leads adults to increasingly prefer spending time with people they're familiar with rather than seeking out new friends and acquaintances. Family and/or longtime friends are those people who will serve positive emotional functions of self-validation and help us manage our emotions. As we get older, we tend to be less interested in meeting new people and broadening our social horizons because we prefer to maximize the emotional and minimize the information functions of our relationships (Lang & Carstensen, 2002).

You may be reflecting on your own friendship patterns and be at a point in your life where spending time with friends and acquaintances is more important than spending time with family. The number of Facebook friends or Instagram followers you have may well be greater than 500 and include many people you have not spoken with for months, even years. As you navigate through adulthood you will most likely find that the number of people in your social network dwindles, and you are left with a much smaller network of close friends and family. As part of this transition, you will go through a "weeding out" process where you focus on maintaining the positive relationships and removing (or "unfriending") the negative ones.

Endings of any kind, whether the end of a friendship or the end of a chapter in your life, bring out strong emotions and cause you to want to spend time with the people you are closest to. Think of times when significant life events have come to an end, such as when you graduated from high school and said goodbye to your classmates or moved away from home for the first time or left a job you held for a number of years. Knowing you did not have much time left to spend with these people, you wanted to make the most out of the time you did have.

**Marriage.** Let's begin with some current facts about marriage. In 2015, 124.4 million adults were married and living with their spouse, a number that represents 51% of the population age 18 and older. Among the entire 18-and-older population, the percentage of those who have ever been married is far higher—approximately 71% (U.S. Bureau of the Census, 2017a). Between the years 2006–2010, the median age of marriage was 25.8 for women and 23.8 for men. Although the age of first marriage is on the increase, by the age of 40, 84% of all women are married, a percentage that has not changed since 1995 (Copen et al., 2012). However, the gap between married and unmarried Americans 15 and older has continued to shrink since 1950 (U.S. Bureau of the Census, 2017d).

FIGURE 9-5 U.S. average age of first marriage.

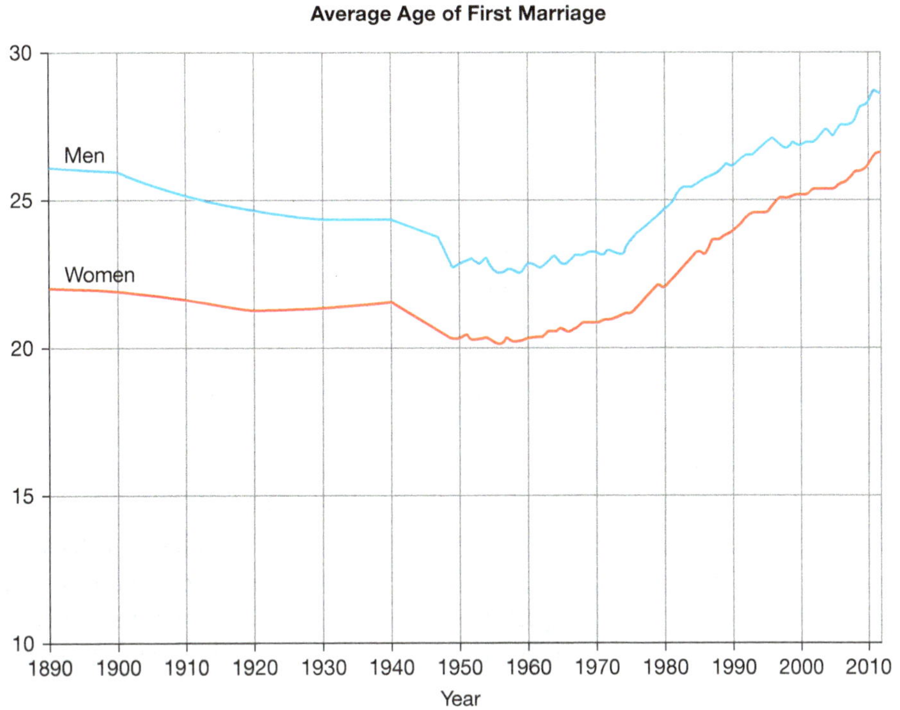


*Source*: https://commons.wikimedia.org/wiki/File:United_States_Average_Age_of_First_Marriage.png.

As a social institution, **marriage** is defined as a legally sanctioned union. Married couples are permitted to file joint income tax returns and are given virtually automatic privileges to share the rest of their finances, as well as other necessities such as health care and housing. Generally, marital partners are entitled to retirement, death, and health insurance benefits as well as the entire portion of the estate when one partner dies. Although marriages need not legally conform to the statutes of a particular religion, many are often performed in a religious context.

Heterosexual couples often share a last name, usually the husband's, although many wives never change their last names. In the 1970s, the trend of couples adopting a new, hyphenated last name emerged, but it now appears to have decreased in popularity. Until 2013, same-sex couples could get married only within certain U.S. states until the Supreme Court ruled part of the Defense of Marriage Act to be unconstitutional in 2015, making same-sex marriages legal throughout the country.

Having explained the legal definition of marriage, you can clearly see what and who is excluded. People who are not legally married are not automatically entitled to the benefits available to those who are. Partners living within a committed and long-term relationship must seek exceptions to virtually all of the conditions set forth for married people.

Obviously, the legal definition of marriage includes no mention of the partners' emotional relationship with each other. People can be legally married and live apart, both literally and figuratively. Most social scientists distinguish between an intimate and a marital relationship because neither is a necessity in these types of partnerships. The legal commitment of marriage adds a dimension to an intimate relationship not present in a nonmarital close relationship in that ending a marital relationship is technically more difficult than ending a nonmarital one. Furthermore, many people view a legalized marriage as a moral and spiritual commitment they cannot or will not violate.

Definitional concerns aside, there is a body of evidence on marriage in adulthood suggesting that married adults have many advantages compared with those who are unmarried. Researchers analyzing the findings of more than 50 studies, including those based on more than 250,000 older adults from a variety of countries, showed a 9 to 15% reduction in mortality risk for married men and women (Manzoli et al., 2007). This protective effect of marriage was greater in countries from Europe and North America compared with studies from Asia and the country of Israel. Marriage also confers with it greater happiness and a variety of other benefits for a person's quality of life, a fact that had come into question (particularly for women) in the 1980s but is now accepted as well established (Wood et al., 2007).

**Cohabitation.** Living in a stable relationship prior to or instead of marrying is referred to as **cohabitation**. Since the 1960s, there has been a steady increase in the number of couples who choose this lifestyle, at least for their first type of long-term, committed union. In 1960, an estimated 439,000 individuals in the United States reported they were cohabitating with a person of the opposite sex. By 2006, there were 6 million, and by 2015 there were an estimated 7.4 million cohabiting couples in the United States (U.S. Bureau of the Census, 2017b). Between 50 to 60% of all marriages are preceded by cohabitation (Stanley et al., 2006); looking at the data on couples who cohabitate, approximately 28% of women age 44 and younger who cohabitate eventually marry their partner (National Center for Health Statistics, 2010). Though the commonsense wisdom is that the experience of living together contributes positively to the success of a marriage, the opposite seems to be true, at least in part. Data on divorce patterns show there is a greater risk of marital break-up among couples who cohabitated before they became engaged. The greater likelihood of divorce among couples who cohabitate before becoming engaged is referred to as the **cohabitation effect** (Cohan & Kleinbaum, 2002).

One explanation for the cohabitation effect is that couples who would not have married "slide" into marriage through inertia; in other words, the fact that they were already living together becomes the basis for entering into marriage even if the fit between the two partners is not all that good. Eventually they divorce due to the fact that they were not well matched to begin with. Not only are they more likely to divorce, but couples with this relationship history experience greater unhappiness during the period in which they remain under the same roof after marrying (Rhoades et al., 2009).

In an attempt to understand causal factors involved in the cohabitation effect, Lu and colleagues (2012) evaluated the likelihood of a cohabiting relationship ending after taking into consideration certain characteristics of the partners prior to their cohabitation. Rather than compare cohabitating with noncohabitating partners, they separated out individuals who had engaged in "serial" cohabitation, meaning they had lived with more than one partner in a cohabiting relationship. This turned out to be important. People who cohabitated only with their spouse prior to marriage did not show the cohabitation effect. It was only those serial cohabitators who showed higher rates of marital disruption. Therefore, cohabitation effect does not appear to apply equally to all couples who cohabitate prior to marriage.

Along with a rise in the overall numbers of couples who cohabitate is a parallel increase in the number of cohabitating adults with children under the age of 15 (Whitbourne & Whitbourne, 2012). In 1960, this number amounted to 197,000. By 2016, there were 3.3 million with a joint biological child and 1.8 million with no joint biological child (U.S. Bureau of the Census, 2018).

**Same-sex couples.** Same-sex marriage was first legalized in the United States by the Commonwealth of Massachusetts in 2004, eventually being legalized by 13 other states prior to the Supreme Court's 2015 action that legalized same-sex marriage across the United States. Around the world, gay marriage is considered legal in 21 other countries as of mid-2015, with the Netherlands the first to legalize same-sex marriages in 2000. Based on the global extent of debate over this issue, it is a topic that will likely remain on political agendas in the coming years.

The U.S. Bureau of the Census (2017c) estimates there are as many as 859,000 same-sex households in the United States, of these 15% are interracial, more than twice the percent of married opposite-sex couples (7.0%), and slightly more than opposite-sex unmarried couples (13.84%). The exact number of same-sex married couples in the United States is not yet available, given the recentness of the Supreme Court ruling and the consequent lifting of bans throughout the majority of states.

In a review of the characteristics of same-sex couples, Peplau and Fingerhut (2007) concluded that there are many similarities in the dynamics of the relationship when compared with heterosexual couples. One notable exception, however, is a greater sharing of household tasks among same-sex couples.

Although there is little research on the factors contributing to the longevity of these relationships and partner satisfaction, the available evidence suggests that because most of the individuals living in these relationships are not legally bound to each other, they are more likely to dissolve when the partnership is not working out. A large study carried out in the United Kingdom of two birth cohorts (1958 and 1970) following same- and opposite-sex cohabitations showed same-sex cohabiting couples were more likely to dissolve than opposite-sex couples (Lau, 2012). It is possible the higher likelihood of break-up among same-sex couples reflects the impact of external forces on the relationship, including discrimination and family pressures. Although such factors can affect both gay and lesbian couples, women in same-sex relationships appear to be at particular risk for partnership dissolution due to these pressures (Khaddouma et al., 2015).

**Attraction.** Two theories contrast the popular notions "like attracts like" and "opposites attract." The **similarity hypothesis** proposes that similarity of personality and values predicts both initial interpersonal attraction and satisfaction within long-term relationships (Gaunt, 2006). Sometimes, similarities may be more superficial than real, however. In one 13-year longitudinal study of marital relationships, researchers found that couples who perceived each other as higher in agreeableness than they actually were in reality were more in love during the early stages of marriage and more likely to remain in love over time (Miller et al., 2006). Partner perceptions also play a role in marital satisfaction, particularly for wives; if they perceive their husband as being supportive, they rate their satisfaction with their marriage as higher (Priem et al., 2009).

The **need complementarity hypothesis**, in contrast, proposes that people seek and are more satisfied with marital partners who are the opposite of themselves (Winch, 1958). Despite the anecdotal evidence you may have about this viewpoint from observing your extraverted cousin happily engaged to a shy introvert, the evidence seems to favor the opposite. This is true particularly in the sensitive area of finances within relationships. People who like to spend money may be attracted to those who like to save, but over the long term, their high level of conflict will detract from the relationship's likelihood of survival (Rick et al., 2011).

**Families.** The transformation of a marriage into a "family" traditionally is thought to occur when a child enters the couple's life on a permanent basis, but there are substantial variations in family constellations (or patterns). Although the average family size in the United States is 2.53 (U.S. Bureau of the Census, 2018), over the past 20 years fewer households include husband and wife families, with increases in the percentages of one-person households, and either one or two people sharing their household with nonfamily members.

In the United States in 2009, there were 3.98 million births, which represented a decline of 1% from just the year before (Martin et al., 2017). However, this decline in births affected women age 15 to 39; rates of childbirth among women in their 30s and older either rose slightly or remained stable. These changes in birth rates reflect larger social influences, including an economic downturn at the end of the 2000s, as well as changes in women's working patterns, which we will discuss shortly.

The arrival of a couple's first child ushers in the **transition to parenthood (TtP)**, the period of adjustment to the new family status represented by the presence of a child in the home. From a biopsychosocial perspective, the TtP can involve biological changes (when the mother bears the child) as her body adapts to rapid hormonal and other physiological alterations. There is evidence for physiological changes in men, too, in particular when it comes to hormones (Saltzman & Ziegler, 2014). Both parents experience psychological changes, including the emotional highs and lows associated with this new status. At the same time, each individual's identity shifts as they begin to incorporate their new status in life into their sense of self. They also undergo social changes due to this new role that alters their status with other family members and the community. Their new role brings changes in what society expects of them, expectations that typically reflect social norms for men and women as fathers and mothers.

Researchers initially became interested in the TtP because they had consistently found that marital satisfaction dips during the childrearing years, a drop-off particularly marked for women. Using different research methods, we know see that although the TtP is not a universal crisis, there are several factors that increase the risk of a couple experiencing major relationship problems when children come into the family, including the younger age of the mother, poor relationships with their own parents, unplanned pregnancy, impulsivity, higher neuroticism, and insecure attachment styles. However, even nonparents show declines in marital satisfaction over a comparable span of time (Mitnick et al., 2009).

Typically, the division of labor in the home becomes more traditional after children arrive. Working women without children already perform more household duties than men do, but after becoming mothers, the situation is exacerbated (Coltrane, 2000). Mothers assume more of the stereotypically roles related to household duties such as laundry, cooking, and cleaning, in addition to providing the bulk of the childcare. Men increase their involvement in paid employment outside the home after the child enters the family (Christiansen & Palkovitz, 2001).

In some heterosexual relationships, marital satisfaction is affected by **doing gender**, a term that refers to the tendency of women and men to behave in stereotypically gendered ways. Parenthood can set up a dynamic that leads the parents to feel they are now a "traditional" family (Vespa, 2009). For a couple who may have shared housework in a more egalitarian fashion before children, this shift into gendered roles can place strain on the relationship (Grote et al., 2004).

With changes in legal status for same-sex marriages, an increasing number of homosexuals are becoming parents, through artificial insemination, adoption, or surrogacy. These couples share many of the experiences of heterosexual couples (Goldberg & Sayer, 2006). However, the social context seems to have a significant impact on same-sex parents. Those who experience homophobia, live in states with unfavorable legal climates regarding adoption by those who are gay or lesbian, and receive less support from their friends and families are more likely to feel depressed and anxious (Goldberg & Smith, 2011). Despite the strains they may experience, however, those who are gay or lesbian provide care for their children that is of comparable quality to that provided by heterosexual parents (Biblarz & Stacey, 2010).

Fatherhood has received more attention in recent decades, in part reflecting the increasing role of fathers in the raising of their children (Marsiglio et al., 2002). Becoming a first-time father can significantly influence a man's patterns of social interaction outside the home. A 7-year longitudinal study of nearly 3,100 fathers of children under the age of 18 described the "transformative" process that occurs as new fathers become more involved with their own parents, grandparents, and other relatives. Fathers also become more involved with service-oriented groups and church. These effects occur along with the birth of each child but are particularly pronounced at the time of the first child's birth (Knoester & Eggebeen, 2006).

**FIGURE 9-6** The transition to fatherhood can affect a man in many ways, including relationships with other family members and social interactions outside the home.

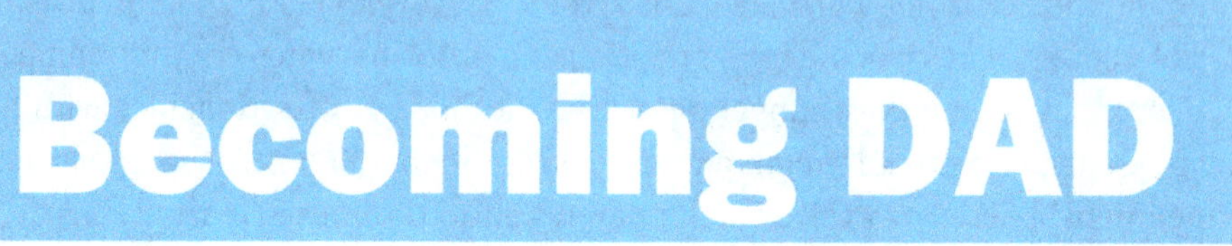


Father's age at birth of first child

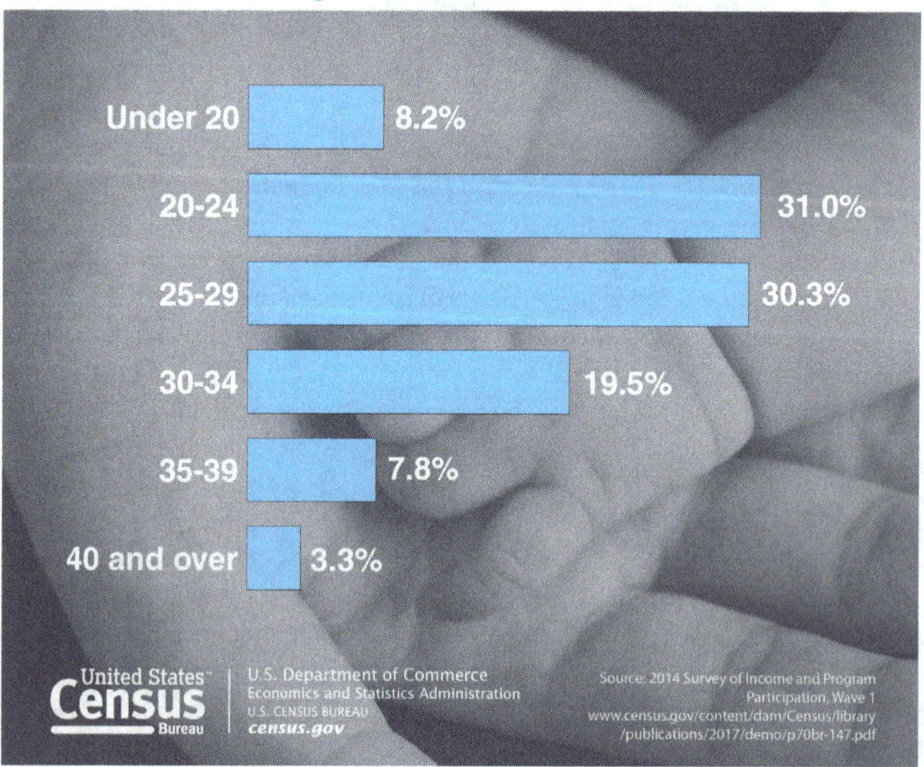


*Source*: Survey of Income and Program Participation, Wave 1, United States Census Bureau, https://www.census.gov/library/visualizations/2017/comm/fathers-day.html.

Men who feel they will be good fathers during the transition to parenthood become more involved in parenting. The way women perceive their husbands in the father role can help shape the way that fathers see themselves. A study of Canadian couples over the first 18 months of first-time parenthood showed that the confidence men had in their parenting was shaped by how competent their wives viewed them that, in turn, shaped both their self-perceptions and their involvement with their infants (Tremblay & Pierce, 2011).

The extent to which a single father adjusts to the role of solo parent is affected by the characteristics of the children, including their age and gender, and his own characteristics, including his age and educational level. The father's adjustment to this role is also affected by his ability to juggle the roles of parent and worker while maintaining a relationship with his ex-wife or partner, as well as by his original desire to have custody (Greif & Deal, 2012). Overall, however, single fathers spend less time caring for their children than do single mothers but more do than married fathers (Hook & Chalasani, 2008).

**Friendships.** Although people's lives change substantially throughout adulthood, many people remain close to their "best" friends. According to a 2002 survey (Fetto, 2002), 65% of American adults have known their best friends for at least 10 years and 36% for 20 years or more. Nearly all (91%) said they would take a vacation with their best friend.

Sticking with our best friends occurs despite pressures of work, children, and romantic partnerships. In fact, as people enter long-term intimate relationships, many engage in **dyadic withdrawal**, which is the process of reducing the individual friendships of each partner and increasing the joint friendships (Kalmijn, 2003). Overall this means a decline will occur in a person's total number of friends. On the other hand, as couples share social networks, they expand their own friendship circles and strengthen their own relationship (Cornwell, 2012). Part of this may occur through "platonic couple love" in which two couples are best friends and emulate the desirable qualities of the other couple (Greif & Deal, 2012).

Friendship patterns at any age may follow a developmental trajectory from formation to dissolution (Adams & Blieszner, 1994). You have probably experienced this trajectory with some your own friends. The friendship formation phase involves moving from being strangers to acquaintances to friends. The maintenance phase encompasses what is usually thought of as "friendship," during which friends sustain an active interest and involvement with each other. They may evaluate the quality of the friendship periodically during this phase, deciding to increase or decrease their level of involvement. Reciprocity levels are highest during the maintenance phase. Friendships may remain in the maintenance phase for years, even decades, at varying levels of closeness. The end of a friendship, which occurs during the dissolution phase, if at all, may be hard to identify. A friendship may end gradually over a period of time as feelings of reciprocity dwindle and the relationship essentially falls by the wayside. Friendships may also end through a conscious decision based on insurmountable disagreements and conflict.

Friendships in adulthood may be distinguished in terms of the closeness of the relationship, which may or may not change over time. People may maintain **peripheral ties** with some friends. These relationships are characterized by a lack of a high degree of closeness, and may go on as such for many years (Fingerman & Griffiths, 1999). Peripheral ties can include people such as neighbors, coworkers, professional contacts, gym buddies, friends of friends, or the parents of one's children's friends. These relationships may be amicable and cordial but never progress beyond this level. Other peripheral ties may be those relationships that are in the friendship formation stage and will later progress to close friendships. A peripheral tie can also be a relationship that was formerly a close friendship but has now moved to the dissolution/disinterest stage.

There may also be variations in friendship patterns in adulthood based on individual differences in approaches toward friends, called **friendship styles** (Matthews, 1986; Miche et al., 2013). Individuals who have an *independent* friendship style may enjoy friendly, satisfying, and cordial relationships with people but never form close or intimate friendships. The type known as *discerning* individuals are extremely selective in their choice of friends, retaining a small number of very close friends throughout their lives. Finally, people with an *acquisitive* friendship style are readily able to make and retain close friendships throughout their lives and therefore have a large social network.

People tend to choose friends who are similar in gender, socioeconomic status, and ethnicity (Adams & Blieszner, 1994). Throughout adulthood, these close social ties serve as buffers against stress and are related to higher levels of well-being and self-esteem. Relationships with friends may even be more predictive of high levels of self-esteem than income or marital status (Siebert et al., 2002). For people who have no family members, friendships serve as important substitutes for keeping an individual socially active (Lang & Carstensen, 1994). Moreover, friendships play a particularly important role in the lives of older gay men and lesbians, who have considerably more elaborated conceptions of their friendship ties than do heterosexual individuals (de Vries & Megathlin, 2009).

Friends are an important influence on you throughout your life. Although you may not realize it, they contribute to our personal narratives, sense of self, and even important life choices (Flora, 2013). The nature of your friendships may change over time, but they continue to serve as a source of self-definition and support.

## The Labor Force

We will start with some basic concepts and statistics about work before we explore the psychological aspects of work in adulthood. The **labor force** includes all civilians age 16 older who live outside of institutions (prisons, nursing homes, and residential treatment centers) and have sought or are actively seeking employment (Whitbourne & Whitbourne, 2012). They are not necessarily the people who are employed.

In 2016, the total size of the civilian labor force age 16 and older was 158.3 million. The unemployment rate was 4.9%, reflecting a continued improvement in the economic situation of the United States since the most recent time of high unemployment (10%) in late 2009. There remain more than 2.1 million unemployed for 27 weeks or longer, but this number is down considerably from the peak of 6.6 million reached in mid-2010. There are at least 7.5 million multiple job holders, equally divided by gender.

The labor force is increasingly comprised of workers age 55 and older. These shifts reflect the continued aging of the "baby boomer" generation who were between 30 and 48 in 1994, and will be 60 to 78 by 2024. Despite the fact that the oldest baby boomers may no longer be alive or in the labor force, they will continue to have an impact on the age distribution of workers until at least 2024 and beyond, depending on how long they continue to work past the age of 60. In fact, in 2018, nearly 80% of the 55- to 59-year-old population were projected to still be in the labor force, an all-time high (Toossi, 2009).

Whites, Blacks, and Hispanics have similar labor force participation rates, ranging at around 60% or slightly higher, meaning they are employed or seek employment to the same extent. However, they differ by unemployment rate. In 2017, the overall unemployment rate was 4.3%, but it was 7.4% for Black or African Americans, 3.8% for Asian Americans, and 5.1% for the Hispanic or Latino population in the United States (U.S. Bureau of Labor Statistics, 2020a).

People with a college education are far more likely to be employed than those with a high school education or less (Whitbourne & Whitbourne, 2012). Even among college graduates, though, there are racial and ethnic disparities in the unemployment rate. As of 2013, Whites with a college degree had a 2.4% unemployment rate, but Blacks or African Americans had a 4.0% unemployment rate. There were also higher unemployment rates compared with Whites for Asian Americans (2.8%) and those of Hispanic or Latino/a ethnicity (3.4%) with a college degree or higher (U.S. Bureau of Labor Statistics, 2016).

Women have differing labor participation rates than men. In 2016, 60.9% of the population of women age 16 and older was in the labor force compared with 72.8% of men (Bureau of Labor Statistics, 2020c). In 2013, nearly 75% of women with children ages 6 to 17 were in the labor force; for women with children under age 6, the rate was 65% and for mothers of 3-year-olds and under, it was 62% (Bureau of Labor Statistics, 2014). Despite their representation in the labor force, however, women still earn less than men. We call this the **gender gap**. It is expressed as a proportion of women's to men's salaries. In 2016, full-time employed women earned 79% of the median for men, even among full-time, year-round workers (Whitbourne & Whitbourne, 2012). This is true despite the higher educational attainment of women and may be accounted for by a range of factors, including gender segregation so that less women are represented in higher-paying jobs and the greater amount of unpaid work in which women engage (U.S. Department of Labor, 2017).

The wage disparity between men and women is particularly pronounced in the area of financial services (56%), real estate brokers (64%), and sales and services (69%) but also in medicine (63%) and teaching (69%) (U.S. Bureau of Labor Statistics, 2017).

The impact of a college education on your paycheck brings generally good news if you're reading this while on your way to completing a 4-year degree. Although students about to graduate from college often worry about whether they will get a job, a college degree is a benefit when it comes to employment status and salary. In 2016, the unemployment rate for college graduates with a bachelor's degree was 2.7%, about half that of those with a high school degree. College graduates, furthermore, earned a median income of $1,156 compared with high school graduates who earned $692 per week (U.S. Bureau of Labor Statistics, 2019).

However, even for college graduates in the United States, there are disparities according to racial and ethnic minority status. For example, in 2014, among men and women with a bachelor's degree or higher, Blacks earned 80% of the salary of Whites, and Hispanic college graduates earned 77% of the income of White men. This disparity remains approximately the same even at the advanced graduate degree level (U.S. Bureau of Labor Statistics, 2017e).

U.S. military veterans represent a population of particular concern from the standpoint of employment statistics. As of 2016, there were 20.9 million adults (9% of the civilian population 18 and older) who had served in the U.S. Armed Forces, 3.9 million who served since 2001 in Operation Iraqi Freedom (the Iraq War) and Operation Enduring Freedom (the war in Afghanistan). For men in the 25- to 34-year-old age bracket, representing nearly half of these veterans, the unemployment rate was 6.6% compared with 4.9% among nonveterans. Prior to 2014, the unemployment rates were even higher, however. With efforts to find employment for these individuals in public sector jobs, the situation is improving even for those with service-connected disabilities (U.S. Bureau of Labor Statistics, 2020b).

**Vocational development in young adulthood.** **Vocation** is a person's choice of occupation. It reflects the individual's personal preferences and interests. However, development in the world of work is influenced in many ways by the social factors of education, race, gender, and age. Because of the realities of the workplace, individuals may not be able to find a job that best matches their vocational interests. Nevertheless, vocational development theories are based on the premise that people are able to choose the career they wish to pursue.

If you have already chosen a desired career path, it is likely you chose it and your college major because of your vocational interests. You may have decided at an earlier point in your life that you wanted to pursue a given field, whether it was music, psychology, nursing, or social work because it suited your personality, values, and skills. These are the factors that vocational development theories take into account when they attempt to explain the career choices people make and determine people's levels of happiness and productivity once they have acted on those choices.

The basis of vocational development theories is the concept of **career**, which is the term that captures the unique connection between individuals and social organizations over time. Many factors shape the individual's career, including personal development, the specific organization for which the person works, and the profession or occupational category that describes the individual's occupation.

According to **Holland's** (1997) **vocational development theory**, people express their personalities through their vocational aspirations and interests. Holland proposed six fundamental types (also called codes) that represent the universe of all possible vocational interests, competencies, and behaviors: realistic (R), investigative (I), artistic (A), social (S), enterprising (E), and conventional (C). The theory is also referred to as the **RIASEC model**, referring to the six basic types that characterize an individual's vocational interests.

**FIGURE 9-7** RIASEC model.

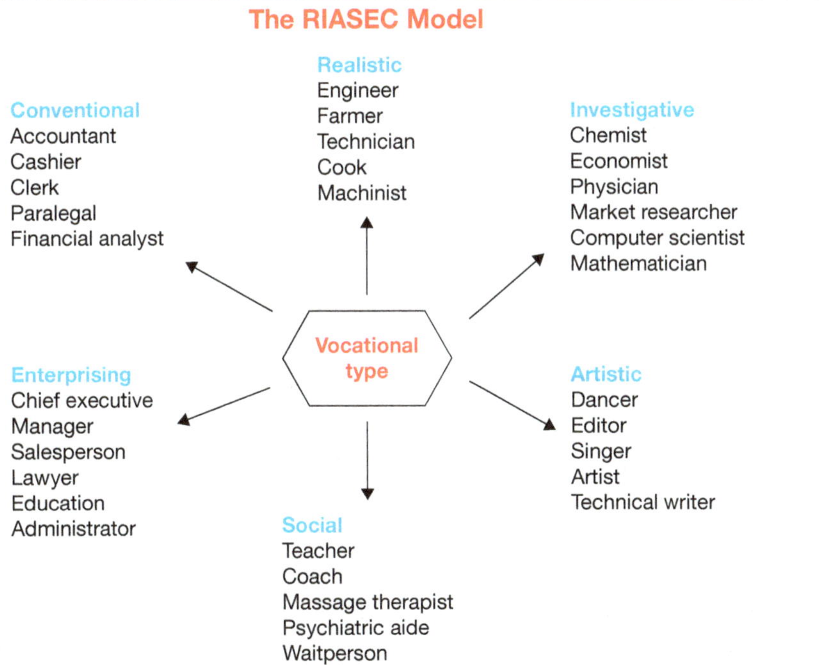


*Source*: Susan Whitbourne

The RIASEC types also apply to the occupational environment because they reflect particular patterns of job requirements and rewards. For example, social occupations involve work with people, and realistic occupations involve work with one's hands. Occupational environments, then, are the settings that elicit, develop, and reward specific interests, competencies, and behaviors of the individuals who work in those environments. If you work in a realistic environment, you are expected to complete activities that make use of your ability to work with things rather than your ability to work with people.

Vocational psychologists typically combine two or three of the codes in the RIASEC model to describe people and occupations. The first letter reflects the primary code into which a person's interest or occupation falls ("S" for social, for example). The second and third codes allow for a more accurate and differentiated picture of the individual or occupation. Both a construction worker and a corrections officer are R code occupations, and both have the RE code designation. They differ in their third code, which is C for the construction worker and S for the corrections officer.

In one variant of the RIASEC model, two underlying dimensions of the six types are identified: interest in people versus things and preference for data versus ideas (Prediger & Vansickle, 1992). The R code reflects the extreme of interest in things, the S the extreme of interest in people, the combination of I and A is at the extreme of ideas, and the combination of E and C is at the extreme of data. Although meant to be comprehensive, the RIASEC model appears to benefit from including these additional dimensions (Deng et al., 2007).

From a personality perspective, the RIASEC types applied to individuals are very much like traits (Armstrong & Anthoney, 2009). Putting the two together, researchers have suggested three underlying dimensions: (1) interest in people versus things, (2) preference for abstract versus concrete ideas, and (3) striving for personal growth versus striving for accomplishment.

The six RIASEC types are organized within the individual in a hexagonal structure. This structure implies that the types have an association with each other based on their distance from each other on the structure. Types that are most similar (such as R and C) are closest; those that are the most dissimilar (such as C and A) are farthest away from each other. The notion of the hexagon is important because it helps define the ways your interests correspond to your environments. You will be the most satisfied in your job if you are in an environment that fits your personality type. **Congruence** or "fit" occurs when your vocational type matches your occupational environment.

Not only does congruence make you feel happier, but it also influences your ability to be effective on the job. According to vocational development theory, if you are happy, you will also be productive. Unfortunately, people cannot always find jobs congruent with their interests, particularly in a tough economy. In these situations, the RIASEC model predicts people will experience low job satisfaction and high instability until they can find fulfilling work environments. When they are unable to do so, their work productivity may suffer.

Supporting this idea, researchers have found that individuals with artistic interests, working in realistic environments, for example, have lower work quality than people whose interests match their environments (Kieffer et al., 2004). Again, when jobs are scarce, people may have to take whatever work they can find and seek congruence elsewhere through leisure pursuits. The artistic type in the realistic job may wait out the hours until the workday is over and then rush home to work on crafts, play a musical instrument, or go to a pottery studio.

The RIASEC theory is derived from the responses of the many thousands of individuals tested over the years of its development. If you want to have your vocational interests assessed using this model, you can complete one or both of the most common assessment instruments. The **Strong Vocational Interest Inventory (SVII)** consists of items that have respondents indicate their preferences for occupations, topics of study, activities, and types of people (Harmon et al., 1994). The SVII is administered by a professional counselor and must be scored through a testing service. The second assessment can be administered and scored on your own. The **Self-Directed Search (SDS)** is a self-administered questionnaire that allows you to assess where you fit on the RIASEC dimensions and rate your strengths. Thus, the SDS allows you to determine the profile of your abilities as well as your interests (Gottfredson, 2002).

Because it's used in occupational interest inventories and classification schemes, the RIASEC model will likely be around for some time to come. Vocational counselors have adopted the RIASEC model as an easily interpretable and user-friendly system. Assessment tools for both people and jobs are readily available and inexpensive, and there is adequate (if not perfect) empirical support for it from large-scale studies (Smith et al., 2001). From the standpoint of vocational counseling for young adults, the codes seem to be relatively stable during the crucial career development years of the late teens and early 20s (Low et al., 2005). However, there are individual differences in patterns of stability, possibly corresponding to variations in personality. For example, people who are more open to new experiences may be more likely to change their career interests over time (Rottinghaus et al., 2007).

Within the field of industrial organizational (I/O) psychology, congruence is now a major focus when it comes to the business of matching people to jobs. At the same time, as anyone who has spent time in a workplace would attest to, it is also important to determine the fit or match among individuals working together as a team (Muchinsky, 1999). Does an RCE type get along better with another RCE, or would their similar styles lead to narrow thinking and lack of productivity among members of a work unit? Perhaps the RCE should be working alongside an SAI, whose "people" orientation will complement the "thing"-oriented approach of the realistic individual.

The notion of congruence between people and jobs has received considerable empirical support, not only in terms of job ratings but also in terms of career change behavior. If at all possible, people will move out of incongruent jobs and into positions more suited to their interests (Donohue, 2006). At the same time, their vocational interests and perhaps even their personality traits may change in response to socialization in their workplace (Wille & De Fruyt, 2014).

Unfortunately for many people, factors outside their control, such as discrimination due to gender, race, and ethnicity, limit these choices. For individuals whose vocational situations are affected by such constraints, the role of identity and the possibility of realizing one's true vocational interests are far less significant than the reality of these sociocultural factors.

**Super's life-span life-stage theory.** As individuals traverse the various stages of their vocational development, their sense of self also undergoes changes. **Super's life-span life-stage theory** focuses on the role of the self and proposes that people attempt to realize their inner potential through their career choices (Super, 1957, 1990). If you see yourself as an artist, then you will desire work in which you can express that view of yourself. In contrast to Holland's theory, which emphasizes vocational preferences (the fact that you prefer artistic work), Super's theory places the focus on the occupation that you see as most "true" to your inner self. Super's theory also takes into account the fact that the constraints of the marketplace mean people are not always able to achieve full realization of their self-concepts. In a society with relatively little demand for artists, the person with the artistic self-concept will need to seek self-expression in a job that allows for a certain degree of creativity but will also bring in a paycheck. Such an individual may seek a career in computer graphic design or teaching, for example, because they are more viable occupations than being an oil painter.

According to Super, the expression of self-concept through work occurs in a series of four stages that span the years from adolescence to retirement. In the exploration stage (teens to mid-20s), people explore career alternatives and select a vocation that can ideally express their self-concept. By the time they reach the establishment stage (mid-20s to mid-40s), people are focused on achieving stability and attempt to remain within the same occupation. At the same time, some people seek to move up the career ladder to managerial positions and higher. In the maintenance stage (mid-40s to mid-50s), people attempt to hold onto their positions rather than seek further advancement. Finally, in the disengagement stage (mid-50s to mid-60s), workers begin to prepare for retirement, perhaps spending more time in their leisure pursuits.

**Occupation as calling.** The role of the self in vocational development forms the core of theories that emphasize people's desires to achieve self-expression through their work and contribute to the larger good. A **calling** is an individual's consuming passion for a particular career domain that serves people in some capacity and contributes to a sense of personal meaning and purpose (Duffy et al., 2013).

Ultimately, your choice of a vocation may reflect a feeling that you are drawn to a particular line of work, either because of the job tasks it entails, the personality needs it fulfills (as in the RIASEC model), or it serves a socially useful purpose. In addition, the notion of calling implies the individual feels the need to pursue the occupation to contribute to the larger social good (Duffy & Dik, 2013). Characteristics an individual may feel about a calling include "being passionate" about your work, enjoying your work more than anything else, being willing to sacrifice everything to do this job, having this job on your mind in some way at all times, and finding the experience of performing your work to be deeply gratifying (Dobrow & Tosti-Kharas, 2011).

A calling is related to identity because when a person pursues a calling, they attempt to express a central feature of the self. A job that fulfills the criteria for a calling has the potential to provide an individual with one of the deepest forms of satisfaction (Hall & Chandler, 2005). People who feel they are pursuing a calling feel more engaged in their work and experience more positive outcomes as a result of this engagement (Hirschi, 2012). For people to experience the benefits of a calling, however, they must actually be living the calling, not just dreaming about it. When they feel their job fulfills the criteria for a calling, they will feel more committed to their work and derive more meaning from it, which will ultimately benefit their overall satisfaction (Duffy et al., 2012).

Furthermore, the process of identifying a calling involves going through a process of intense reflection about life values and priorities. Individuals can promote this process through meditation, introspection, and reflection. Ultimately, people's ability to pursue a calling requires self-understanding, an adaptability to changing economic and social circumstances, and the belief they can be successful at their chosen career path (Hall & Chandler, 2005). The model also provides a useful framework for career counselors, as it suggests ways their clients can be helped to find more fulfilling career choices that, in turn, have a positive impact on their sense of meaning in work and life (Dik & Duffy, 2015).

# CHAPTER 10 Midlife

Midlife brings with it a host of physical changes for some, from the way our bodies look, the way the feel, and underlying changes that may be undetectable. Additionally, a greater sense of psychological control over one's life may appear as we settle into our adult lives and responsibilities. Still many things can change, in our relationships as children age and as parents may have greater needs that the midlife adult is called on to fulfill. The balance between home life and work life also influences each of those aspects of our day-to-day functioning. In other words, there's a lot going on for midlife adults!

# Biological Functioning

**LO 10-1** **Describe some of the physical changes that take place during midlife.**

**LO 10-2** **Identify the benefits of treatments for menopause and andropause.**

**LO 10-3** **Identify the syndromes and diseases that can be affected by diet and exercise during midlife.**

It can be easier to see the aging process and its effects on some individuals as opposed to others. Some 50-year-olds begin to slow down; age may show on the body and how it moves, and aches and pains may emerge. Others may look, feel, and be healthier than those who are 10 and 15 years younger. Regardless of how the body looks and feels to you and others, there are changes to our bodily systems and functions that may require a retooling of certain behaviors (such as diet and physical activity levels) and more monitoring both by the individual and by health professionals.

## Physical Changes

**Vision.** By the end of middle age, most people will require corrective lenses or procedures to address vision loss. The loss of the ability to focus vision on near objects is referred to as presbyopia and is the primary culprit in a 40- or 50-something-year-old's need for reading glasses. Presbyopia is caused by the thickening and hardening of the lens, which is the focusing mechanism of the eye (Sharma &

### What Would You Do? Gary's Story

I spent 25 years as an auto mechanic, working full time while a member of the Army Reserves, pretty much straight out of high school. I've always been a physical guy, who likes doing things.

When I was younger, I didn't go to college, but getting my degree was something I thought a lot about during my adult life, and I felt for a long time it was something I missed out on earlier in life. Regardless, I was a talented and successful mechanic, and I made my way up through the ranks in the Army to a command sergeant major position, with significant management duties. I was deployed once to Iraq when I was in my late 30s and was mobilized again for a year when I was 43. At that time, I was stationed in state and not overseas. I knew this was my opportunity to finally go to college, because I would be employed full time with the Army, I wouldn't be overseas, and I could use the post-9/11 GI Bill and tuition assistance. I also saw this as my way out of the automotive industry, which had always been physically demanding and something I might not be able to keep up with for the rest of my life.

I got some college credits for the work I had done in the Army and finished my degree in 22 months, but I walked away from the experience not really feeling much smarter than when I went in. In hindsight, I think the school I chose did not force me to challenge myself enough, and if I had I to do it over again I would have gone to a more challenging school that would've taken me more time.

Being 45 years old and in a classroom was aggravating at times. I was always the student to raise their hand, while everyone else was silent. Very frequently, the professors would say, "Someone other than Gary." I also felt the environment was different. I was used to classroom settings where if you wanted to talk, you'd have to raise your hand, but in this case it seemed like if you knew the answer, you'd just blurt it out. I felt like showing up and being on time was an option for some students, while I always felt you have to be there on time and be ready to do what you're supposed to do.

I'd always look forward to seeing someone who felt more similar to me, someone who looked like they were working 40 hours a week and going to college, and thankfully I found a group of people I got along with. Sometimes we'd intentionally register for the same classes. But if that weren't the case, we'd still try to seek each other out at the start of a new class or semester. We'd quickly find each other for group projects, because there's always group projects, and because we always knew together we'd get the work done. I also developed some good relationships with most if not all of the instructors. It felt like they, too, they were my peer group.

I was lucky going back to school when I did because while I was mobilized, my commander in the Army, who was for all intents and purposes my boss at that time, gave me lots of flexibility, and I never took a heavy course load because I was mobilized. Then I came off mobilization and, for a year and a half, I was essentially unemployed, but I still volunteered very regularly with the Army to take up some of my free time. I needed to keep busy because the only other thing I had to do was go to school. I was always at school early. I could always stay late if I had to, but I knew I had this finite amount of time to get the degree done. I wanted that degree so I could get a job. And once I graduated I wasn't overly proud. I felt like I did it, checked the box. It wasn't like I graduated from a university or something. It wasn't a colossal journey for me like it is for a younger person, it was just a thing I had to get done.

So then I was 48 and looking for a job. I honestly didn't think it was going to be that hard, plus I thought I had a pretty good resume. I had 25 years of experience. I had a degree. I took placement tests and passed them with high marks. I felt like I did everything, but employers just weren't interested.

Still I was lucky yet again because money wasn't really an issue. I could always take another mobilization with the Army if I had to. I recognize that's a lifeline that not many people have at their disposal. There's a lot of people who have been in the same situation, with nothing to fall back on. My wife also provided a stable source of income for our family, and because of that I wasn't out looking for a job in a more panicked fashion. It's probably the reason I didn't end up working in a $10 or $15 an hour job at the local hardware store. Getting a job was more a mental thing than a monetary thing. Waking up with a purpose every morning is what gives me energy. That's one of the things that was wearing on me during the year and a half I was unemployed. I could feel it sucking the life out of me, not feeling a purpose, laying back down at 9:30 in the morning to take a nap if I felt like it. It's wired in me to wake up and do something. It's part of who I am.

It seemed that getting a job, or even getting my foot in the door wasn't about how good my resume was. It wasn't the school I went to. It wasn't what I did before. It was all about who I knew. I felt frustrated. There were probably 10 rejections and 20 no responses to resumes I sent out over a year's time. In that time, I got a vocational teacher's certificate to teach automotive. As I interviewed over the course of the summer it seemed like breaking into the system is

Santhoshkumar, 2009). Due to these changes the lens cannot adapt its shape when needed to see objects up close to the face. By the age of 50, presbyopia affects the entire population.

Bifocals had been the only correction for presbyopia, available since the time of Benjamin Franklin (who invented them), as there is no cure. Several alternatives to bifocals are available, but none at present provide an ideal solution (Davies et al., 2016). Smoking has been known to accelerate the aging of the lens, which contributes to presbyopia (Kessel et al., 2006).

**Skin.** The first signs of aging generally appear in the 30s, and by one's 50s the skin shows distinctive marks of the passage of time. These changes are most apparent in the exposed areas of the skin, which include the face, hands, and upper arms. The age-related changes to the skin we can see reflect changes that occur beneath the surface.

The outermost layer of the skin, known as the **epidermis**, consists of a thin covering of cells that protects the underlying tissue. Over time, and not visible to the naked eye, the epidermal skin cells lose their regular patterning. The most significant changes occur in the **dermis**, the middle layer of the skin, which is made up of connective tissue, among which nerve cells, glands, and the hair follicles reside. The connective tissue in the dermis changes over time. This is because the two types of protein molecules that comprise the dermis, collagen and elastin, are changing. Collagen undergoes cross linking, as we described in the previous chapter. This causes the skin to become more rigid and less flexible. Elastin, a molecule that contributes to skin flexibility, becomes less able to return to its original form after it is stretched during a person's movements. As a result of these changes in collagen and elastin, the skin can no longer return to its original state of tension and begins to sag. At the same time, the sebaceous glands, which normally provide oils that lubricate the skin, become less active. Consequently, the skin surface becomes drier and more vulnerable to damage from being rubbed or chafed. The subcutaneous fat layer is the bottom-most layer of skin gives skin its opacity and smooths the curves of the arms, legs, and face. In middle adulthood, this layer starts to thin and provides less support for dermis and epidermis. This exacerbates the wrinkling and sagging caused by changes in the dermis, and blood vessels beneath the skin become more visible.

The skin's coloring changes across adulthood, most visibly in fair-skinned people. People develop discolored areas often referred to as "age spots" (also known as lentigo senilis). These areas of brown pigmentation are more likely to occur in the sun-exposed areas of the face, hands, and arms. Pigmented outgrowths (moles) and elevations of small blood vessels on the skin surface (angiomas) also appear.

The general changes that occur in the skin contribute to the aging of the face. This can affect the appearance of the eyes, which develop bags, small lines at the creases (crow's-feet), areas of dark pigmentation, and puffiness. The face's underlying structure also changes as a result of bone loss in the skull, particularly in the jaw. The nose and ears can become longer because of changes in cartilage. The muscles of the face also lose their ability to contract, meaning a face that is frowning or smiling looks more similar to a face at rest (Desai et al., 2009). Nails are a part of the skin that undergoes age-related changes, as well. Toenails, especially, grow more slowly and may become yellowed, thicker, and ridged.

Certain antiaging treatments for the face, such as laser resurfacing, chemical peels, injections of artificial fillers, and microdermabrasion, can only be administered by a plastic surgeon,

very much like trying to get into a club, and if you're not already in the club you're not getting in the club. I had an interview at one school and the vice principal told me "I've got 10 other resumes from other instructors. This is going to be tough for you." That was really deflating.

I did eventually find a job, and it's the job that I'm working at today, in manufacturing management. I work for a company that makes 3D printers. I would not have that job if it weren't for a former colleague of mine from the Army, but it wasn't easy getting in either. The position came up and he told me to apply for it. Two weeks later he asked whether I applied because the hiring managers never saw my resume. I told him I applied the very day he told me about it. Apparently my resume didn't even make it through the initial human resources review, so he personally took it to the hiring managers, who agreed I was a good fit.

I've been with the company now almost 2 years and I love it. I love the never-ending chase of trying to do better than I did the day before, and the new challenges that come along. There's always going to be something that goes wrong, from the equipment to personnel. There's no such thing as an average day. It's also exciting to me that in the 21st century I work for a company that actually makes something and sells it. Every day we ship out of our backdoor the things we made that weeks or months earlier came in as components through that backdoor. We make things. And I've always been in a career where we make things or we fix things we made. It's tangible. Every day there's something I can put my hands on that we did or I fixed. There's something I can point at and say "I did that." That's part of who I am, too.

That's even how I like to spend my free time. Last weekend I pulled an engine out of my plow truck that's been sitting in my garage for a year. I've had tremendous difficulty with it but I felt such a sense of satisfaction when I had that engine strung up on a chain, at the top of a crane, over the engine compartment. I did that. It's interesting and maybe this ties into the fact that I don't like to do things like texting or e-mails. There's nothing tangible there. It doesn't feel like I did anything. God, I'm turning into an old curmudgeon.

I do recognize, though, that it's necessary to adapt to changes in technology. I have to force myself to do it. Sometime in my life I will probably get a smart phone. And I admit I am probably a little more resistant to changes in technology than others, and that may be something that has come with age. When I was younger and in the automotive business, and all the changes came out with computerized mechanisms in cars, I was the first person to learn all that stuff. Maybe as we age we become more resistant to change. Maybe it's because I get comfortable with things that work. And maybe the reality is that the new things don't work the same.

I also know that if I need to learn a new technology to get to where I want to be, I absolutely will. I'm motivated to learn because if I see some of my peers do it, I know I can do it. It's just like the engine stuck in the plow truck. I think, "I can do this." And I see my coworkers using these new technologies and I say to myself, "If I want his job I've got to learn how to do it." I will learn it as I need it, and that may limit me. As I get older I'm going to be competing for jobs that younger people will be going for, too, and they probably will have more ability than I will. But it doesn't make me nervous. I'll beat them on determination.

And in 10 years I'll probably still be working on the career path I'm on now, which is some sort of production. I've got to make things or be involved with making things or moving things. Will I be at the same company I'm at now? I hope so. I don't leapfrog from job to job. I'm more inclined to stay within an organization, to do well for the organization and expect the organization to do well for me. But I know that's not necessarily the reality of today's business environment.

In terms of physicality, and pulling that engine out of the plow truck, I can see myself physically declining a bit. In my late 20s and early 30s, I was on top of my game. In my mid-30s, late 30s, and early 40s, I was holding my own. It's like I'm on a cross-country flight from California to Boston, and now I'm about over Albany on the descent. I can't eat what I used to eat, or in the volume that I used to eat it, I can't stay up as late as I used to, and I can't do two jobs anymore, which is kind of why I'm getting out of the Army completely this year. Something's got to give.

I'm okay with all these changes, but I'm trying to not give up on anything. I still do the same things, I just go about them differently. My mentality about aging is to adapt. This whole age gracefully, I don't care what I look like. It's going to happen, just adapt. I'm not going to be the 62-year-old with a six pack. I'm just not that guy. I'm probably the last person you'll ever see get some sort of elective surgery to make something look this way or that. I'm going to run with what I've got until I can't go anymore, and when it gets to the point where hurts every day, then I might get a knee done or something like that. I don't feel like any of these things have changed who I am. After all, I still yanked that motor out of my truck last weekend.

Think about what you would do in this situation after reading the chapter, and then decide the following:

- If you were Gary, would you have pursued a more challenging university? Why or why not?

dermatologist, or other trained medical professional. Others, such as topical retinoids used to treat photoaging and fine wrinkles or skin lightening creams for age spots, are available by prescription. One of the most popular anti-aging treatments for the face is the injection of botulinum toxin (Botox®). In a Botox® treatment, a syringe containing a small amount of a nerve poison is injected into the area of concern, such as around the eyes or in the middle of the forehead muscle. This procedure paralyzes the muscle, relaxing the skin around it and causing a temporary reduction in the appearance of wrinkles. Increasingly, products that simulate these procedures are being introduced into the market as affordable, effective, and convenient alternatives.

**Teeth.** Loss of enamel on the surface of the teeth leads to yellowing, and stains can build up over time due to coffee and tea, certain types of food, and—for smokers—tobacco. Teeth loss is not uncommon as we age, a process that affects not only a person's appearance but aspects of their health in general. Middle-aged adults may suffer less from problems related to tooth loss than previous generations because of improvements in dental hygiene, particularly increased rates of flossing. Nevertheless, some changes in the teeth and gums are bound to occur as we age (Deng et al., 2009).

**Hair.** Melanin is a natural pigment that gives hair its color. Eventually melanin production stops, and it is very likely by the time a person reaches the age of 75 or 80, there are virtually no naturally colored hairs left on the scalp or other hair-covered areas of the body. Of course, there are variations in the rate at which this change takes place. You may have an older relative or friend whose hair is only slightly gray or know people in their 20s who have a significant amount of gray hair already.

- If you were Gary's career counselor, how would you have advised him in his job search?
- If you were Gary, how would you adapt to changing technologies?
- If you were Gary's doctor, would you be concerned about his level of physical mobility?

The thinning of the hair occurs for both sexes, although it's more visible in males. Hair loss is generally a result of the destruction of the germination centers that produce hair in the hair follicles. The most common form of hair loss with increased age is androgenetic alopecia, known as **patterned hair loss**, and is classified differently for males and females. This is a condition that affects 95% of adult males and 20% of adult females, to some degree. Patterned hair loss causes the hair follicles to stop producing the long, thick, pigmented hair known as terminal hair and instead produce short, fine, unpigmented, and largely invisible hair known as vellus hair. Eventually, the vellus hair becomes invisible, because it no longer protrudes from the follicle, which itself has shrunk. Although hair stops growing on the top of the head where it is desired, it may appear in larger amounts in places where it is not welcome, such as the chin on women, the ears, and in thicker clumps around the eyebrows in men.

**FIGURE 10-1** Male patterned baldness.

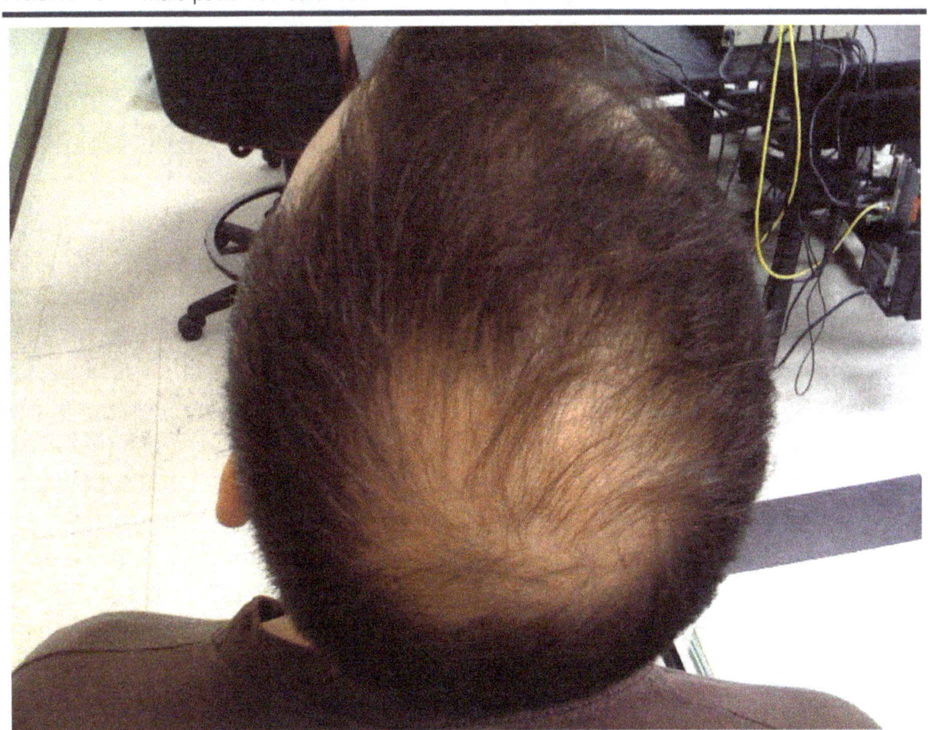

*Source*: Copyright © Welshsk (CC BY-SA 3.0) at https://commons.wikimedia.org/wiki/File:Alopecia.jpg.

Pharmaceutical companies are working to find a solution for unwanted hair loss. There are a number of products designed to stop or mask hair loss, from chemicals applied directly to the scalp, most notably topical minoxidil (Rogaine), to herbal remedies and surgically implanted hair plugs. Oral finasteride (Propecia) is another alternative considered effective against hair loss, but it is available by prescription only and has side effects that can interfere with male sexual functioning (Chiriaco et. al., 2016).

**Body build.** Cross-sectional and longitudinal studies demonstrate people get shorter as they age, a process that is more pronounced for females. For example, if you're 5 feet, 8 inches tall, you may think of yourself as remaining at that height for the rest of your life. However, chances are you will lose as much as an inch of height over the coming decades. This is because of the loss of bone material in the vertebrae. With the weakening of the vertebrae, the spine collapses and shortens in length (Pfirrmann et al., 2006). The weight gain during middle adulthood often represents the accumulation of body fat around the waist and hips, commonly referred to as the "middle-aged spread" (Ding et al., 2007).

**Mobility.** Every component of your mobility undergoes significant age-related losses, occurring as early as in your 40s (or earlier if you have sustained certain types of injuries). One result is walking more slowly as we age, although we can make up for a slower gait by taking longer steps more frequently (Jerome et al., 2015; Shumway-Cook et al., 2007).

Bone changes in adulthood involve a higher rate of bone destruction compared with renewal and greater porosity (volume of empty space) of the calcium matrix. This leads to loss of bone mineral content. These changes are partially controlled by a set of protein-like substances that act on the bone cells. These substances are, in turn, influenced by the sex hormones estrogen (in females) and testosterone (in males). Therefore, as people experience decreases in sex hormones, they also lose bone mineral content (Cao et al., 2005; Maltais et al., 2009; Sigurdsson et al., 2006; Travison et al., 2009).

Heavier people tend to have higher bone mineral content so they lose less in adulthood, particularly in the weight-bearing limbs involved in mobility, but obese individuals are at greater risk for bone loss. Bone loss is also greater in females, especially White females, who lose bone density at a higher rate than African American females. Conversely, African American males seem to lose bone mineral density at a higher rate than White males. People living in rural areas have higher bone density than those in cities, perhaps reflecting their greater mobility (Cauley et al., 2008; Pongchaiyakul et al., 2005; Sheu et al., 2009).

Muscle strength remains at a plateau in our 40s and 50s, but after that it declines at a rate of 12 to 15% per decade, with more pronounced decreases for men. In contrast with the declines in speed and strength, people retain their muscular endurance, as measured by isometric strength involved in exercises such as holding a plank position. There are also relatively minor effects of age on eccentric strength, the action involved in activities such as lowering arm weights (in other words, the downward motion of a bicep curl) or going down the stairs. Changes in muscle mass strongly, but not entirely, predict age-related reductions in strength in adulthood. Another contributor to loss of muscle strength comes from disrupted signals the nervous system sends to the muscles telling them to contract. Tendons also become stiffer, which makes it more difficult to move the joint and thus exert muscular strength (Carroll et al., 2008; Klass et al., 2006; Kostka, 2005; Raj et al., 2010; Roig et al., 2010).

Regarding joint function, exercise can lessen some effects of aging if you use caution. Strength training, in which you build the muscles that support the joints while avoiding putting stress on impaired tendons, ligaments figments, and arterial surfaces, is particularly good. Resistance training, in which people use weight machines, can increase the flexibility of the tendons, allowing joints to move more comfortably and through a greater range. Flexibility training, such as stretching or practicing gentle forms of yoga that expand range of motion, is also important. An exercise program should also focus on lowering body fat, as increased weight associated with obesity contributes to joint pain and stiffness and loss of cartilage volume. Certain types of exercise also stimulate circulation to the joints, enhancing blood supply and promoting the repair process in the tendons, ligaments, and surfaces of the areas being exercised (Boling et al., 2006; Hunter & Eckstein, 2009; Oken et al., 2006; Reeves et al., 2006; Teichtahl et al., 2009).

## Vital Bodily Functions

**Cardiovascular system.** Changes in the cardiovascular system related to the normal aging process described in the previous chapter become noticeable during middle age, and our risk of developing cardiovascular disease during middle age becomes high. Research on cardiovascular health during this stage focuses quite a bit on lifestyle factors such as exercise and how aerobic training can contribute to the health of our cardiovascular system. These behaviors can set the stage during middle and age impact subsequent health habits and general health as we grow older.

**Respiratory system.** Aging affects all components of the respiratory system. Respiratory muscles lose their ability to expand and contract the chest wall, and lung tissue is less able to expand and contract during respiration. As a result, starting at about age 40, all measures of lung functioning in adulthood tend to show age-related losses. These losses are more severe in females and are particularly pronounced during exercise, when people place the most stress on their respiratory systems (Adachi et al., 2015; Harms, 2006; Zeleznik, 2003).

**Digestive system.** Aging can lead decreases in the strength of esophageal contractions, the stomach lining's ability to resist damage and the rate at which the stomach empties food. Some people can become lactose intolerant due to changes in the small intestine, and excessive bacteria growth in the small intestine can cause digestive complaints, and the rectum can enlarge to a certain extent. People also increasing experience heartburn, ulcers, hemorrhoids, and irritable bowel syndrome as they age.

**Endocrine system.** The endocrine system's **basal metabolic rate** (BMR) begins to slow in middle age and is responsible for the weight gain that occurs even when a person's caloric intake remains stable. When you think of your "metabolism" and whether yours is slow or fast, you're actually talking about your BMR, which is the number of calories your body needs to function while at rest. BMR decreases pretty reliably with age, due to changes in physiology, including decreases in muscle mass and accumulation of abdominal fat that become common as we age. One easy way you can increase your BMR, or metabolism, is to increase the amount of exercise you do.

Dehydroepiandrosterone (DHEA) is a steroid hormone that circulates in the body in abundance. It is higher in males than females and shows a pronounced decrease over the adult years, decreasing by 60% between the ages of 20 and 80 (Feldman et al., 2002). This phenomenon, termed adrenopause, is greater in males, although males continue to have higher levels than females throughout later life, simply because they start at a higher baseline. Extremely low levels of DHEA are linked to cardiovascular disease, some forms of cancer, immune system dysfunction, and obesity (von Muhlen et al., 2007).

**Menopause.** **Menopause** refers to the point when female menstruation stops permanently. However, many people often think of it as a phase of middle adulthood covering the years during which female reproductive capacity diminishes. The more accurate term for the gradual winding down of reproductive ability and sexual activity is **climacteric**, a term that applies to both males and females. For females, this period typically unfolds over a 3- to 5-year span called **perimenopause**, which concludes with menopause, after a menstrual period has not occurred for 1 year. The average age of menopause onset is 50 years, but timing varies. Menopause occurs earlier in those who are thin or who are malnourished or who smoke.

During perimenopause, there is a diminished production of estrogen, the primary female sex hormone, in the ovarian follicles. Progesterone, the other female hormone, also begins to decline because it is produced in response to ovulation. Estrogen decline begins roughly 10 to 15 years before menopause, at some point in the mid-30s, and by the mid-40s the ovaries have begun to function less effectively and produce fewer hormones. Menstrual cycles typically end altogether by the early to mid-50s, but the ovaries continue to produce small amounts of estrogen and the adrenal glands stimulate the production of estrogen in fat tissue. Follicle-stimulating hormone (FSH) and luteinizing hormone (LH) levels rise dramatically during perimenopause period, as the anterior pituitary gland sends out signals to produce more ovarian hormones. In turn, the hypothalamus produces less gonadotropin-releasing factor (GnRH). Like puberty, the progression toward menopause varies considerably from person to person. There are certain characteristic symptoms, such as the occurrence of "hot flashes." A hot flash is a sudden sensation of intense heat and sweating that can last from a few moments to a half-hour. It is the result of decreases in estrogen levels, which cause the endocrine system to release higher amounts of other hormones that affect the temperature control centers in the brain (Whitbourne, 2001). Fluctuating estrogen levels can also lead to fatigue, headaches, night sweats, and insomnia, among other physiological symptoms. During this time, psychological symptoms such as irritability, mood swings, depression, memory loss, and difficulty concentrating are not uncommon. However, evidence supporting a connection between physiological changes and psychological symptoms is far from conclusive.

Menopause is also associated with alterations in the reproductive tract. There is a reduction in the supply of blood to the vagina and surrounding nerves and glands due to lower estrogen levels. The tissues become thinner, drier, and less able to produce secretions to lubricate before and during intercourse, resulting in potential discomfort during intercourse (da Silva Lara et al., 2009). Urinary problems, such as infections and stress incontinence, can also become more common.

Other effects of menopause associated with the impact of decreasing estrogen levels include weaker bones, high blood pressure, and cardiovascular disease for those who are postmenopausal. There are changes in cholesterol levels in the blood associated with menopause, causing postmenopausal women to be at higher risk of atherosclerosis and associated conditions.

To counteract the negative effects of decreased estrogen production, estrogen-replacement therapy (ERT) was introduced in the 1940s, and later combined with the hormone progestin, to reduce cancer risk. Administration of both hormones is referred to as hormone replacement therapy (HRT). Initial studies on HRT yielded support, citing positive impacts on skin tone and appearance, bone mineral density, immune functioning, thickness of the hair, sleep quality, prevention of accidental falls, and improvements in memory and mood. However, starting in 2002, HRT became hotly debated by researchers due to its possible relation to breast cancer and deep vein thrombosis (blood clots). The United Kingdom's National Health Service (2017) published a lengthy report documenting the risks and benefits of HRT for a variety of physical and psychological symptoms associated with menopause. Those interested in HRT should consult a health professional before determining whether and when to begin HRT as well as method of HRT administration, as there are differing risks for transdermal (skin) applications compared with those associated with oral ingestion (Stuenkel et al., 2015). Alternatives to HRT are available, including exercise, quitting smoking, lowering cholesterol in the diet, and perhaps having one alcoholic drink a day.

## Changes in the Brain

There is a growing body of evidence for how aging affects the normal brain. The areas most affected include the prefrontal cortex, the area of the brain most involved in planning and the encoding of information into long-term memory, and the temporal cortex, which is involved in auditory processing (Fjell et al., 2009). The hippocampus, the structure in the brain responsible for consolidating memories, becomes smaller with increasing age, although this decline is more pronounced in abnormal aging such as in Alzheimer's disease (Zhang et al., 2010). Nevertheless, evidence exists in support of the plasticity model within the cells of the hippocampus (Lister & Barnes, 2009).

In the frontal lobe, abnormalities known as white matter hyperintensities (WMH), which are thought to be made up of parts of deteriorating neurons, can occur as a result of aging. Their presence seems to interfere with long-term memory as they disrupt the integrity of white matter (Charlton et al., 2009). Some speculate that WMHs are a result or co occur with hypertension, as their presence is more common in those diagnosed with hypertension. Therefore, WMHs may not necessarily exist for (Burgmans et al., 2010).

## Lifestyle and Health

Midlife provides the opportunity to maintain or develop healthy habits related to diet, exercise, and other lifestyle behaviors such as smoking and alcohol consumption.

**Cardiovascular disease.** We begin our discussion of health with cardiovascular disease, a set of abnormal conditions that develop in the heart and arteries. Cardiovascular disease is the number one cause of death worldwide and can cause chronic disability. The distribution of blood throughout the body is essential for the normal functioning of all other organ systems. Therefore, cardiovascular disease can have a widespread range of effects on the individual's health and everyday life.

As we described previously, fat and other substances accumulate in the walls of the arteries throughout the body as part of the normal aging process. One of the most pervasive chronic diseases is **atherosclerosis**, a form of. Recall that arteriosclerosis is a general term for the thickening and hardening of arteries. In atherosclerosis, fatty deposits collect at an abnormally high rate, substantially reducing the width of the arteries and limiting the circulation of the blood. Everyone experiences some degree of arteriosclerosis as part of normal aging. It is possible to live with atherosclerosis and not encounter significant health problems. However, atherosclerosis can eventually lead to a build-up in plaque in particular arteries, blocking the blood flow to that part of the body. The organs or tissues fed by that artery then suffer serious damage due to the lack of blood supply. When this process affects arteries that feed the heart muscle, the individual is said to have coronary (or ischemic) heart disease. The term "myocardial infarction" refers to the acute condition in which the blood supply to part of the heart muscle (the myocardium) is severely reduced or blocked.

An individual with **hypertension** suffers from chronic abnormally elevated blood pressure. The technical definition of hypertension is based on the two measures of blood pressure. Systolic is the pressure exerted by the blood as it is pushed out of the heart during contraction, and diastolic is the pressure when the blood is relaxed between beats. Blood pressure is measured in units of "mm Hg," or millimeters of mercury, referring to the display on a blood pressure scale. Several medication bodies and organizations have put forth criteria for hypertension; in general a person is diagnosed with hypertension when their blood pressure is 130–140 mm Hg systolic pressure or greater, or 85–90 mm Hg diastolic pressure or greater.

Atherosclerosis contributes to hypertension via the accumulation of plaque that forces the blood to be pushed through narrower and narrower arteries. Because of this, the pressure on the blood as it is being pumped out of the heart becomes greater and greater. The more pressure that the blood exerts when it passes through the arteries, the greater the strain on the arteries' delicate walls. Over time, these walls become weakened and inflamed. As they do, they accumulate even more plaque, which tends to settle into those cracks and weak areas. Consequently, hypertension becomes even more pronounced. This problem is more severe in the larger arteries, particularly the ones leading from the heart, which take the full force of the heart's pumping action.

Hypertension also increases the workload of the heart. Because of the narrowing of the arteries, the heart must pump harder and harder to push out blood. The heart muscle in the left ventricle (the part that pumps out the blood) becomes thickened and overgrown. This further compromises the health of the cardiovascular system.

**Congestive heart failure** (or heart failure) is a condition in which the heart is unable to pump enough blood to meet the needs of the body's other organs. Blood flows out of the heart at an increasingly slower rate, causing the blood returning to the heart through the veins to back up. Eventually, tissues become congested with fluid. This condition can result from a variety of diseases, including coronary heart disease, scar tissue from a past myocardial infarction, hypertension, disease of the heart valves, disease of the heart muscle, infection of the heart, or heart defects present at birth. Congestive heart failure limits a person's ability to exert themselves without becoming exhausted and short of breath. Their legs may swell due to **edema**, a condition in which fluid builds up in their bodies. They may also experience fluid build-up in their lungs along with certain kidney problems.

The term "cerebrovascular disease" refers to disorders of circulation to the brain, such blockages in one or both carotid arteries that bring oxygenated blood to the neck, head, and brain, which can lead to increased risk for stroke. A "stroke" or "brain attack" is an acute condition in which an artery leading to the brain bursts or is clogged by a blood clot or other particle. The larger the area of the brain deprived of blood, the more severe the deterioration of the physical and mental functions controlled by that area. Another condition caused by the development of clots in the cerebral arteries is a transient ischemic attack (TIA), also called a ministroke. TIA and strokes are caused by the same processes, but the blockage of the artery is temporary in a TIA. The tissues that were deprived of blood soon recover, but chances are another TIA will follow. People who have had a TIA are also at higher risk of subsequently having strokes.

In the United States, stroke rates are in general elevated for African Americans. There is ongoing extensive research being conducted to better understand the health disparities we see according to race and ethnicity in terms of disease rates and factors such as health literacy and access to care. Stroke rates are also higher for the stroke belt, a region including the states of Alabama, Arkansas, Georgia, Indiana, Kentucky, Louisiana, Mississippi, North Carolina, South Carolina, Tennessee, and Virginia. The higher risk present in the stroke belt may be a result of lower levels of education, poorer diet, and less access to health care than other areas within the United States.

**Diabetes mellitus** (DM) causes blood glucose (sugar) levels to remain elevated over longer periods of time than usual. DM affects the body's ability in some cases to produce insulin and in other cases to use insulin to convert dietary glucose to a form that can be used by the body's cells for energy. Normally, the digestive process breaks food down into components that can be transported through the blood to the cells of the body. The presence of glucose in the blood stimulates the pancreas to release insulin, a hormone that acts as a key to the cell receptors within the body that "opens the cell doors" to let in the glucose. Excess glucose then is stored in the liver or throughout the body in muscle and fat, at which point its level in the blood returns to normal.

There are three common types of DM: type 1 diabetes, type 2 diabetes, and gestational diabetes. What causes people to develop type 1 diabetes is not fully understood, but there is a genetic basis for certain. **Type 1 diabetes** occurs as a result of the pancreas's inability to produce insulin, and onset typically occurs in childhood. Type 2 diabetes seems to be caused by obesity, diets high in sugar, saturated and trans fats, and lack of physical activity, and there appears to be a genetic component that predisposes certain people rather than others. **Type 2 diabetes** is a result of the body's inability to use the insulin it produces appropriately. Its onset typically occurs in adulthood. However, people are being diagnosed with type 2 diabetes at younger and younger ages. In type 2 diabetes, the pancreas produces some insulin, but the body's tissues fail to respond to the insulin signal, a condition known as insulin resistance. Because the insulin cannot bind to the cell's insulin receptors, the glucose cannot be transported into the body's cells to be used (Whitbourne, 2001). As a result, large amounts of glucose remain in the blood. Lastly, **gestational**

**diabetes** is characterized as elevated blood glucose levels during pregnancy and can be harmful to the fetus and the mother.

The symptoms of diabetes include fatigue, frequent urination (especially at night), unusual thirst, weight loss, blurred vision, frequent infections, and slow healing of sores. Monitoring diabetes requires frequent testing, usually by measuring blood glucose levels. Many people treat diabetes with insulin injections or other oral medications that help lower blood glucose levels. Insulin must be used under the guidance of a health care professional and blood sugar levels must be monitored with its use, because if blood sugar levels dip too low (a condition known as **hypoglycemia**), the individual can become nervous, jittery, faint, and confused. Alternatively, in **hyperglycemia**, when blood glucose levels become too high, the person can also become seriously ill. Type 2 diabetes is associated with long-term complications that affect almost every organ system and can contribute to blindness, heart disease, stroke, kidney failure, and nerve damage that can lead to limb amputations.

According to the World Health Organization (n.d.), global prevalence of diabetes is roughly 9%, having doubled since 1980 along with obesity rates. Approximately 1.5 million deaths in 2012 were estimated to be due to diabetes. The United States is third, following India and China in the number of people who suffer from diabetes.

Diabetes can be understood from the biopsychosocial perspective because it involves some of the same physical, behavioral, and sociocultural risk factors for heart disease noted earlier. Echoing the findings of other research on the benefits of moderate consumption of alcohol, research on diabetes risk also suggests that people can protect themselves against diabetes by drinking 1 to 2 ounces per day as long as this doesn't conflict with other medications or conditions people may have (Baliunas et al., 2009).

**Cancer.** Certain screenings for a wider range of cancers including breast and colon cancers become more standard clinical practice in certain regions of the world. There are risk factors associated with different cancers that may affect when cancer screenings should start to carefully balance the risks and benefits. People at risk based on their age, sex, and lifestyle should undergo screenings as recommended by health care professionals and depending on known risk factors (including genetics, lifestyle, occupational hazards) present for each individual. Organizations such as the American Cancer Society in the United States and the Canadian Cancer Society in Canada publicize the need for tests, such as breast self-examination, mammograms, prostate examinations, and colon cancer screenings. In each case, patients and their physicians must weigh the risks incurred by undergoing screening (and possibly receiving a false positive) against the failure to detect a treatable cancer. Your best advice as a patient is to keep up with the literature for your own sex and age group, and advise your relatives to do the same, especially given that a relative's cancer diagnosis could increase your risk of being diagnosed, too.

**FIGURE 10-2** A map of melanoma and other skin cancers according to prevalence rates across the globe, with higher prevalence rates appearing in darker shades.

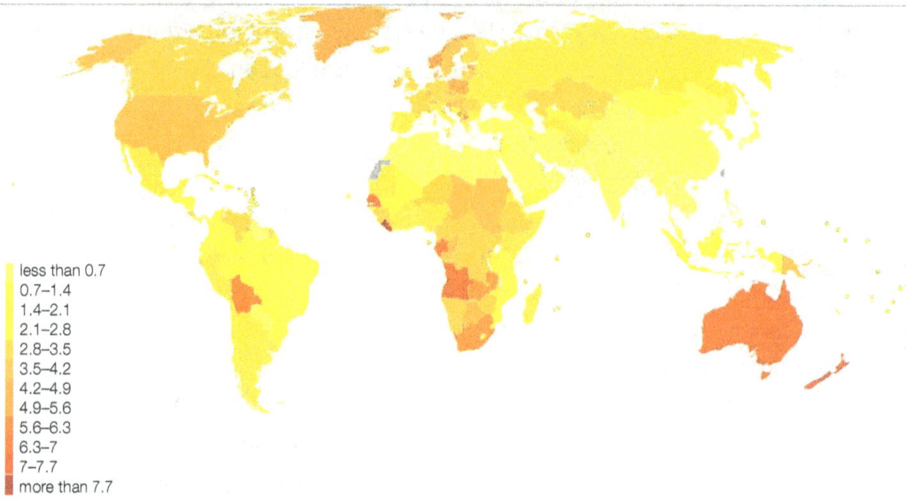

less than 0.7
0.7–1.4
1.4–2.1
2.1–2.8
2.8–3.5
3.5–4.2
4.2–4.9
4.9–5.6
5.6–6.3
6.3–7
7–7.7
more than 7.7

*Source:* https://commons.wikimedia.org/wiki/File:Melanoma_and_other_skin_cancers_world_map_-_Death_-_WHO2004.svg.

The best ways to minimize your cancer risk are to avoid known carcinogens and maintain a healthy lifestyle. There are environmental toxins in the air, food, and water that make certain people more vulnerable to cancer, including asbestos, arsenic, beryllium, cadmium, chromium, and nickel. Exposure to these compounds significantly increases a person's risk of cancer in various sites in the respiratory system, including the lung and nasal cavity. In addition, people exposed to leather, silica, and wood dust are more likely to develop respiratory cancers (Straif et al., 2009). People exposed to arsenic are at risk for bladder cancer, and those to asbestos more likely to develop ovarian cancer. Certain occupations are more exposed to these types of carcinogens and place individuals at greater risk, for example those who work in iron and steel founding or who manufacture isopropyl alcohol, paint, and rubber (Baan et al., 2009).

Being overweight is linked to a variety of cancers of the gastrointestinal system. Those with the highest body mass indexes (BMIs) have death rates from cancer that are 52% higher for males and 62% higher for females compared with those of normal BMI. The types of cancer associated with higher BMIs included cancer of the esophagus, colon and rectum, liver, gallbladder, pancreas, and kidney. Increasing risk with higher BMIs has been observed for deaths from cancers of the stomach and prostate in males and for deaths from cancers of the breast, uterus, cervix, and ovary in females (Calle et al., 2003). This provides even more support for the benefits of maintaining a low BMI as a critical preventive step in lowering your risk of cancer.

Eating specific foods seems to play a role in cancer risk. Stomach cancer is more common in some parts of the world, such as Japan, Korea, parts of Eastern Europe, and Latin America, where people eat foods that are preserved by drying, smoking, salting, or pickling. The risk of developing colon cancer is thought to be higher in people whose diet is high in fat, low in fruits and vegetables, and low in high-fiber foods such as whole-grain breads and cereals. Red meat consumption is also related to colorectal cancer risk (Aykan, 2015). In contrast, fresh fruits and vegetables may help protect against stomach cancer.

Race and sex are also associated with certain types of cancers. Skin cancer is more likely to develop in people with fair skin that freckles easily, whereas people with dark skin are less likely to develop skin cancer. Uterine cancer is more prevalent among Whites, and prostate cancer is more prevalent among Blacks. Stomach cancer is twice as prevalent in males and is more common in Blacks, as is colon cancer. Rectal cancer is more prevalent among Whites (Whitbourne & Whitbourne, 2012).

Certain hormones may increase the risk of cancer. Although the exact causes of prostate cancer are not known, testosterone stimulates the growth of both cancer cells and normal cells in the prostate. Estrogen taken as part of HRT in postmenopausal women is thought to increase their likelihood of developing uterine cancer. However, other factors, such as the endocrine-disrupting chemicals found in bisphenol A (BPA) can also increase a woman's risk of developing cancer (Rachon, 2015).

Should a person be diagnosed with cancer, various treatment options are available depending on the extent of a cancer's progression at the time of diagnosis. Surgery is a common treatment for most types of cancer when it is probable that all of the tumor can be removed. **Radiation** therapy may also be used and involves the use of high-energy X-rays to damage cancer cells and stop their growth. **Chemotherapy** uses drugs to kill cancer cells. Patients are most likely to receive chemotherapy if the cancer has spread beyond the primary site to other areas of the body. When this happens, the cancer is said to **metastasize. Biological response modifiers** are substances that improve the way the body's immune system fights disease and may be used in combination with chemotherapy to treat cancer that has metastasized.

As more information is gathered through rapidly evolving research on cancer and its causes, new methods of treatment and prevention will likely emerge. Furthermore, as efforts grow to target populations at risk for the development of preventable cancers (such as lung cancer), we hope cancer deaths will decrease even further in the decades ahead.

**Diet.** As we've emphasized, maintaining a healthy lifestyle is key to successful aging. A diet high in fruits and vegetables significantly lowers susceptibility to certain chronic conditions and is linked to lower mortality rates. The effect on mortality is mainly due to lower rates of cardiovascular disease, particularly **ischaemic heart disease** (Crowe et al., 2011). Ischaemia means reduced blood supply and ischaemic heart disease is also known as coronary artery disease. It's characterized as a sudden and severe narrowing or closure of the coronary artery or other large arteries that can lead to a number of heart-related events including stable angina, unstable angina, myocardial infarction, and sudden cardiac death.

Research highlights the benefits of the "Mediterranean style diet" as a way of lowering one's risk of cardiac death (Nordmann et al., 2011). It includes a diet of minimally processed fruits, vegetables, nuts, seeds, grains, olive oil as the main source of fat, low amounts of red meat and dairy foods, with moderate amounts of wine during meals. People who follow the Mediterranean diet have a lower risk of metabolic syndrome, higher levels of HDL cholesterol, and reduced cognitive decline and risk of dementia (Féart, Samieri, et al., 2013; Kastorini et al., 2011).

We've also emphasized that exercise is a vital component of all preventive programs aimed at reducing the prevalence of heart disease (Haskell et al., 2007). Research suggests referral to exercise programs for patients with coronary heart disease is underutilized and greater emphasis should be placed on encouraging these patients to attend such programs (Swift et al., 2013). There is also some evidence that suggests adults with hypertension can benefit from relaxation training; in one study, even a 12-session audio relaxation training program was shown to have beneficial effects (Tang et al., 2009).

As we noted earlier, there are significant differences in the United States in terms of rates of cardiovascular disease. In Central and Eastern Europe poor dietary habits contribute significantly to high rates of morbidity and mortality (Boylan et al., 2009). This is likely the case for the United States as well. If we are to lower rates of cardiovascular disease, we will need to address the levels of fats and salt in our diets, as well as smoking and physical activity (O'Flaherty et al., 2016). Still, we should acknowledge that people are reluctant to change their lifestyle habits, particularly when they must make these changes after decades of unhealthy habits. Health care professionals must, therefore, educate high-risk individuals and give them encouragement that change is possible (Resnick et al., 2009).

**Sleep.** A sedentary lifestyle is a major contributor to sleep problems, another reason why exercise in adulthood is so important. A variety of psychological disorders can also interfere with the sleep of middle-aged and older adults, including depression, anxiety, and bereavement (Kim et al., 2009). Seeking help may not only help symptoms related to the disorder, but could have benefits for a person's sleep, which could also help alleviate symptoms. Reading late at night with an e-reader, tablet, or smart phone may also interfere with the quality of anyone's sleep, regardless of their age, because of an impact on circadian rhythms (Chang et al., 2015) but may be particularly detrimental as we age because of decreases in melatonin levels and changes in sleep-wake timing. There are a number of illnesses and chronic conditions that can disrupt sleep, including arthritis, osteoporosis, cancer, chronic lung disease, congestive heart failure, and digestive disturbances (Bloom et al., 2009; Spira et al., 2009). People with Parkinson's disease or Alzheimer's disease also suffer serious sleep problems (Gabelle & Dauvilliers, 2010).

As we age we also experience normal age-related changes in the bladder that lead to more frequent urges to urinate during the night and can contribute to sleep disruptions. Urine production may also undergo alterations in timing throughout the night due to changes in circadian rhythms (Duffy et al., 2015). Menopausal symptoms can lead to frequent awakenings during the night, although exercise seems to help minimize the impact of menopause on aging (Chedraui et al., 2010). Periodic leg movements during sleep (also called nocturnal myoclonus) also contribute to nighttime waking (Ferri et al., 2009).

Nighttime sleep disruptions can lead to daytime sleepiness and fatigue. This creates a vicious cycle: The individual starts to establish a pattern of daytime napping, which increases the chances of sleep interruptions occurring at night (Foley et al., 2007) or cause a person to be too tired to exercise. Sleep problems also can increase the risk of falling, cause difficulty concentrating, and lead to negative changes in quality of life (Ancoli-Israel & Cooke, 2005).

Although changes in sleep occur as a normal feature of the aging process, severe sleep disturbances do not. Exercise can help improve disturbed circadian rhythms (Benloucif et al., 2004), and sleep specialists can offer innovative approaches (for example, light therapy "resets" an out-of-phase circadian rhythm) and encouragement of improvements in sleep habits (Klerman et al., 2001).

# Psychological Functioning

Psychological development and functioning in midlife reflect both positive and negative stereotypes about aging. Many feel a greater sense of control, more than any other period in their lives, and some hit their stride when it comes to coping with stressors. Some report memory challenges, even this early in life, but it's unclear how aging stereotypes affect our beliefs versus actual memory performance. Popular beliefs as opposed to empirical research also seem to challenge the existence of the midlife crisis.

**LO 10-4** **Explain how aspects of adult attachment patterns and personality affect health.**

**LO 10-5** **Argue why you believe a midlife crisis does or does not exist.**

## Cognitive Perspective

**Memory.** Evidence supports in part the commonly held belief that at least some forms of memory suffer as people get older—what varies is perhaps how much, exactly which type, and when. However, there is also evidence to suggest that how you think about your memory may play just as important a role as your actual age or state of the brain.

The identity process model, mentioned in previous chapter, predicts that undue concern about memory loss can translate into an "over-the-hill" attitude. Believing one's memory is failing, and experiencing such embarrassing situations as forgetting someone's name, adults can come to believe that their minds are on a hopeless downhill course. Middle-aged adults are highly sensitive to age-related changes in memory (Whitbourne & Collins, 1998), and as we age, we can be affected by the notion that memory functioning suffers an inevitable decline in later life (McDonald-Miszczak et al., 1995). The confidence a person has in his memory and his abilities to successfully perform memory-related tasks is called **memory self-efficacy**. This should, in turn, affect how well you actually perform. Unfortunately, people feel less and less confident about their memory and consequently, their memory, self-efficacy suffers (West et al., 2003),

**Control.** One's sense of personal **control** is of interest to researchers in part because of the common belief that adults start to feel a loss of control over what happens to them as they with age. Studies carried out within the National Survey of Midlife Development in the United States (MIDUS) showed that contrary to the popular myth, as we age, even into older adulthood, many of us retain the feeling of being in control of our lives despite being aware of the constraints we may encounter. We tend to do so by viewing our potential and our resources in a positive light rather than focusing on losses (Plaut et al., 2003).

**Stress and coping.** The cognitive approach to stress emphasizes the role of our perceptions and how they determine whether an event will be viewed as a threat that, in turn, determines whether it is viewed as stressful. Along these lines, the experience of **stress** occurs when you perceive that a situation is overwhelming your ability to manage effectively in that situation. **Coping** refers to the actions people take to reduce stress. There are two main forms of coping. In **problem-focused coping**, people attempt to reduce their stress by changing something about the situation, often by taking some sort of action to solve the problem at hand and reduce the stress. Conversely, in **emotion-focused coping**, people attempt to reduce their stress by managing the emotions of a stressful situation and potentially changing the ways they think about the situation, rather than trying to change the situation itself. Other methods of coping fall in between these two, such as seeking social support, a coping method that involves both taking action (by talking to other people) and changing ways of thinking (which may result from talking to other people).

There is no one best way to cope for stressful situations that cannot be changed. People can become more stressed if they *only* use problem-focused coping, because repeatedly taking action against something that cannot be changed (for example, a terminal illness) can deplete one's resources over time. For situations that can be changed, however, using emotion-focused coping *alone* might mean you fail to take steps to improve the situation. For example, if you have a number of pressing deadlines, simply wishing they would go away and taking deep breaths will not be an effective means of coping, because by missing the deadlines you create further problems for yourself.

When you cope successfully with a stressful situation, your mood improves and you have a higher sense of well-being (Lachman et al., 2009). The process seems to be reciprocal—people who feel better also cope more successfully. One longitudinal investigation of coping in midlife adults found that people who were less depressed were more likely to resolve problematic situations successfully.

## Psychodynamic Theory

**Generativity.** Midlife adults must also come to terms with issues relating to generativity, according to Erikson's theory of ego development we've discussed in earlier chapters. Erikson defined **generativity** as showing care and concern for guiding the next generation. Often we think about generativity in terms of good parenting, but there are other ways adults can be generative and contribute to the well-being of future generations, for example, through other family relationships, mentor relationships, and even giving back to the community. Generativity goes beyond good parenting and one's family to extend to concern with larger society. Matsuda and colleagues (2012) found that midlife adults high in generativity were also more likely to be concerned with environmental issues. Similarly, people scoring high on generativity are more likely to believe in, and engage in, environmentally responsible behavior (Urien & Kilbourne, 2011).

Successfully parenting children, not simply having them, seems to be more consistent with Erikson's views. Peterson (2006) found that parents higher in generativity not only felt closer to their college-age children but also had children who were happier and more likely to be able to plan for the future and had higher prosocial personality attributes and higher social interest, as indicated by their interest in politics, a characteristic of generative midlife adults, as well (Hart et al., 2001). Grandparenting is another way to express generativity by being involved in mentoring, spending time with them, and strengthening the bonds of mutual family ties (Hebblethwaite & Norris, 2011).

Generativity is not entirely selfless. According to McAdams (2008), generative behaviors expand and enrich one's ego through the "redemptive self." In other words, by being generative, your own development benefits, in addition to those you help. In truly generative behavior, though, the balance shifts more toward concern about others rather than concern about your own personal accomplishments.

**Defense mechanisms.** The psychodynamic theory proposed by George Vaillant (2000) emphasizes the development of defense mechanisms over the course of adulthood. **Defense mechanisms** help protect the conscious mind from knowing about unconscious desires and are strategies that people use almost automatically as protection against morally unacceptable urges and desires. Women are generally more likely to avoid unpleasant or stressful situations, to blame themselves when things go wrong, and to seek the support of others as defense mechanisms. Men are more likely to externalize their feelings and to use reaction formation, a defense mechanism in which people act in a way that is opposite to their unconscious feelings (Diehl et al., 1996; Labouvie-Vief & Medler, 2002). Unlike Freud, who proposed that personality doesn't change after childhood, Vaillant believes ego defense mechanisms become increasingly adaptive in adulthood, helping people cope with life's challenges, ranging from stress at work to discrimination to marital unhappiness. Over time people use increasingly mature and adaptive defenses and fewer immature and maladaptive ways of minimizing anxiety.

You can understand these differences by considering these two scenarios. In acting out (an immature defense), you react when you are angry by throwing something, slamming a door, or hitting your fist against a wall. These actions may temporarily relieve your anger but can also cause you (or your possessions) harm. You also will look quite ridiculous to your friends if you throw such a fit of rage in front of them. Using a more mature defense mechanism, such as humor in the face of anger, would help you feel better and avoid the social and practical costs of rash action. Using mature defense mechanisms can help us manage emotions by controlling negative feelings and putting a difficult situation into perspective.

Studies have shown that men who used immature defenses are more likely to experience alcohol problems and have unstable marriages, antisocial behavior, poorer health, and higher rates of mortality in old age (Malone et al., 2013; Soldz & Vaillant, 1998). People who use immature defense mechanisms are also more likely to drive other people away, leading to long-term consequences such as lack of social support, and with less social support, a person can become isolated and more prone to both mental and physical health problems.

**Adult attachment theory.** Recall our earlier discussions of developing attachments; an internal working model sets the stage for the characteristics and quality of future attachment relationships, including those we maintain in adulthood with our spouses and children. Our early relationships with our primary caregivers create an underlying, reliable understanding or mental representation of the world. These mental representations form models not only of relationships but also of the self. In adulthood, these attachment representations are ways of thinking that are supported by interactions with those who provide secure base support, typically our adult partners.

**FIGURE 10-3** Attachment styles in adulthood.

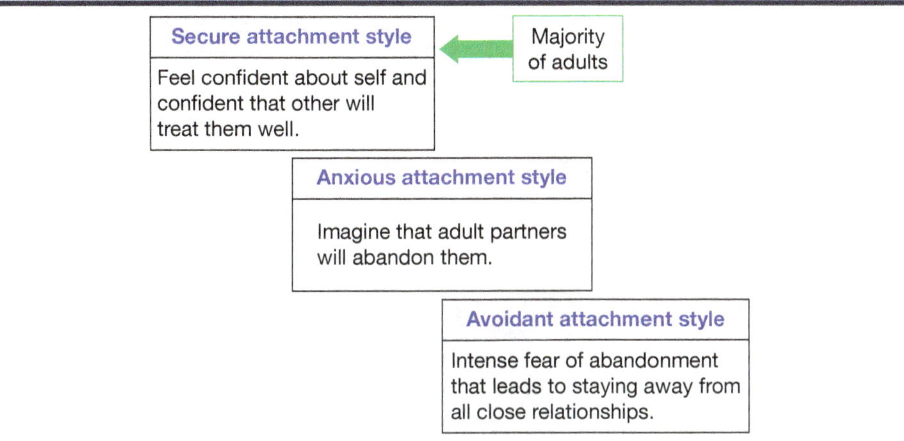


*Source:* Susan Whitbourne

**Adult attachment and parenting.** From a parenting perspective, attachment representations include a person's evaluations of their own caregiving in terms of their willingness to respond to the child and the child's needs, the effectiveness of their caregiving strategies, and their ability to read and understand the child's signals (George & Solomon, 1996). A parent should also consider their ongoing needs associated with partnerships, friendships, and other social roles (for example, occupational roles), in addition to the responsibilities associated with taking care of a child (George & Solomon, 1999, 2008). Optimal caregiving, then, requires the flexibility of the parent to view caregiving in relation to, and prioritize it alongside, other personal and developmental needs and goals (Solomon & George, 1996).

**Adult attachment and health.** Some believe adult attachment representations have implications for health (Ciechanowski et al., 2003; Feeney & Ryan, 1994; Fricchione, 2011; Glanz & Schwartz, 2008; Maunder & Hunter, 2009). The most adaptive (secure) attachment representation should enhance one's ability to accurately evaluate stress and lead to flexible, adaptive, and effective care seeking with respect to one's health. This translates to a person's adaptive use of resources, more rapid resolution of arousal associated with stress, and, consequently, lower allostatic load (refer to Chapter 5 for a discussion of allostatic load) (McEwen & Getz, 2013). Insecure adult attachment representations (dismissing/avoidant and preoccupied/anxious) are hypothesized to lead to less accurate assessments and less flexible and adaptive coping strategies, as well as more prolonged arousal under stressful conditions (Kidd & Sheffield, 2005). In terms of health, dismissing/avoidant attachment representations would be associated with poor identification of stressful experiences, including avoiding and/or dismissing cues and symptoms, overrating or idealizing one's well-being, and/or avoiding the use of close others as supports when stressed (Davis, Usher et al., 2014). A preoccupied/anxious attachment representation may lead to heightened detection of and response to stress, and active, even "hyperactive" care seeking, but with decreased "soothability" and sustained arousal (Crowell et al., 2002; Feeney & Ryan, 1994). Both of these insecure patterns would theoretically lead to greater allostatic load.

## Personality

We've discussed personality in previous chapters, ways we measure it, and how it affects other aspects of our lives. People's personalities influence their life choices, and many of those life choices in turn affect their personalities. According to the **correspondence principle**, people experience particular life events that reflect their personality traits; once these events occur, they further affect people's personalities (Roberts et al., 2013). A person who is high on extraversion, for example, is more likely than a person who is more introverted to choose social pursuits at night or on weekends. Being in these social situations may, in turn, promote further growth in extraversion. According to this principle, then, personality stability is enhanced by the active choices that people make rather than by any internal factors that may cause personality to remain stable over time.

**Personality and health.** The idea that personality traits are related to significant health problems and health-related behaviors originated when researchers discovered what became known as the "type A" behavior pattern, a collection of traits that include being highly competitive, impatient, feeling a strong sense of time urgency, and being highly achievement-oriented. First identified by cardiologists Meyer Friedman and R. H. Rosenman (1974), the type A behavior pattern became known as a major risk factor for heart disease, particularly when people high in the type A behavior pattern also had high levels of hostility (Suarez et al., 1991). Indeed, hostility and anger appear to be important personality traits to add to the equation in predicting heart disease. In one study, researchers concluded that men higher in hostility and more prone to experience anger also showed increases in coronary heart disease risk (Boyle et al., 2007).

Anxiety at high levels may also serve as a risk factor for cardiovascular disease. In comparing personality factors including anxiety, general levels of distress, and anger, researchers found that people high in trait anxiety were more likely to develop subsequent illness, even taking into account their other risk factors such as smoking, cholesterol, BMI, and blood pressure (Kubzansky et al., 2006).

**Five factor model.** Recall the five factor model of personality with the traits of openness, conscientiousness, extraversion, agreeableness, and neuroticism. Links between these traits and health have been established. For example, researchers have observed relations between low scores on conscientiousness in childhood and higher death rates in adulthood (Friedman et al., 1995). Being low in conscientiousness might lead people to be more careless about many aspects of life, including control over diet and exercise patterns, leading them to develop higher BMIs. In turn, they are more likely to gain weight during adolescence and early adulthood (Pulkki-Raback et al., 2005). Conscientiousness relates to greater weight gains during adulthood, particularly in women, placing them at risk for weight-related diseases. People low in conscientiousness and high on neuroticism are also more likely to smoke cigarettes (Terracciano & Costa, 2004). One study showed a relation between women's scores on neuroticism and weight gain (Brummett et al., 2006). High neuroticism scores, particularly on the facet of vulnerability, relate to high rates of heroin and cocaine use among adults.

The MIDUS showed that people high in conscientiousness and neuroticism had lower levels of a particular inflammatory marker (IL-6) linked to diabetes, atherosclerosis, and depression. Researchers believe the link between these personality traits and health is due, in part, to lower rates of obesity (Turiano et al., 2013). Being high on neuroticism may, then, have health benefits when paired with high levels of conscientiousness.

Conscientiousness may exert its positive effect on health through its link with prevention-related behaviors. Lodi-Smith and colleagues (2010) analyzed relations among conscientiousness and engagement in preventive and risky health-related behaviors and self-reported health. People higher in conscientiousness engaged in more preventive behaviors and fewer high-risk health behaviors (smoking, excessive drinking). Because self-report bias may lead people to rate themselves high in conscientiousness and positive health-related behaviors, the researchers also obtained ratings from other observers, namely a person who had a close relationship with the participant. People high in observer-rated conscientiousness actually did engage in fewer risky health-related behaviors.

Lower mortality is related to other personality traits, such as high scores on conscientiousness, low scores on neuroticism, and high scores on the activity facet of extraversion (Terracciano et al., 2008). High levels of openness, particularly emotional awareness and curiosity, also seem related to lower mortality rates, even after eliminating any potential influences of educational levels (Jonassaint et al., 2007).

# Social Contexts and Functioning

Midlife adults say their positive relationships with others, especially family, are what matter most. These relationships also contribute in important ways to a person's sense of well-being (Markus et al., 2005; Stansfeld et al., 2013). There is substantial research on adults' feelings of solidarity, conflict, and ambivalence toward parents, adult siblings, children, spouses, and friendships (Birditt et al., 2012; Fingerman, et al., 2004; Magai, 2008). As far as overall well-being is concerned, supportive relationships are generally viewed as positive influences on development, health, and functioning, whereas problematic relationships are negative influences (Birditt et al., 2005; Crowell et al., 2014; Stansfeld et al., 1998; Uchino et al., 2006). Social support is a well-established protective factor for many physical health outcomes and longevity.

Work demands tend to increase across midlife as job responsibilities change. As with personal relationships, the work environment, including work demands, pace, and social support contributes to midlife well-being (Selvarajan et al., 2013; Stansfeld et al., 2013). Although the work environment and personal relationships are both important independent predictors of well-being in midlife, work and home life can feed off of each other in positive ways that promote well-being or be at odds with one another in ways that affect well-being, mental health, health behaviors such as alcohol use, and perceived physical health. How we organize our roles and responsibilities and the expectations that are placed on us in midlife can lead to conflicting demands, in competition for time, energy, and mental effort. These conflicts can have additional negative influences on health and well-being (Marks, 1998).

**LO 10-6** **Describe key aspects of theories on partner relationships that explain why people stay satisfied and remain in committed relationships.**

**LO 10-7** **Consider jobs you've held in the past or may have today. Was your job satisfaction impacted by intrinsic or extrinsic factors in vocational satisfaction?**

## Relationships in Midlife

**Quality of relationships.** Gender differences in the relations among social support, stress, health, and well-being present a complex picture. Compared with men, women in midlife tend to have more positive extended family relationships and receive more personal social support rather than work-based social support (Taylor et al., 2017). Women also experience less distress upon job loss compared with men (Paul & Moser, 2016). Yet work stress appears to have a greater negative impact on health for women than for men (Heraclides et al., 2012). The same can be said for low levels of spousal support (Donoho et al., 2013). Among certain populations, extended family stress leads to greater health problems for women whereas extended family cohesion leads to greater health problems for men (Penedo et al., 2015), suggesting social demands can place a certain physical burden on us during midlife.

**Social exchange theory** attempts to predict why some relationships succeed and others fail in terms of whether the relationship's rewards exceed the costs of the alternatives. The rewards of marriage include love, friendship, and feelings of commitment. When considering a break-up, partners weigh these benefits against legal, financial, social, and religious barriers or constraints. Children will also factor into this equation, adding both to the perceived benefits such as coparenting and to the costs, which include child custody. When the balance shifts so that rewards no longer outweigh costs, one or both partners will initiate a break-up. Over time, exchange theory predicts the intrinsic rewards of being in the relationship, including the reliance the partners develop toward each other, increase to the point where the attractiveness of alternatives tends to fade. Researchers find the earning potential of young women is becoming more important in determining their desirability as mates.

With women making strides in the labor market, their income is now sometimes seen by husbands as an important asset in their own movement up the occupational career ladder (Sweeney & Cancian, 2004). However, there are still some very traditional determinants of what makes men happy, at least in the early years of marriage. In a 3-year longitudinal study of characteristics important in a mate, men placed higher value on good looks, a pleasing disposition, and a dependable character over time rather than financial prospects or favorable social status (Shackelford et al., 2005).

For cohabitating couples, sexual aspects of relationship seem to follow the principles of social exchange theory. In one study, comparisons of relationship dissolution among cohabitating and married couples showed that cohabitators were more likely to end relationships in which the partners only rarely engaged in sex. Presumably, those who are cohabitating perceive fewer barriers to ending a relationship if the sexual dimension of the relationship no longer proves to be satisfactory (Yabiku & Gager, 2009).

Similar to exchange theory, **equity theory** proposes that partners are satisfied in a relationship if they feel they are getting what they deserve (Walster et al., 1978). This means they seek getting no more, and certainly no less, than they put into the relationship (Hatfield & Rapson, 2012). Equity theory seems to apply particularly well for couples in the early stages of a relationship when couples are deciding whether to build further ties with each other (Hatfield et al., 2008).

The behavioral approach to marital interactions emphasizes the actual behaviors that partners engage in with each other during marital interactions as influences on marital stability and quality (Karney & Bradbury, 1997). According to this perspective, people will be more satisfied in long-term relationships when their partners engage in positive or rewarding behaviors (such as expressing affection) and less satisfied with their partners when they are critical or abusive. Conflict increases when a partner either turns away from or turns against a partner who is trying to make an emotional connection (Gottman & Driver, 2005).

Finally, the latest approach to understanding marital satisfaction emphasizes the role of individual fulfillment within the context of the couple. According to Finkel and colleague's (2015) **suffocation model** of marriage, contemporary adults place more emphasis on marriage as a source of self-expression and fulfillment but have less time to devote to maintaining their marriages than ever before. For those married couples who do invest in their marriages, however, the best marriages are becoming better than they were before at any previous time in history.

**Relationship pathways.** A 13-year longitudinal study by University of Texas family psychologist Ted Huston (2009) provides some useful insights into the course of long-term marriages. The surprising feature of Huston's work was his discovery that the seeds of marital bliss, or trouble, are often sown even before the couple walks down the aisle. In the **enduring dynamics pathway**, the way a couple interacts early in their relationship will characterize the course of the relationship over time. They either get along well with each other and resolve conflict easily, or they don't.

**FIGURE 10-4** Relationship pathways in adulthood.

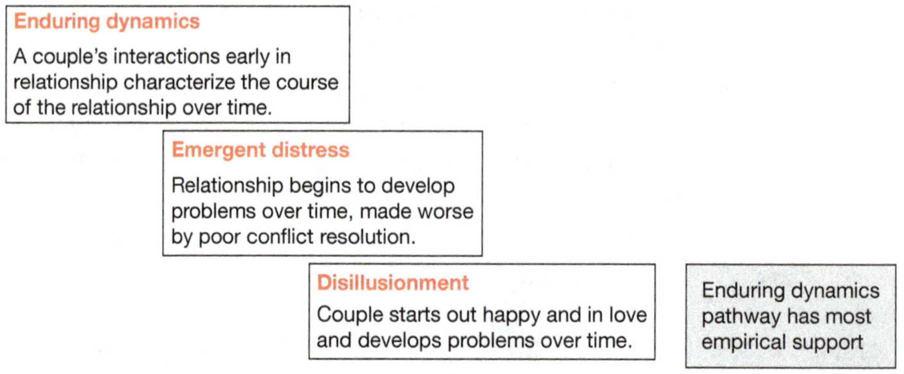

**Enduring dynamics**
A couple's interactions early in relationship characterize the course of the relationship over time.

**Emergent distress**
Relationship begins to develop problems over time, made worse by poor conflict resolution.

**Disillusionment**
Couple starts out happy and in love and develops problems over time.

Enduring dynamics pathway has most empirical support

*Source:* Susan Whitbourne

There are, however, couples whose problems evolve over time. Those who fit the emergent distress pathway develop relationship problems over time as they find they are unable to cope with the inevitable arguments that occur when people live together. Instead of resolving their problems with adaptive tactics such as communicating openly and working out compromises, they become defensive, withdraw, stonewall, and become blatantly vicious toward each other. It's unclear whether their distress causes these dysfunctional coping behaviors or whether their behaviors lead to distress. The upshot is that these couples become increasingly unhappy over time until they finally decide to end things entirely.

Like couples who experience emergent distress, those who fit the disillusionment pathway start out happy and in love when they first tie the knot. Over time, they gradually fall out of love and develop mixed feelings about their partners. Part of what happens is they take each other for granted. They become less and less interested in seeking their partner's love and approval than they are at the beginning of the relationship, and as the initial allure fades, they drift further and further apart.

Both the emergent distress and disillusionment models assume couples start out as hopeful and optimistic their relationship will work out; it is only after the months or years go by that they find themselves arguing constantly or just losing interest.

Returning to Huston's work, after following couples for 2 and 13 years after marriage, Huston and his team concluded their data gave the most support to the enduring dynamics model of distress. Rather than newlyweds being head over heels in love, only to have the relationship unravel over time, the dynamics that characterize the beginning of a relationship persist over time. Two key features seem to differentiate the happy from the unhappy couples: positive expressions of affection and love and negative behaviors of being critical, angry, and impatient toward the partner. The happy couples expressed their love through affectionate behaviors, enjoyed being together, and made sure that they spent time together. The unhappy ones created a negative emotional climate and avoided being with each other. The more in love the couple were, the more they expressed their positive feelings toward each other, including initiating sexual activity (Schoenfeld et al., 2012).

Such marital discord for unhappy couples takes its toll on individual well-being. Couples in their later years who are constantly in conflict are at risk for experiencing higher levels of depression and anxiety and lower levels of self-esteem and life satisfaction (Whisman et al., 2014).

For couples who want to work on a relationship, couples therapy is a known effective method for promoting positive change (Davis et al., 2012). Couples therapy shares many features of individual therapy, but there are important differences. Couples therapists are trained to examine the interactive patterns that lead couples into conflict and then, more importantly, help them break these dysfunctional patterns. They tend to be more "take charge" than individual therapists, actively intervening when they see problems unfolding before them during therapy sessions. As the couple learns to see their strengths and feel change is possible, they can come to new understandings of themselves and their (Benson et al., 2012).

Changes in family living situations are often discussed in terms of blended families, also known as reconstituted families. Within these family situations, at least one adult is living with a child who is not a biological or adopted child of that adult. Often, these family situations develop after a divorce and remarriage (or cohabitation), in which two adults establish a household together. The dynamics within these relationships, though the subject of many fictional accounts, are only beginning to receive empirical attention in the literature. Some evidence suggests these relationships are more stressful in the case of stepmothers and stepchildren than between stepfathers and stepchildren (Ward et al., 2009).

**Divorce and remarriage.** Remaining relatively stable over time, approximately 10% of the adult population in the United States is divorced (U.S. Bureau of the Census, 2018); the rate of divorce is 3.2 per 1,000 in the total population (Centers for Disease Control and Prevention, 2020). Taking into account all marriages that end in divorce, the average length of a first marriage prior to divorce is roughly 8 years (Kreider & Ellis, 2011). Divorce statistics show important variations by race. Black women between the ages of 25 and 44 have higher divorce rates than White or Hispanic women (Goodwin et. al., 2010). Research on children of divorced parents suggests parental divorce is a stronger indicator of a lack of commitment and confidence in the marriage for women, but not men (Whitton et. al., 2008; Whitbourne & Whitbourne, 2012).

**FIGURE 10-5** Marital status trends since the early 1900s.

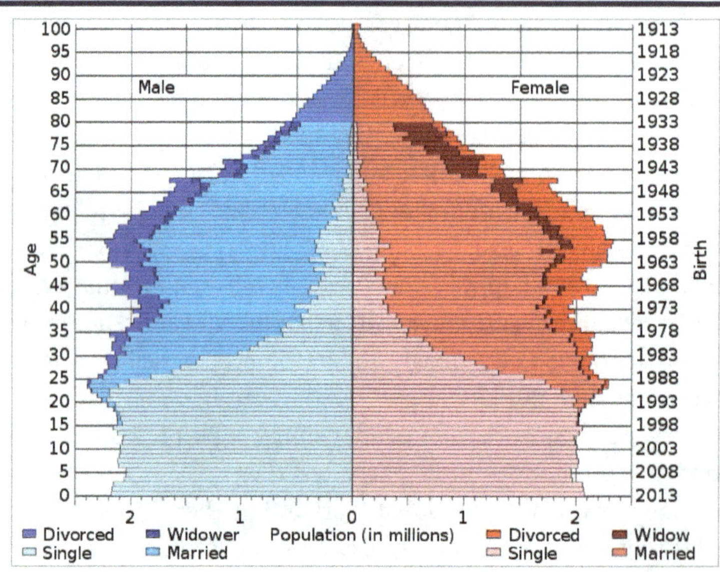


*Source:* https://commons.wikimedia.org/wiki/File:United_States_Population_by_Age_Sex_and_Marital_Status.svg.

Divorce rates have been declining steadily since peaking in 1980. Many factors combine to account for this decreasing divorce rate. One factor is people are marrying at later ages; the older a woman is when she marries, the lower the probability she will become divorced (Bramlett & Mosher, 2002). Second, the previously skyrocketing divorce rates increased consciousness in society about the need for prevention. Suggesting such efforts can pay off, a study of more than 2,200 households in the Midwest of the United States showed that couples who participated in premarital education had higher levels of marital satisfaction, lower levels of conflict, and reduced chances of divorce (Stanley et al., 2006). Research on second marriages suggests that couples are less likely to engage in premarital education compared with couples entering into first marriages—a trend linked to decreased marital happiness and increased rates of divorce (Doss et. al., 2009).

The dissolution of a marriage is often perceived by those involved as a disappointment and a sad or even tragic event. One or both partners may be relieved to end an unsuccessful relationship, but they are still affected in many ways by the consequences of the divorce on their daily lives, the lives of children, and the lives of extended family members. The couple must resolve a range of practical issues, such as changes in their housing and financial affairs—but the greatest toll is the emotional one. For many couples, child custody arrangements present the most significant challenge caused by their altered status as a family.

Studies on divorced (compared with married) individuals show they have lower levels of psychological well-being, poorer health, higher mortality rates, more problems with substance abuse and depression, less satisfying sex lives, and more negative life events (Amato, 2000). The negative consequences of divorce are more severe for those with young children, especially women (Williams & Dunne-Bryant, 2006). These effects may persist for many years, particularly for individuals who remain psychologically attached to their ex-partner, those who experience conflict in coparenting, or those who have unusual difficulty living on their own (Sweeper & Halford, 2006). Divorced or widowed adults who do not remarry are in poorer health (including chronic conditions and depressive symptoms) than those who remarry (Hughes & Waite, 2009).

Although technically divorce rates in the population as a whole have declined, the media frequently cite the disturbing statistic that one out of every two marriages will end in divorce. However, the divorce statistics are much more complicated than this simple formula would imply. Those who divorce in a given year are generally not the same people as those who marry, so the number of divorces cannot simply be compared with the number of marriages to determine the odds of divorcing. Furthermore, the divorce rate in any given year includes those people who are divorcing for a second or third time. Second and third marriages tend to have a higher divorce rate than first marriages. Including these individuals artificially inflates the divorce rate for all marriages.

The divorce rate is influenced in part by the number of people in the population of marriageable age, which itself is influenced by birth and death rates. In the United States, approximately 13% of all marriages are second marriages, and 4% are third marriages (Lewis & Kreider, 2015). The average duration of a second marriage that ends in divorce is about the same as that for a first marriage (Kreider & Ellis, 2011). The probability of a second marriage ending in divorce after 10 years is 0.39, slightly higher than the ending of a first marriage, which is 0.33 (Bramlett & Mosher, 2002).

Another way to view divorce statistics is by looking at the subset of people who are still married within a given category based on number of marriages. In other words, about 60% of men and women in their 40s were married once. Among these, about 48 to 50% are still married. Slightly fewer 40- to 49-year-olds married twice (17%) and are still married (about 14%), and the same is roughly true for those married three or more times. Thus, even among those marrying multiple times, the majority are currently married.

People who are more likely to contemplate divorce when their marriage is in trouble are said to be high on divorce proneness. These individuals are also more likely to have extramarital affairs (Previti & Amato, 2004). Those high in divorce proneness may have a long history of difficulties with intimacy. Data show that women who had low intimacy scores in college are more likely to divorce by their late 50s; the same is not true for men, though (Weinberger et al., 2008).

Separated and divorced individuals often cite infidelity as the cause of their break-up. Data from a national U.S. survey conducted between 1991 and 2008 reveal that more than one half of men and women who engage in extramarital affairs also become separated or divorced from their spouses (Allen & Atkins, 2012). People who are in troubled marriages may become unfaithful because they are unhappy with their spouses. For these individuals, the extramarital affair is the final push toward divorce, particularly if it is the other partner who has the affair. By the same token, people who engage in an affair and then say their marriage was unhappy may be using identity assimilation, seeking to protect their identities as good individuals.

Identity may also play a role in how individuals cope emotionally with divorce. There are a wide range of negative emotional outcomes associated with divorce. People who are divorcing experience feelings such as loss of trust, low self-esteem, anxiety, worry about being hurt in future relationships, anger, depression, and preoccupation with what others think. For some individuals, however, divorce provides relief from a highly conflictual situation.

You may think the initiator of the divorce has fewer negative emotions than the noninitiator, but the individual's role in the divorce does not always relate to emotions. Some divorced couples seem to transition well into postdivorce relationships, remaining friends, sharing parenting, or operating a joint business. Examining these factors, Frisby and colleagues (2012) proposed that one of the most difficult aspects of divorce is loss of "face," meaning that divorce represents a threat to the individual's identity. Individuals who divorced within the prior 2 years had more positive emotions if they were able to see the divorce as a way to gain independence and were supported by their partner in protecting their identities.

**Children of divorced parents.** As difficult as it is for children to be caught between parents who are divorced, it may be just as hard, if not harder, to be caught between parents who are in a high-conflict marriage. In one longitudinal study of marriage, children (age 19 and older) of divorced parents were asked to state whether they felt they had been caught in the middle of parental arguments. The children of parents whose marriages were characterized by a high degree of conflict were most likely to feel caught in the middle. Not surprisingly, these feelings were related to lower subjective well-being and poorer relationships with their parents (Amato & Afifi, 2006).

Among divorced couples, mediation is increasingly viewed as an effective means to reducing conflict and hence improving children's adjustment. Mediation is based on a model of cooperative dispute settlement rather than the more adversarial approach that occurs when lawyers become part of the scene. In a 12-year longitudinal study, divorced couples were randomly assigned to either mediation or legal assistance. Conflict significantly declined, particularly in the 1st year after divorce, among couples who participated in mediation (Sbarra & Emery, 2008).

Following the dissolution of the marriage, either through divorce or widowhood, there is approximately a 14 to 20% chance a person will marry again or their partner will. As may be expected, these odds go up among increasingly older age groups. The odds of remarrying are higher for people with a college degree or higher, and for those making incomes of $100,000 or more (Lewis & Kreider, 2015).

## Caregiving

**The sandwich generation.** Midlife can bring forth social stressors and strains as our social roles typically experience considerable restructuring as we move from being part of what's considered a less experienced generation during young adulthood to a more experienced generation during midlife. This is especially true within families as many midlife adults have both children and older living parents who require emotional and practical support and find themselves part of the sandwich generation. Midlife adults' children are growing, some into adults themselves, yet still require support, and their aging parents may have a new set of attention and resource needs. In 2013, 71% of those between the ages of 40 and 59 were considered part of the sandwich generation (Parker & Patten, 2013). These adults often report feeling pressed for time and "squeezed" between the two generations, with the need to more broadly distribute one's logistical, financial, and psychological resources (Pierret, 2006). The good news is self-reported happiness does not differ between adults who find themselves sandwiched between children and parents requiring support and those who do not. And many characterize the relationships within the "sandwich" in a positive light, highlighting ways that positive relationships can nevertheless still be a source of stress or strain in midlife.

**Caregiving for aging relatives.** Providing care for aging relatives, particularly when a person is no longer able to function independently, largely falls on their spouse and children. Caregivers are those individuals, usually family, who provide support to people with chronic diseases. They have been the focus of considerable research efforts over the past 30 years. We now know that caregivers are very likely to suffer adverse effects from the constant demands placed on them. The term "caregiver burden" is used to describe the stress that caregivers experience in the daily management of their afflicted relative. As the disease progresses, caregivers must provide physical assistance in basic life functions, such as eating, dressing, and toileting. As time goes by, the caregiver may experience health problems that make it harder and harder to provide the kind of care needed to keep a person with a disease like Alzheimer's at home.

Given the strain placed on caregivers, it should come as no surprise that health problems and rates of depression, stress, and isolation are higher among these individuals than among the population at large. For example, research suggests that daughters caring for parents with neurocognitive disorders suffer significantly more cardiovascular stress compared with wives caring for their spouses (King et al., 2002).

Fortunately, support for caregivers of people with Alzheimer's disease is widely available. Local chapters of national organizations in the United States such as the Alzheimer's Association provide community support services for families and caregivers. Caregivers can be taught ways to promote independence and reduce distressing behaviors in the patient, as well as to learn ways to handle the emotional stress associated with their role (National Institute of Aging, 2009). We'll discuss Alzheimer's disease in greater detail as it relates to the individual diagnosed with the disease in the next chapter.

**Caregiver strategies for managing Alzheimer's symptoms.** An important goal in managing the symptoms of Alzheimer's disease is to teach caregivers behavioral methods that will help maximize the patient's ability to remain independent for as long as possible. The idea behind this approach is that, by maintaining the patient's independence, caregiver burden is reduced to a certain extent. For example, the patient can be given prompts, cues, and guidance in the steps necessary to get dressed and then be positively rewarded with praise and attention for having completed those steps. Modeling is another behavioral strategy, much like we discussed in earlier chapters, in which the caregiver performs the desired action (such as pouring a glass of water) so that the patient can see this action and imitate it. Again, positive reinforcement helps to maintain this behavior once it is learned (or, more properly, relearned). The caregiver then has less work to do, and the patients are given cognitive stimulation by actively performing these tasks rather than having others take over their care completely.

Caregivers can also use behavioral strategies to reduce or eliminate the frequency of actions such as wandering or aggressive behaviors. In some cases, these strategies may require ignoring problematic behaviors. By eliminating the reinforcement of those behaviors in the form of attention, the patient will be less likely to engage in them. However, a more active approach will likely be needed, especially for wandering. In this case the patient can be provided with positive reinforcement for not wandering. Even this may not be enough, however, and the caregiver may need to take precautions such as installing protective devices in doors and hallways.

Operating according to a strict daily schedule can be helpful. The structure provided by a regular routine of everyday activities can give the patient additional cues to use as guides for which behaviors to carry out at certain times of day. Identifying situations in which the patient becomes particularly disruptive, such as during bathing or riding in the car, is also important. In these cases, the caregiver can learn how to target those aspects of the situation that cause the patient to become upset and modify them accordingly. For example, a simple alteration such as providing a terry cloth robe rather than a towel after bathing can help reduce the patient's feeling of alarm at being undressed in front of others.

It is also important for caregivers to understand the disease progression and what to expect as it unfolds. In a study of more than 300 nursing home patients with an advanced neurocognitive disorder, fewer interventions considered burdensome, such as tube feeding, were used when those responsible for the patient's treatment were aware of the prognosis and typical course of the disease (Mitchell et al., 2009).

Creative approaches to managing the recurrent stresses involved in the caregiver's role may help to reduce the feelings of burden and frustration that can become part of daily life. Along with the provision of community and institutional support services, such interventions can go a long way toward helping the caregiver and ultimately the patient (Callahan et al., 2006).

**The empty nest.** We examined the factors that influence the transition to parenthood when their first child arrives. Now we will look at what happens during the reverse process. The empty nest describes the period in a person's or couple's life that occurs when their children permanently depart from the home.

For many years, the common belief was the empty nest is an unwelcome change, particularly for women. However, the reality is the empty nest may be a positive step, at least in a couple's relationship. Much of the research on the empty nest dates back to earlier decades, when women were less likely to maintain continuous employment outside the home than is currently true. Furthermore, much of the earlier research was conducted at a time when children were more clearly launched out of the home, compared with present day when children often take longer to leave the parental home and may "boomerang" back if economic circumstances take a turn for the worse. Many parents, then and possibly now, regard their children's leaving as a mark of their own success in preparing their children for adulthood.

With the children gone from the home, couples potentially have the opportunity to enjoy more leisure-time activities together, a change that should bring them closer together (Gagnon et al., 1999). Being able to spend time with each other may also allow them to enjoy greater marital satisfaction and improved sexual relations. Perhaps for these reasons, the empty nest may have some advantages in helping keep a couple's sexual relationship alive. When children do return home for whatever reason, the quality of a couple's sexual relationship may decline, at least in terms of frequency of sexual activities (Dennerstein et al., 2002). In fact, a survey of more than 15,000 midlife Canadian women showed that the predictors of sexual activity within the past 12 months included age, marital status, race, income, alcohol use, smoking, and empty nest status (Fraser et al., 2004). Women whose children were still living in the home were less likely to have intercourse than women who were empty nesters.

However, among certain couples, the empty nest can pose challenges. Mitchell and Lovegreen (2009) identified a pattern they called the "empty nest syndrome" (ENS). The interviews showed that mothers were slightly more likely than fathers to report ENS; however, the percentages of despondent parents were very low overall, ranging from 20 to 25% in most of the groups studied. Parents of Indo/East Indian ethnicity, whose culture emphasizes continuing bonds between parents and adult children, had far higher rates of ENS (50 and 64% for fathers and mothers) than the parents of Chinese or Southern European or British ancestry. In addition to the role of culture, this study identified key social psychological factors that seemed to place these midlife parents at risk of experiencing ENS. These include having an identity wrapped up in their parental role, feeling they are losing control over their children's lives, having few or only children, and lacking a support network. Parents who worried about their children's safety and well-being in the world outside the home also were more vulnerable to ENS. For the most part, however, the parents in this study were more likely than not to adapt well to the empty nest transition.

Although the empty nest is viewed as the norm when discussing adult children and their parents, there are a growing number of adult sons and daughters living with their parents (ages 25 to 34), a situation referred to by the term "boomerang" children in the United States and "kids in parents' pockets eroding retirement savings" (KIPPERS) or "kidults" in the United Kingdom. In part, the return of children back into the empty nest is associated with the economic downturn of the late 2000s (Palmer, 2009). Since 2000, there has been an uptick in the number of emerging adults living with their parents, particularly for men 25 to 34 years old, but the percentage is approximately the same (8 to 10% of men and 15 to 17% of women) (Vespa et al., 2013).

As is true for the empty nest, there is surprisingly little research on boomerang children. One Canadian survey reported cultural differences in the tendency of parents and young adult children to live together, with Asian- and Latin American-born parents most likely to host their 20- to 24-year-old children (Turcotte, 2006). Parents with live-in children were more likely than those whose children did not live at home to experience feelings of frustration over the time spent taking care of their adult children, but the percentage of these negative feelings was very low (8% with live-in children versus 4% whose children did not live at home). The parents of children living at home also reported more couple conflicts about money, the children themselves, and the distribution of labor in household responsibilities.

The situation seems more negative with boomerang children compared with children who never leave the home, particularly as mothers are likely to resent the fact they are losing some of the freedom they gained when their children initially left home. These parents are less likely to say their children make them happier (57%) compared with the parents of nonboomerang children (68%). On the other hand, a larger percentage of parents of children living at home (64%) say they are satisfied with the amount of time they spend with their offspring than are parents whose children have moved out (49%).

Parents and children transition together, then, over the course of their relationship, from the children's entrance into the home until their eventual exit, whether permanent or not. The dynamics of these relationships over time may be understood in terms of identity and sociocultural factors. Many parents highly value their identities as parents and see the development of their children as reflections of their own competence. Meanwhile, children try to detach from their parents to establish their own identities. All these changes happen in a sociocultural context that, as we have seen in empty nest research, may affect the normative expectations parents and children have regarding their positions in the family.

## Work and Career

Recall the discussion of Super from the previous chapter, and his work on career development. When he first put forth his ideas, the job market was much more stable than today. In the 1950s, many people were employed by one company for their entire careers. Climbing up the career ladder was seen as a fairly typical goal, particularly for workers in white-collar occupations, but also for blue-collar workers employed in industries such as steel or car manufacturing. This model began to change substantially in the 1980s, when large corporations began programs of downsizing, particularly after the advent of computerized technology.

The modern workplace is likely to promote recycling, the process through which workers change their main field of career activity partway into occupational life (Sullivan et al., 2003). In recycling, middle-aged workers may find themselves once again in the establishment stage they thought they left behind in their late

20s. People can recycle back through Super's stages several times throughout their work lives (Hall, 1993). People may also experience career plateauing, in which they remain static in their vocational development. They may experience structural plateauing, in which they do not advance up to higher-level positions, or content plateauing, in which they feel they have mastered their work and no longer see it as a challenge (Lapalme et al., 2009). People may reach a plateau at a young age if they enter so-called dead-end jobs or their moves within or between companies involve lateral changes rather than vertical advancement. At that point, the individual may decide it is time to seek another job (Heilmann et al., 2008). However, some employees are content to remain in the status quo, particularly if they have achieved success and are satisfied with their current position (Smith-Ruig, 2009).

**Vocational satisfaction.** The concept of vocational satisfaction is the extent to which people find their work to be enjoyable. For our purposes, we will consider vocational satisfaction to be equivalent to job satisfaction, as both terms are used in the literature. We can assume that workers who are satisfied are more committed to the organizations for which they work (Hoffman & Woehr, 2006). Therefore, both employees and employers benefit when workers are high in vocational satisfaction.

**Intrinsic and extrinsic factors related to job satisfaction.** People can be satisfied with their jobs either because they love the work they perform, they value the salary and other perks it provides, or both. Intrinsic factors in vocational satisfaction refer to the tasks required to perform the work itself. The central defining feature of an intrinsic factor is it cannot be found in precisely the same fashion in a different type of job. For example, the sculptor engages in the physical activities of molding clay or stone, and the accountant must perform the mental activities of manipulating numbers. Although each job involves other activities, these are the ones that serve to define the work required to perform each. Intrinsic factors involve or engage your sense of identity because the work directly pertains to your feelings of competence, autonomy, and stimulation of personal growth. Your ability to express autonomy and self-direction in the daily "doing" of your job are also part of the intrinsic aspects of work because these factors are directly tied to your sense of self. Having work that is a calling also fulfills your intrinsic motivation, but you can have intrinsic motivation for your work without feeling it is a calling.

Extrinsic factors in vocational satisfaction are the features that accompany the job but are not central to its performance. You can receive extrinsic satisfaction from many different jobs regardless of the work tasks they require. The easiest extrinsic factor to understand is salary. Although some jobs pay more than others, you can earn the same amount of money by performing very different work tasks. A professional athlete and a real estate tycoon may earn the same six- or seven-figure paycheck for performing a very different set of job activities. Therefore, salary is not intrinsic to work. There are a number of additional extrinsic factors associated with the conditions of work, such as the comfort of the environment, demands for travel, convenience of work hours, friendliness of coworkers, amount of status associated with the job, and adequacy of the company's supervision and employment policies. These aspects of work are "psychological," in a sense, but they do not directly engage your sense of personal identity and competence. Although a high salary may certainly reinforce your sense of worth (particularly in Western society), you can earn that high salary in many ways that are not necessarily tied to your true vocational passions. The racial climate is another important condition of the workplace that can affect worker satisfaction but is not intrinsic to the job itself (Lyons & O'Brien, 2006).

At this point in your life, you may or may not have had a job yet that you felt was intrinsically satisfying. However, you can probably think of people you know who do feel connected to their work at an intrinsic level. Perhaps you have encountered a customer service representative who seemed genuinely interested in helping you solve a problem and was willing to work with you until you found the satisfactory solution. This may have been an employee who found the job to be intrinsically rewarding, feelings she expressed in the apparent pride she took in helping you with your situation. Intrinsic factors provide a sense of active engagement in work and contribute to sense of self. The customer service representative who provided you with such kind and gracious help may not see her job as one that represents her life's work; however, she may nevertheless enjoy the part of her job that allows her to get people what they need.

Personality traits can influence the ways in which people interpret what happens to them at work. You might think people high in agreeableness are better able to bounce back from negative interactions at work. However, in a study of university employees, researchers found that those high in agreeableness actually have more negative affect following interpersonal conflict than those low in agreeableness. Highly agreeable employees are also more likely to experience negative affect when they perceive their work environments are low in social support (Ilies et al., 2011).

Personality traits may also interact with changes in job satisfaction over time. Looking at the intrinsic–extrinsic dimension of vocational satisfaction, researchers found that people with high neuroticism scores are less likely to feel their jobs are intrinsically rewarding. Perhaps for this reason, neuroticism is negatively related to job satisfaction; by contrast, people high in the traits of conscientiousness and extraversion are more satisfied in their jobs (Furnham et al., 2009). In one longitudinal study of adults in Australia, although personality changes were found to predict changes in work satisfaction, changes in personality were also found to result from higher job satisfaction. Over time, workers who were more satisfied with their jobs became more extraverted (Scollon & Diener, 2006).

**Age and vocational satisfaction.** The question of whether job satisfaction increases, decreases, or stays the same over adulthood is a surprisingly difficult one to answer. This is because, as you learned earlier, more and more working adults recycle through their jobs. As a result, it is job tenure, the length of time a person has spent in the job, rather than age that may relate to job satisfaction. Gender, level of employment, and salary also interact with age differences in job satisfaction

(Riordan et al., 2003). Ng and Feldman (2010) examined the relation between age and 35 different measures of job attitudes. Across these studies, age was related only weakly to overall job satisfaction, satisfaction with the work itself, satisfaction with pay, job involvement, and intrinsic work motivation.

One factor that may affect an older worker's commitment to and involvement in the job is exposure to age discrimination in the workplace. Although older workers are protected by federal law prohibiting discrimination, negative stereotypes about the abilities and suitabilities of older persons in the workplace persist (Rupp et al., 2006). Older workers may begin to disengage mentally when they feel they are subject to these age stereotypes, pressures to retire in the form of downsizing, and the message that their skills are becoming obsolete (Lease, 1998). These pressures can lead older workers to be less likely to engage in the career development activities that would enhance their ability to remain on the job or find a new one when their job is eliminated due to downsizing. Furthermore, older workers who feel that their contributions are not valued, or who experience ageism on the job, will have lower vocational satisfaction regardless of how confident they feel in their abilities (Foley & Lytle, 2015).

Support from employers is a key factor in the association between age and job satisfaction. Older workers can be more fully engaged in their job and hence achieve higher satisfaction if they feel their employer values their contributions. Providing training and development programs specifically geared for older workers is a part of this process. Important to keeping the older worker motivated and satisfied is providing job assignments to keep the work fresh and interesting (Armstrong-Stassen & Ursel, 2009).

Age-related changes in physical and cognitive functioning must also be taken into account. If these changes interfere with the ability to perform the job satisfactorily, then the older worker will be unable to perform their duties or may only be able to do so with difficulty. If the aging process alters fit between the individual and the job, the worker will feel increasingly dissatisfied and unfulfilled. The role of the supervisor may be particularly important in this regard. For example, a manager who is sensitive to an older worker's physical limitations may be able to lessen the physical demands placed on the employee.

**Work stress.** Work stress can be a major threat to people's feelings of well-being and can eventually take its toll on physical health. There are many forms that work stress can take, ranging from negative interactions with coworkers to difficulties dealing with clients, customers, and supervisors. People may also experience stress when they feel their job is not compatible with their needs, interests, values, and personal dispositions. The Whitehall II study provided compelling data to show the links between work-related stress and the risk of metabolic syndrome (Chandola et al., 2006). Men under high levels of work stress over the course of the study had twice the risk of subsequently developing metabolic syndrome. Women with high levels of stress had more than five times the risk of developing this condition.

More recent research suggests that Whitehall II men who reported higher justice at work (such as perceived job fairness) had a far lower risk of metabolic syndrome compared with men who experienced lower work justice (Gimeno et al., 2010). For women, stress encountered at work independently predicted type 2 diabetes, even after taking into socioeconomic position and stressors unrelated to work (Heraclides et al., 2009). Thus, maximizing workplace satisfaction, in addition to helping maintain worker productivity, can make a key difference in promoting the health and long-term well-being of the individual (Olsson et al., 2009).

## Connections Between Work and Family Roles

One of the great challenges of adult life is dividing your time, energy, and role involvement across your many commitments. The two areas many people find most difficult to integrate in terms of competing demands are their occupation alongside family life. Both carry with them major obligations and responsibility, and both contribute heavily to the individual's sense of identity. However, they do not necessarily need to be in conflict, as research is increasingly demonstrating.

According to the work-family enrichment model, experiences in one role improve the quality of life in the other. This model is based on the theory of conservation of resources, which proposes that organizations can protect their workers against stress by providing them with support to maintain both their work and family roles (Hobfoll, 2002).

There are five categories of resources people can acquire through their role experiences that can improve performance in the other area (Greenhaus & Powell, 2006). For example, parents may gain networking experience with other parents who help them on their job. Researchers also use the term "positive spillover" to describe this transfer of skills from one domain to the other (Masuda et al., 2012). Role experiences can be enriching through their effect on mood. If you have a good day at work, you bring your good mood home. In addition, employees who feel their work supports their ability to carry out their family roles feel more obligated to reciprocate with favorable attitudes toward their job and their company.

Using the work-family enrichment model, McNall and colleagues (McNall et al., 2010) examined the two directions of work-family enrichment: from work-to-family (WFE) and family-to-work (FWE). They considered variables such as job satisfaction, affective commitment (emotional attachment to the organization), turnover intentions, family satisfaction, life satisfaction, and physical/mental health. Both WFE and FWE were positively associated with the work-related outcomes of job satisfaction and affective commitment. WFE had a positive influence on the nonwork-related outcomes of family and life satisfaction. FWE had a positive association with family satisfaction. Both forms of enrichment were related to physical and mental health. The findings also showed stronger effects for women than men, reflecting the fact that women are more likely to integrate the two sets of roles (Whitbourne & Bookwala, 2015).

Alternatively, the work-family conflict model proposes that people have a fixed amount of time and energy to spend on their life roles. This model is based on a scarcity perspective (Edwards & Rothbard, 2000): the more time and energy people invest in one area, the less they have for the other set of demands and activities. The workaholic, according to this view, has little energy or time for family relationships. Conversely, high involvement with family should limit commitment to one's job.

When work-family conflict occurs, it takes causes emotional strain, fatigue, perception of overload, and stress (van Hooff et al., 2005). There are variations in the extent and impact of work-family conflict, however, and not all workers feel the same degree of conflict. Conflict is most likely to occur among mothers of young children, dual-career couples, and those who are highly involved with their job. Workers who devote a great deal of time to their job at the expense of their families ultimately pay the price in terms of experiencing a lower overall quality of life (Greenhaus et al., 2003).

Age also plays into the work-family conflict equation. Younger workers (under age 45) typically experience more conflict than older workers (age 46 and older); though when older workers experience conflict, the effects seem to be stronger (Matthews et al., 2010). Feelings of self-efficacy regarding the ability to manage competing work and family demands can play a role. Workers who feel they can navigate successfully and who feel good about maintaining a balance between these two worlds may have more favorable experiences in both realms (Tement, 2014). Organizations are increasingly recognizing the importance of providing a "family-friendly" environment, which may include support and schedule control (McNall et al., 2010). There are tangible benefits to these situations. When managers provide support to employees through policies such as accommodating work schedules, employees actually become more productive and less likely to leave the organization (Odle-Dusseau et al., 2012). In addition, when workers feel a strong sense of engagement with their jobs in family-friendly organizations, their work-family enrichment increases (Siu et al., 2010). Conversely, a strong family identity can promote feelings of satisfaction and commitment to the job (Wayne et al., 2006) Social support from an individual's workgroup also plays a role because many potentially positive or negative interactions at work involve coworkers (Bhave et al., 2010). Moreover, supervisors who themselves experience work-to-family enrichment promote similar outcomes in their subordinates.

# Later Life

## Biological Functioning

There is so much to be experienced during later life, especially if we maintain our good health. Still, like midlife, there are important things to be on the watch for. Declines in physical health and the increased prevalence of certain diseases must be considered. The importance of maintaining a healthy diet and staying physically active to the best of one's abilities cannot be emphasized enough.

**LO 11-1** **Explain why people tend to lose weight in their 60s and beyond.**

**LO 11-2** **Explain why urinary incontinence occurs for some in later life.**

**What Would You Do? Dana's Story**

I guess I'm having a hard time totally retiring but the desire is there. I had two different jobs to do for other people today, and I said to myself on the way out the door, "I thought I was going to retire." During the last few years at my job as a tour operator, I went from full time to 2 days a week, so I've cut back, but when you think about it, the job was seasonal work. It gave me 4 to 6 months off every year. If I worked 2 years total, I'd have a year off total, so that's semi-retired right there. The company I worked for started to change a bit though, and I did get tired of driving into the city. I wanted a little change.

Because I loved my job and the people I worked with, it was hard to leave. It's much easier if you don't love a job. And a lot of people find their personalities defined by their jobs, so when they give it up, they give up who they are. But I decided I wanted to do things for myself and other people, which had a lot to do with me cutting back. Even so, if you're really active and love working, it's hard to retire completely. For me, it's hard to sit still. It's my personality.

So today after a hectic start I said, "Wait a minute, I'm retired," and at 3 o'clock I stopped everything I was doing and took the boat out on the lake. My wife thinks I work too much, too. Yesterday she declared a holiday, so we took off, went up the mountain near our house, hiked, and had a wonderful day together. That's one of the glorious things; I don't have to work every minute now. I can have a day off because I'm not forced to work. Still I find myself working a little more than I want to.

My favorite thing to do is to go to a place I've never been. And so this is what my wife and I want to do with our retirement. Every year we're going to try to do some kind of mission trip with a Christian organization, whether it's helping in a foreign country or doing something in this country helping with hurricane or tornado victims. I don't want retirement to be all about myself. I want to be an encouragement for people. I want to drive friends to their doctors' appointments. I want to visit them if they're going through cancer treatment and talk to them. I want it to be about helping others and doing fun things. And so we'll do some traveling for ourselves. We have a bucket list of countries. Most recently we've been trying to figure out how to get to New Zealand. Next winter we may go to Cuba or to Montreal for a few days, and next spring we're thinking about renting a van and going up to Alaska. Where else do we want to go? Wherever we haven't been.

My wife and I have been dealt a good hand in life, but that doesn't mean the future won't be difficult and potentially

**LO 11-3 Compare the neuronal fallout model with the plasticity model in terms of changes in the brain.**

## Physical Changes

**Vision.** Older adults are likely to experience the loss of visual acuity, or the ability to see details at a distance. The level of acuity in an 85-year-old individual is approximately 80% less than that of a person in their 40s. Turning up the lights is one effective strategy to compensate for loss of acuity, but at the same time older adults are more sensitive to glare. For example, older drivers are more vulnerable to the glare caused by the lights of oncoming traffic on a dark road at night or the light of the setting sun shining directly on the windshield. Making lights brighter may actually impair rather than improve an older person's visual acuity. In addition to experiencing normal age-related changes in vision, older people become increasingly vulnerable to visual disorders. In fact, about one half of adults over the age of 65 report they have experienced some form of visual impairment. Common impairments include **cataracts**, a clouding or opacity in the lens that results in blurred or distorted vision because the retina cannot clearly focus the images; **age-related macular degeneration**, caused by damage to the photoreceptors in the macula, the central region of the retina used in reading, driving, and other visually demanding activities; and **glaucoma**, a group of conditions that lead to blindness due to the destruction of the neurons leading from the retina to the optic nerve by increased pressure inside the eyeball.

FIGURE 11-1

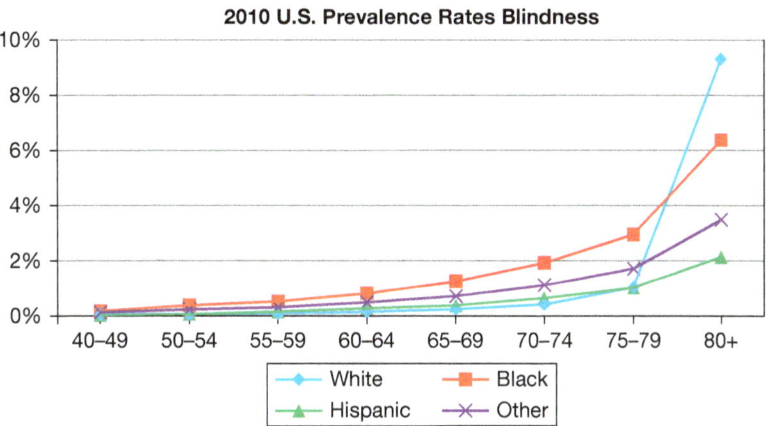


*Source*: National Eye Institute, https://nei.nih.gov/eyedata/blind.

**Hearing.** Age-related hearing loss occurs progressively during later adulthood. The most common form of age-related hearing loss is **presbycusis**, which is associated with loss of high-pitched sounds. The loss is continuous across increasingly older ages (Allen & Eddins, 2010). Another hearing disturbance that is relatively common in older people is **tinnitus**, a condition in which the individual perceives sounds in the head or ear (such as a ringing noise) when there is no external source of the sound. Hearing aids can help adults with hearing loss overcome many hearing-related problems. Given increasing improvements in the quality of hearing aids, as well as reductions in their size, people no longer need to rely on devices that are clearly visible to others. Miniature devices considerably reduce the social stigma many associate with the need to wear a hearing aid in older adulthood. They are also more effective, and particularly because people are more likely to use them given they are small and generally out of sight.

Hearing loss clearly has an effect on the older adult's ability to engage in conversation (Murphy et al., 2006). In turn, older adults may be more likely to avoid potentially noisy

filled with some tough times. A wise person once said, "Life is like a box of chocolates; you never know what you're going to get." The older you get the more you think about what the future will bring, because you're on the sled going down the back side of the hill, and the sled is accelerating. As you get older you think about these things a lot. Am I going to die first; will my wife go to go first? And these thoughts, you don't have many of these thoughts when you're 45. So you start thinking about your beliefs and I'm glad that I have my faith and my religion, and I count my blessings, but I also think about what would it be like if I were in a wheelchair. I thank God for the good times in my life. If we died tomorrow, my wife and I have lived a full wonderful life. And we've rolled an awful lot into 70 years when I think about some of the things we've done and where we've been, and we're still rolling.

During my off months at the tour company, we would always take off to a foreign country. We've gone many places without knowing the language, figuring out the best things to see, and take it on for 2 and 3 months at a time. Despite the fact that we're 70, I think our only limitation is not knowing the language in some places; you still can communicate with people but maybe not to the depth you would if you spoke the same language. You just have to smile a lot.

I don't feel any physical limitations now but some of us guys tend to live on the edge. There was one occasion when we were hiking and I felt some pressure in my arms. When I got back home and told my doctor, he said, "You know, maybe you shouldn't hike." But I think I know my body better than my cardiologist in some ways. So when we were in Peru and at 13,000 feet altitude, I told myself I'd stop if I felt pressure, but I didn't, so I went on another 2,000 feet. When we were in Thailand and we slept on hard, one-quarter-inch thick mattresses, I could feel my bad hips. But usually the only time I feel them is when I travel. We don't let it stop us.

I've also learned that when I get back, all this traveling makes me appreciate home and my family even more. There was one time when we were traveling in Thailand over the Thanksgiving holiday and video messaging our family at the Thanksgiving dinner table. I said then and there that I don't want to spend another holiday away from family.

I've learned there is spectacular beauty in every country and every group of people we've ever seen or met. I've learned that I love adventure. I love meeting new people. I love eating different foods. And I'm fortunate that I married a woman who likes adventure. We've learned how to travel together over the years. When we first traveled we learned to make concessions because I'd want to go in one direction and she'd want to go in another, but we solved it because we want to be together. So now we take turns. One day we do what I want to do. The next day we do what she wants to do, and the next day we rest. I actually really enjoy being with my wife at these times, because remember it's not a vacation, it's an adventure. Our traveling is an adventure. And as a side note, I don't think there's anyone on the face of this Earth who could travel with us.

There is such an education in traveling. We have learned so much about different countries and people and cultures. Despite the fact that I'm 70 years old, I'm still learning things. People are so different and they're worth studying. I love seeing how different people and cultures live and react to things. I think if you can live with the people, not stay at a big hotel, but stay with these people for a week and learn what their culture's like, that's where it's at. I've learned that you can go to places like Mexico and Costa Rica and Peru and meet people who may have so much less "stuff" than we do, but they're just as happy if not happier. And they don't think they've been dealt a bad hand.

One thing I've learned is that lots of people I've met along the way do things or think things that, to me, are strange, but then I realize, I'm probably strange to them. I love going to different places. Other people will go to the same place for 20 years, because they don't like change. They want to open the chocolate and know exactly what they're going to get. Me? I'd rather have 150 chocolates. You get a couple bad ones, who cares? And I know in the future that if I bite into a bad chocolate I'll have my faith and my family right there for me. So it's okay.

situations, such as eating at a restaurant. Yet even without a hearing aid, however, it's possible for older adults with hearing impairments to improve their ability to understand speech if they take advantage of various communication strategies. The first is to look directly at the person speaking to them and to make sure that there is enough light so they can clearly see the person's face. Older adults may also turn down background noise that can interfere with the audio stream they are trying to follow, whether it's another person, the television, or the radio. At restaurants and social gatherings, they may wish to find a place to talk that is as far away as possible from crowded or noisy areas. They may also ask the people speaking to them not to chew food or gum while talking and not to speak too quickly (Janse, 2009).

When talking to an older adult (with or without hearing loss), many people tend to overcompensate and raise their voices unnecessarily high, but this interferes with the speech signal. It is important for the speaker to enunciate clearly, speak in a low tone (to offset presbycusis), and look straight at the older adult. Most importantly, if you're the speaker, you should avoid talking to the person as if he or she were a child. This includes referring to the individual in the third person or leaving the person out of the conversation altogether (based on the assumption that they can't hear). Providing context is useful because this gives additional cues to the listener about the topic of conversation. You can gauge whether you are understood by paying careful attention to how the other person is responding to you, both verbally and nonverbally. Finally, rather than becoming frustrated or upset with the listener, maintaining a positive and patient attitude will encourage the listener to remain more engaged in the conversation.

Think about what you would do in this situation after reading the chapter, and then decide the following:

- If you were Dana, would you have a similar approach to retirement and aspects of later life, such as mortality? Why or why not?
- If you were Dana, would your attitude about your physical limitations differ?
- If you were Dana's doctor, how would you counsel him on his leisure activities that may put a strain on his physical health?

**Skin.** We expect to see further changes in the skin, much like what we discussed in the previous chapter, including the thinning of skin, the development of age spots, and varicose veins. Medications that older adults may be taking can also affect the hair, skin, and nails, further exacerbating changes due to the aging process. **Actinic purpura** is the more noticeable and severe-looking bruising we see in older adults that are often due to only minor bumps. Actinic purpura occurs as a result of cumulative sun damage over time. This leads to the fine capillaries of sun-exposed skin, typically on the forearms and legs, to be more fragile and easily broken. Many older adults develop fungal infections in their toenails, causing the nails to thicken and separate from the nail bed. Older adults with limited joint movement and flexibility experience more difficulty caring for their own feet and lower extremities (Mitty, 2009).

**FIGURE 11-2** Skin features of older adults.

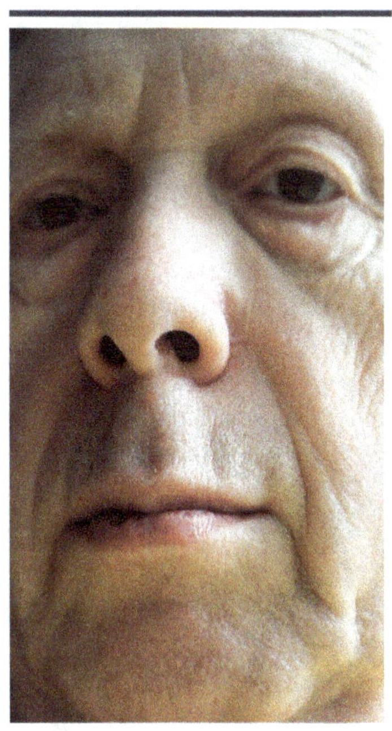

*Source*: https://www.publicdomainpictures.net/en/view-image.php?image=184094&picture=sad-man.

**Teeth.** In the United States, roughly 26% of adults over the age of 65 have lost all their natural teeth (Schoenborn & Heyman, 2009). These rates double for those in lower income brackets or without private medical insurance. To prevent tooth decay, the National Institute of Dental and Craniofacial Research (2019) recommends that adults use fluoride toothpaste, brush twice daily, floss regularly, and maintain routine dental checkups.

**Body build.** For most people, when they lose body weight in their 60s and beyond, it's not due to a loss of body fat but to a loss of muscle. Older adults lose pounds because they suffer a reduction of **fat free mass** (FFM), or all the components of your body that are not fat. This includes muscle, bone, connective tissue, and water. The loss of FFM and sarcopenia, or the loss of muscle mass, can occur even if a person maintains high levels of activity (Manini et al., 2009). Some older adults, however, continue to gain weight as they age to the point of developing a body mass index (BMI) that places them in the overweight or obese classifications. Between the mid-1990s and mid-2000s, the percentage of older adults classified as overweight increased from 60 to 69%, and as obese from 22 to 31% (Houston et. al., 2009).

As we continue to highlight, many of the effects of aging on body build and composition can be countered by exercise. On the basis of extensive research on both short- and long-term exercise benefits, the American College of Sports Medicine and the American Heart Association (ACSM/AHA) (Chodzko-Zajko et al., 2009) both recommend specific amounts and forms of exercise for older adults. The ACSM/AHA states that the intensity and duration of physical activity should be low at the start for older adults who are functionally limited or who have chronic conditions that affect their ability to perform physical tasks. The progression of activities should be tailored to the individual and strength and/or balance training may need to precede aerobic training until the individual gains some strength to be able to perform aerobic exercise.

Even if a person is unable to engage in the minimum amount of activity, they should perform some type of physical activity to avoid being sedentary. For example, older adults who have impaired balance and mobility can be given chair aerobics to perform, such as raising and lowering their arms. Individuals who have mobility problems or are frequent fallers can be given balance training that includes progressively difficult postures, dynamic movements—such as turning in circles, heel stands, toe stands—and standing with their eyes closed.

**Mobility and strength.** Loss of muscle mass can lead to negative consequences, including increased risk of falling, limitations in mobility, and reduced quality of everyday life. Unfortunately, sarcopenia can become part of a vicious cycle: the greater the loss of muscle mass, the greater the difficulty a person has undertaking exercise, which leads to more muscle loss and greater weakening (Lang et al., 2009). If sarcopenia occurs in the presence of gains in fat, a condition known as **sarcopenic obesity** may develop, in which the individual both loses muscle and gains body fat (Zamboni et al., 2008). Strength training with free weights or resistance machines is the top preventative measure in counteracting the process of sarcopenia in adulthood (Sanchis-Gomar et al., 2014). Although older adults do not achieve as high a degree of improvement as younger adults, even a program including resistance training that's as short as 16 weeks can build certain muscle fiber numbers to match those found in young adults (Kosek et al., 2006). There seems to be no age limit on who can benefit from this type of exercise, as adults in their 90s also show improvements in muscle strength after training (Kryger & Andersen, 2007).

Effective muscle strength training typically involves 8 to 12 weeks, three to four times per week, using multiple repetitions of weights that are 70 to 90% that of the most weight a person can do in one repetition. For these benefits to be maintained, the individual has to keep exercising. It's not enough to exercise for a year or two and then stop. Aerobic exercise can provide additional benefits to boost the effects of muscle training (Harber et al., 2009).

One of the major benefits of muscle training is that the stronger muscles become, the more pull they exert on the bones, which contributes to bone strength. Loss of bone strength is an equally significant limitation on the health and well-being of older adults. Estimates of the decrease in bone mineral content over adulthood are about 0.5% per year for males and 1% per year for females (Emaus et al., 2006), although the rates become higher for females as they age, 3 to 5% per year (Ferrucci et al., 2014). Further weakening occurs because of microcracks that develop in response to stress placed on the bones (Diab et al., 2006). Part of the older bone's increased susceptibility to fracture can be accounted for by a loss of collagen, which reduces the bone's flexibility in response to (Saito & Marumo, 2009). The problem is particularly severe for the upper part of the thigh bone right below the hip, which does not receive much mechanical pressure during walking and therefore tends to thin disproportionately (Mayhew et al., 2005).

People lose bone at varying rates as the result of a number of causes. Genetic factors are estimated to account for as much as 70% of bone mineral content in adulthood (Ferrari & Rizzoli, 2005). Consequently, not all older adults experience loss of bone mineral. In fact, one longitudinal study of aging and bone mineral density showed a subset of older adult females showed no significant bone loss (Cauley et al., 2009).

These changes in body mass lead to changes in mobility, such as walking speed. Older adults may find it hard to adapt to a slower walking speed, leading them to be more likely than younger people to make mistakes when predicting how long it will take them to cross the street (Lobjois & Cavallo, 2009). Thus, these changes have far-reaching consequences on the older adult's life and health.

**Balance.** The **vestibular system** includes parts of the inner ear and the brain and helps process information from the environment so we can maintain our balance. Two symptoms frequently associated with age-related vestibular dysfunction are dizziness and vertigo. Dizziness is an uncomfortable sensation of feeling light-headed and even floating. Vertigo refers to the sensation of spinning when the body is at rest.

Because the vestibular system is so intimately connected to other parts of the nervous system, people may experience symptoms of vestibular disturbances that result in headaches, muscular aches in the neck and back, and increased sensitivity to noise and bright lights. Other symptoms include fatigue, inability to concentrate, unsteadiness while walking, and difficulty with speech. Increased sensitivity to motion sickness is another common symptom. Some of these changes may come about with diseases that are not part of normal aging; others may occur as the result of normative alterations in the vestibular receptors. People who are more likely to fall have compromised balance, are weaker, have an impaired gait, are more likely to be on medications, and have a history of previous falls (Tinetti & Kumar, 2010). Older individuals who have more difficulty detecting body position are more likely to lose their balance or fail to see a step or an obstacle in their path on a level surface.

Exercise can help older adults learn to compensate for factors that increase their chance of falling (Kim et al., 2010). The most beneficial forms of exercise include learning how to step with assistance (Hanke & Tiberio, 2006) and strengthening the leg muscles (Takahashi et al., 2006). Tai chi can help older adults improve their balance and lessen the likelihood of falling (Harmer & Li, 2008). People who are concerned about falling should also cut back on medications they may take for other conditions that can cause confusion or disorientation (Kannus et al., 2005).

**Pain.** The question of whether older adults are more or less sensitive to pain is a topic of considerable concern for health practitioners. Changes in pain perception with age could make life either much harder or much easier for individuals with illnesses (such as arthritis) that cause chronic pain.

There is no evidence that older adults become somehow immune to or at least protected from pain by virtue of age changes in this sensory system. Most older adults are able to maintain regular functioning despite the presence of chronic pain. However, as one would expect, the pain makes it more difficult for them to carry out their everyday activities (Covinsky et al., 2009).

Psychological factors may also interact with the experience of pain in older adults. Symptoms of benign pain may diminish along the aging process because older adults have become habituated to the daily aches and pains associated with changes in their bones, joints, and muscles. It is also possible that cohort factors interact with intrinsic age changes to alter the likelihood that complaints about pain will be expressed. The experience of pain is associated with the personality trait of stoicism (the tendency to suffer in silence) (Yong, 2006). Older adults may simply not wish to admit to others, or even themselves, that they are feeling some of those aches and pains. This tendency to deny pain may be more likely to occur among older adults who ascribe more strongly to negative aging stereotypes (Bernardes et al., 2015).

People can reduce their risk of pain in later adulthood can by controlling for factors related to greater pain prevalence. Obesity is highly associated with chronic pain even after controlling for education and related conditions such as diabetes, hypertension, arthritis, and depression (McCarthy et al., 2009). Thus, weight management would seem to be an important and effective intervention. At the same time, rather than relying on pain medications alone, which carries the risk of abuse and/or interactions with treatments for other conditions, it is advisable that older adults learn to manage their pain through holistic methods that consider biological, psychological, and social factors (McCleane, 2007).

**Temperature control.** An older adult is generally less able to adjust their internal bodily temperature, even under normal conditions. This is because sweat output is reduced, which causes a person's core temperature to rise (Dufour & Candas, 2007). Adding to this is the fact that the dermal layer of the skin becomes thinner as we age, making it more difficult to cool the skin (Petrofsky et al., 2009).

**Touch.** Well-established evidence supports a link between aging and the loss of the ability to discriminate touch. Research shows age differences in the ability to differentiate the separation of two points of pressure on the skin and the detection of the location of a stimulus applied to the skin. One estimate places the loss at 1% per year from age 20 to 80. However, the rate of loss varies according to body part. The hands and feet are particularly susceptible to the effects of aging compared with centrally located areas, including the lips and tongue. These losses can compromise the ability to grasp, maintain balance, and perform delicate handwork and can interfere with speech (Wickremaratchi & Llewelyn, 2006).

**Smell and taste.** Approximately one third of all adults over the age of 65 suffer some form of olfactory impairment (Shu et al., 2009) with almost half of those age 80 and older having virtually no ability to smell at all (Lafreniere & Mann, 2009). The loss of olfactory receptors reflects intrinsic changes associated with the aging process, as well as damage caused by disease, injury, or exposure to toxins. In fact, environmental toxins may play a larger role in olfactory impairment than changes due to the aging process. And chronic diseases, medications, and sinus problems may be more significant sources of impairment than age itself over the life span (Rawson, 2006).

Tobacco smoke is a major cause taste and smell impairments. Although people who quit smoking eventually experience an improvement in their sense of smell, this can take many years (equal to the number of years spent smoking). Dentures are another cause of loss of taste sensitivity, given they may block the receptor cells of the taste buds. Certain medications also interfere with taste disorders (Schiffman, 2009). However, it is difficult to determine whether aging brings with it inherent changes in taste.

Some believe cognitive changes are associated with a loss of smell sensitivity. Older adults who experience the greatest levels of cognitive impairment may also be the most vulnerable to loss of odor identification abilities. In one longitudinal study that followed older adults over a 3-year period, researchers observed that those with the most rapid decline in cognitive processes had the greatest rate of decline in the ability to label various odors (Wilson et al., 2006).

Although nothing can be done to reverse age-related losses of smell and taste once they occur, people who suffer from severe losses may benefit from medical evaluations and treatments for underlying conditions (Welge-Lussen, 2009). Apart from such interventions, older people can also take advantage of strategies to enhance the enjoyment of food, such as expanding their food choices, planning meals in pleasant environments, and finding good dining partners.

## Vital Bodily Functions

**Cardiovascular system.** Exercise helps maximize the heart's functioning, and it can counteract the increased stiffness of the arteries that can occur over time. In one training study, a simple program of daily walking for 12 weeks was sufficient to have beneficial effects on health (Teichtahl et al., 2009). Other short-term training studies further reinforce conclusions about the value of exercise for both middle-aged and older adults (Chodzko-Zajko et al., 2009). To be maximally effective, exercise must stimulate a person's heart rate to 60 to 75% of maximum capacity, and should occur three to four times a week. People benefit from many forms of aerobic activities, including walking, hiking, jogging, bicycling, swimming, and jumping rope. However, even moderate or low-intensity exercise can have positive effects on sedentary older people (Whitbourne, 2001).

**Respiratory system.** The normal age-related changes contribute to **lung age**, which is a mathematical function showing how old your lungs are based on a combination of your age and a measure obtained from a spirometer called forced expiratory volume. By calculating lung age, individuals can understand the extent to which they place themselves at risk by engaging in behaviors such as smoking that are known to compromise respiratory function.

If you want to minimize the effects of aging on your lungs there are two main strategies to follow. The first may be the most obvious—stay away from or quit smoking cigarettes. People who smoke lose more forced expiratory volume in later adulthood than those who do not (Yohannes & Tampubolon, 2014). Of course, it is better to quit smoking than to continue smoking; still there are deleterious changes in the body's cells that remain for at least several decades after a person has quit smoking (Masayesva et al., 2006).

It may come as little surprise that the other lifestyle changes involve diet and exercise. Researchers have determined that obesity is related to poor respiratory functioning (Harrington & Lee-Chiong, 2009). Exercise, even in people who have never exercised before, can strengthen the muscles of the chest wall, and, in the process, compensate at least in part for lost elasticity of lung tissue (Abrahin et al., 2014).

**Urinary system.** Researchers once believed kidney function inevitably declined steadily due to loss of nephrons over time. Remember nephrons are the kidney cells that filter metabolic waste from the blood. However, the jury is still out on this question. There do appear to be age differences in kidneys (Lerma, 2009), but many factors other than age can compromise nephrons, for example cigarette smoking. This can lead to serious kidney disease in older adults with other risk factors (Stengel et al., 2000), perhaps through its effect on changes within the nephron's ability to filter wastes (Elliot et al., 2006). Older studies may have exaggerated estimates of the effects of normal aging on the kidneys, reflecting instead the fact that a large percentage of the population smoked cigarettes for much of their adult lives. However, this doesn't account for the entire effect of age on the kidneys. Illness, extreme exertion, and extreme heat all serve as stresses that greatly compromise the kidneys' and bladder's ability to do their jobs that can lead to incontinence (Fuiano et al., 2001). According to one estimate (Anger et al., 2006), for females the prevalence of daily incontinence ranges from 12% in those age 60 to 64 to 21% in those age 85 or older. Of those reporting incontinence, 14% experience it on a daily basis and 10% on a weekly basis. Among the risk factors for urge incontinence in females are being of White race; having diabetes treated with insulin; experiencing symptoms of depression; and currently using estrogen (Jackson et al., 2004).

**Digestive system.** You've no doubt heard about digestive aids, such as treatments for heartburn (acid reflux), gas, bloating, and bowel irregularity. Surprisingly though, the reality is most older people do not experience significant compromises in their ability to digest food. Still, there are physiological changes to consider. Changes in the esophagus are relatively minor (Achem & Devault, 2005), as are changes (for people in good health) in the stomach and lower digestive tract (Bharucha & Camilleri, 2001). There are decreases in saliva production (Eliasson et al., 2006); fewer gastric juices are secreted; and the stomach empties more slowly in older adults (O'Donovan et al., 2005). There are also decreases in liver volume and blood flow through the liver (Serste & Bourgeois, 2006). However, these changes vary tremendously from person to person, in part because of variations in one's overall health status (Drozdowski & Thomson, 2006). Smoking status and medications also affect digestive system functioning in older adults (Greenwald, 2004).

Fecal incontinence affects only 4% of the population over the age of 65 (Alameel et al., 2010). Though rare, it is certainly troubling when it occurs. One individual described it as "trying to control the daily life that is out of control" (Olsson et al., 2009, p. 141). As is true with urinary incontinence, behavioral control training can help manage the condition (Byrne et al., 2007). Increasing the amount of fiber in one's diet can also help older adults maintain bowel regularity and prevent incontinence (Markland et al., 2009).

In general, the best way for older adults to maintain their digestive health is to eat a diet that includes a balance among foods containing protein, complex carbohydrates, and fats.

**Endocrine system.** Changes in the endocrine system continue across older adulthood, affecting several areas. Recall our discussion of basal metabolic rate, or BMR in the previous chapter. Changes in BMR over adulthood are at least in part related to age-related decreases in thyroid hormones (Meunier et al., 2005). Subclinical hypothyroidism can affect as many as 15 to 18% of adults over the age of 60 (Diez & Iglesias, 2004) and can be associated with cognitive impairment (Hogervorst et al., 2008).

A decline in growth hormone (GH) activity, called **somatopause**, is thought to account for a number of age-related changes in body composition across adulthood, including increases in fat tissue and bad cholesterol levels, decreases in bone mineral content and muscle mass and losses in strength, exercise tolerance, and general quality of life (Lombardi et al., 2005). Age differences exist in the activity of GH. In young people, GH production shows regularly timed peaks during nighttime sleep; in older adults, this peak is smaller, a pattern that may contribute to the changes we see over time (Espiritu, 2008). GH also rises during exercise, but this response is weaker in adults age 60 and older (Weltman et al., 2006).

It appears increases in cortisol negatively affect memory and other forms of cognitive functioning in older adults (Comijs et al., 2010); the glucocorticoid cascade hypothesis contends that aging causes dangerous increases in cortisol levels (Angelucci, 2000). According to this view, increased cortisol levels accelerate the loss of neurons in the hippocampus, and repeated (cascading) increases in cortisol over the time lead to further degeneration. This is called into question, though, by a fascinating study in which older and younger adults were compared on the relation between hippocampal volume and cortisol levels under differing conditions of environmental stress. It was only when testing conditions were stressful for an individual's particular age group that the relation appeared (Sindi et al., 2014). This suggests environmental stress and not aging contributes to differences we see in age groups on hippocampal volume.

Some believe changes in circadian rhythms that occur throughout middle and later adulthood correspond to declines in melatonin production across adulthood (Mahlberg et al., 2006). There is the belief that melatonin supplements reduce the effects of aging and age-associated diseases, especially in the brain and immune system. It is true melatonin supplements for females can lead to improved pituitary and thyroid functions (Bellipanni et al., 2001) and reduce sleep problems (Gubin et al., 2006). However, melatonin use can produce significant side effects including confusion, drowsiness, headaches, and constriction of blood vessels (which is dangerous for those with high blood pressure). Typical dosages in over-the-counter medications may be as high as 40 times the amount normally found in the body, and the effects of large doses taken long term are unknown (National Library of Medicine, 2010).

In addition to concerns about safety, melatonin supplements can interfere with sleep cycles if taken at the wrong time of day. If older adults nevertheless wish to take melatonin supplements, they are advised to take amounts as small as possible to mimic normal physiological circadian rhythms (Vural et al., 2014).

**Immune system.** The two primary types of immune cells found in the blood are "T cells" and "B cells," both of which are involved in destroying bodily invaders known as antigens. Researchers believe that there are widespread age-related declines in immune system functioning, a process known as **immune senescence**. As a result of immune senescence, these cells lose their ability to perform effectively, causing older adults to be less resistant to infections (Grubeck-Loebenstein, 2010). Therefore, although children are more likely to develop an influenza infection during flu season, mortality from such a disease occurs almost entirely among older adults unless the flu virus was one to which the older adult was exposed as a child or young adult. Conversely, other cells in the immune system show certain damaging changes, including those associated with age-related chronic diseases (Valiathan et al., 2016).

**FIGURE 11-3** A T helper cell in the immune system.

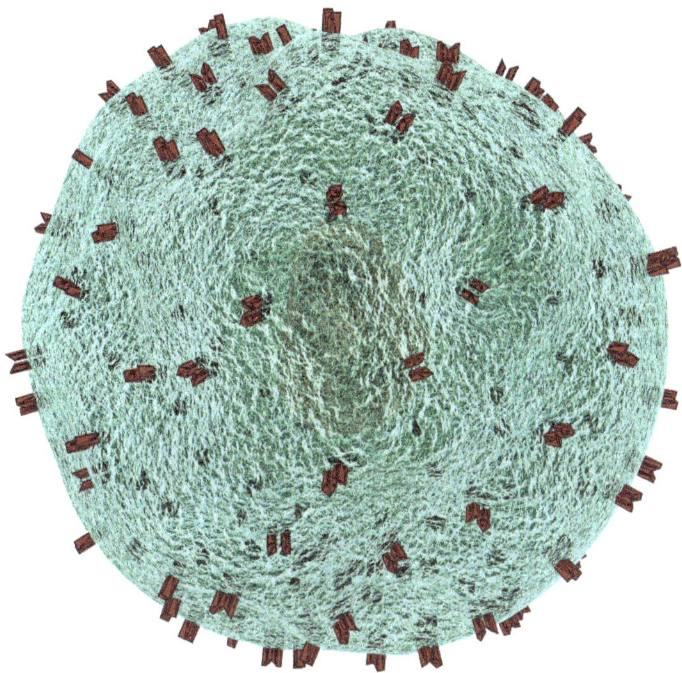

*Source*: https://pixabay.com/en/t-helper-cell-cell-immune-system-1123292/.

Age-related changes in the immune system may be affected by diet, exercise, and exposure to stress. Zinc is an important nutrient related to the functioning of the immune system, and decreases in zinc intake can therefore exacerbate immune senescence (Maywald & Rink, 2015). Similarly, deficient protein intake can lower immune functioning in older adults (Aoi, 2009). Obesity in later life can negatively also alter immune functioning and accelerate harmful changes (Garg et al., 2014), but lifetime patterns of high-intensity exercise can offset age-related declines in immune system functioning in later adulthood (Moro-Garcia et al., 2014). Chronic stress also has deleterious effects on the immune system and can therefore accelerate its rate of aging, whether experienced later in life (Gouin et al., 2008) or during early development (Dich et al., 2015). Furthermore, older adults who are clinically depressed may be more likely to experience more pronounced rates of immune senescence (Vogelzangs et al., 2014).

There may be some protective mechanisms not completely understood at present that help maintain the immune functioning of certain healthy agers. For example, studies of centenarians show that some of the basic cells in the immune system were as healthy in this hardy group of older adults as in young adults (Alonso-Fernandez et al., 2008).

### Theory Then and Now

**Theory then:** The **neuronal fallout model** contended individuals progressively lose brain tissue over the life span because neurons do not have the ability to replace themselves when they die. This model was based on data from autopsy studies in which neuroanatomists counted the number of neurons in the brains of people of different ages. These studies did not always take into account the cause of death, the fact that brain tissue may be destroyed after death by the methods used to study it, and the possible diseases that the individuals suffered from while alive. All these factors may have biased the results and caused an exaggerated picture of the extent to which nerve cell populations change later in life.

**Theory now:** Newer findings present a more optimistic view of the effect of aging on the nervous system. It now seems clear that in the absence of disease, the aging brain maintains much of its structure and function. Not only that, it is possible that neurons may actually gain in both structure and function even until late in life. The **plasticity model** proposes that neurons that remain alive are able to take over the function of those that die (Goh & Park, 2009).

Conflicting studies on aging and the immune system support the principle of interindividual variability in the aging process. This variability may reflect different samples being studied in addition to the fact that health, diet, and exercise, not to mention biological differences, all play a role in affecting the rates at which any one individual experiences immune system changes.

## Changes in the Brain

Extensive research has shown how aging affects the normal brain. The areas most affected include the prefrontal cortex, most involved in planning and the encoding of information into long-term memory, and the temporal cortex, involved in auditory processing (Fjell et al., 2009). In those over the age of 60, white matter hyperintensities, discussed in the previous chapter, seem to account for a significant amount of the variation in cognitive functioning (Vannorsdall et al., 2009). The hippocampus, the structure in the brain responsible for consolidating memories, becomes smaller with increasing age, although this decline is more pronounced in abnormal aging such as in Alzheimer's disease (Zhang et al., 2009). Nevertheless, evidence exists in support of the plasticity model within the cells of the hippocampus (Lister & Barnes, 2009).

## Lifestyle and Health

**Cardiovascular disease.** Heart disease is the number one killer in the United States, resulting in 19% of all deaths in the year 2014. Together, heart disease and cerebrovascular disease, including various types of strokes, accounted for 25% of all deaths in the United States of people age 65 and older (Kochanek et al., 2016), making deaths from heart disease and stroke proportionately highest among the oldest segment of certain populations. In addition, heart disease accounts for 14% of all health expenditures, more than any other diagnostic group, with an estimated cost from 2012 to 2013 of $361 billion. Adding to this figure the cost of nursing home care, it rises to $396 billion, and by 2013 will be $918 billion (Benjamin et al., 2017). Cardiovascular disease is the leading cause of death worldwide, causing 17.7 million deaths in 2015, or 31% of all deaths (World Health Organization, n.d.).

There are four major risk factors for cardiovascular disease: smoking, excessive alcohol intake, a sedentary lifestyle, and an unhealthy diet.

Although it is not known exactly why smoking increases the risk of heart disease, most researchers believe the smoke itself damages the arteries, making them more vulnerable to plaque formation and leading to the harmful changes presented earlier. Though having long-lived parents is related to lower levels of cardiovascular risk, the benefits of heredity don't seem to help females who smoke (Jaunin et al., 2009). Excessive alcohol intake is another major risk factor for cardiovascular disease. This is partly because alcohol is high in calories, and in excess it damages the cardiovascular system and the brain.

A sedentary lifestyle is the next major risk factor for heart disease. There is a well-established relation between exercise and heart disease (Yung et al., 2009), with estimates ranging from a 24% reduction in the risk of myocardial infarction among individuals engaging in nonstrenuous exercisers to a 47% reduced risk among those engaging in a regular pattern of strenuous exercise (Lovasi et al., 2007). In addition to aerobic exercise, muscle strengthening is essential to a healthy lifestyle. As it happens, the majority of adults at highest risk for heart disease (i.e., those 75 and older) are the least likely to exercise. Only 12% of people age 65 and older met the U.S. government's recommendations for aerobic activity and muscle strengthening and 59% met neither criteria for these two healthy categories of physical activity (Centers for Disease Control and Prevention, 2017a).

An unhealthy diet places a person at risk for developing a BMI in the overweight or obese range. An analysis of 57 longitudinal studies conducted in Western Europe and North America showed a causal relation between a high BMI and mortality due to vascular disease (Whitlock et al., 2009; Whitbourne & Whitbourne, 2012). According to the Centers for Disease Control and Prevention (CDC, 2017a), dramatic increases in the number of overweight and obese individuals have occurred among United States adults over the past 20 years. Currently, 36% of the U.S. population is considered obese by government standards. This is far higher than the worldwide rate of adult obesity, which is 13% (World Health Organization, 2020).

**COPD.** The main form of respiratory disease affecting adults in middle and late life is **chronic obstructive pulmonary disease** (COPD), a group of diseases that involves obstruction of the airflow into the respiratory system. Two related diseases—chronic bronchitis and chronic emphysema—often occur together in this disease. People with COPD experience coughing, excess sputum, and difficulty breathing even when they carry out relatively easy tasks, such as putting on their clothes or walking on level ground. According to the World Health Organization (2017c), 5% of all deaths globally are due to COPD, with more than 90% of deaths occurring in low- and middle-income countries.

Although the exact cause of COPD is unknown, most who study the disease generally agree a significant contributor is cigarette smoking. Exposure to environmental toxins such as air pollution and harmful substances in certain work environments may also be contributing causes. The specific mechanism in the link between smoking and emphysema is thought to involve an enzyme known as **elastase**, which breaks down the elastin found in lung tissue. Cigarette smoke stimulates the release of elastase and results in other changes that make the cells of the lung less resistant to elastase. Normally there is an inhibitor of elastase found in the lung that minimizes its impact known as alpha-1 antitrypsin (AAT). However, cigarette smoke also inactivates AAT and allows elastase to destroy more lung tissue.

Of course, not all smokers develop COPD, and not all people with COPD are or have been smokers. Heredity may also play a role. There is a rare genetic defect in the production of AAT in about 2 to 3% of the population that is responsible for about 5% of all cases of COPD. For smokers, quitting is a necessary first step in prevention and management of COPD. At the same time, individuals with COPD can additionally benefit from medications and treatments. These include inhalers that open airways to bring more oxygen into the lungs or reduce inflammation, machines that provide oxygen, or, in extreme cases, lung surgery to remove damaged tissue.

**Diabetes.** A large portion of the population age 65 and older (an estimated 11.2 million or approximately 25% of adults in this age category) suffers from type 2 diabetes (Centers for Disease Control and Prevention, 2020). Black females aged 65 to 74 have the highest rates of diabetes among the adult U.S. population. The highest rates of diabetes in the world are found among Native Americans. Half of all Pima Indians living in the United States have adult-onset diabetes. Having diabetes doubles a person's risk of death compared with others in one's own age group who don't have diabetes. Rates of type 2 diabetes among children due to the increase in childhood obesity rate will no doubt have important health implications for future generations of older adults.

**Musculoskeletal diseases.** **Arthritis** is included in a group of musculoskeletal diseases and is a general term for conditions affecting the joints and surrounding tissues that can cause pain, stiffness, and swelling in joints and other connective tissues. **Osteoarthritis**, the most common form of arthritis in older adults, affects joints in the hips, knees, neck, and lower back. Many active forms of treatment for osteoarthritis are increasingly available. One approach is via an injection of a synthetic material into an arthritic joint to replace lost synovial fluid, which reduces friction between joint cartilage so joints can move more smoothly and easily. Another option is an injection of sodium hyaluronate directly into the joint, which also acts as a lubricant.

When treatments no longer produce relief, the individual with osteoarthritis may undergo the total replacement of the affected joint. Although hip or knee replacement surgery may seem like a drastic measure, it is one that typically proves highly satisfactory. Following surgery, many individuals can lead pain-free lives and resume some of their former activities. Exercise also helps reduce the pain of osteoarthritis, particularly when the disease is in its early stages (Kujala, 2009). The best exercises for osteoarthritis will strengthen the muscles around the joint and stretch the tendons (Verweij et al., 2009). Swimming is a great form of exercise that can offset pain and the limitations of osteoarthritis (Alkatan et al., 2016). Osteoarthritis can be worsened by obesity, so exercise programs that focus on weight loss can be helpful for these individuals. Exercise can also help alleviate mood symptoms associated with the chronic pain that often accompanies osteoarthritis.

**FIGURE 11-4** Normal bone compared to osteoporosis.

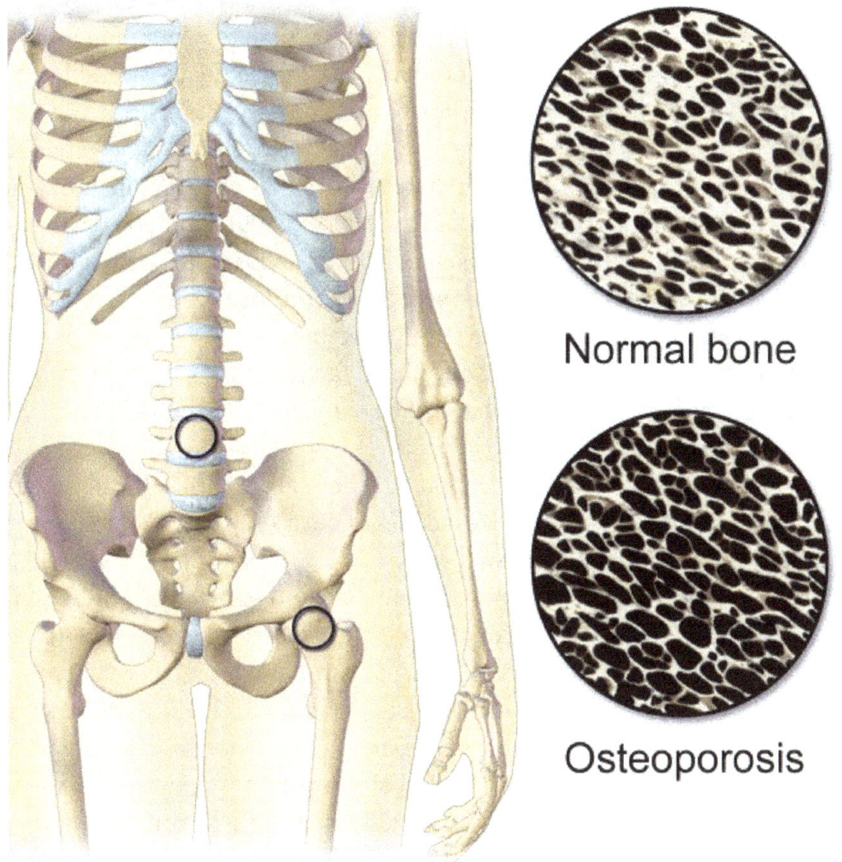


*Source*: Copyright © BruceBlaus (CC BY-SA 4.0) at https://commons.wikimedia.org/wiki/File:Osteoporosis_Locations.png.

As discussed earlier, people steadily lose bone mineral content throughout adulthood. These losses are due to an imbalance between the rates of bone resorption (a breakdown on bone tissue and loss of calcium in the bone) versus bone growth. This can result in bones becoming weak and brittle, a condition known as **osteoporosis** (literally, "porous bone"). As many as 8 million females and

2 million males in the United States suffer from osteoporosis. Females (particularly postmenopausal females) are at higher risk than males of developing osteoporosis because they have lower bone mass in general. However, osteoporosis is still a significant health problem in males. Females vary by race and ethnicity in their risk of developing osteoporosis; White females are twice as likely (15.8%) as Black females (7.7%) to have osteoporosis; Mexican American females have the highest rates of all subgroups (20.4%). About half of all females and 35% of all males age 50 and older in the United States have low bone mass (Wright et al., 2015). In addition, females who have small bone structures and who are underweight have a higher risk for osteoporosis than heavier females.

Excessive alcohol use and a history of cigarette smoking increase an individual's risk of osteoporosis. People can reduce their risk with diets containing adequate amounts of calcium present in dairy products, dark-green leafy vegetables, tofu, salmon, and foods fortified with calcium such as orange juice, bread, and cereal (similar to recommended diets to prevent heart disease). Other dietary measures include eating foods high in protein and nutrients such as magnesium, potassium, vitamin K, several B vitamins, and carotenoids (Tucker, 2009). Vitamin D, in the form of exposure to sunlight (most dermatologists agree that 30 minutes of unprotected sun exposure, twice a week in the morning or afternoon, is sufficient) or as a dietary supplement, is another important preventative agent (Bischoff-Ferrari et al., 2009). Exercise and physical activity are also significant factors in reducing a person's risk of osteoporosis, particularly when that exercise involves resistance training with weights (Guadalupe-Grau et al., 2009).

Once an individual develops osteoporosis, there are a variety of medications that can slow or stop bone loss, increase bone density, and reduce fracture risk. Some medications, though, can have serious side effects, for example bone loss in the jaw. In severe cases, some people may have no choice but to take these medications. To minimize their side effects, such individuals can benefit from a "drug holiday" by taking a short amount of time off the medications, as the medications tend to have long-lasting effects (Villa et al., 2016). A deficiency of sex hormones, in both males and females, may contribute to osteoporosis; as discussed in the previous chapter, the risks of hormone replacement therapy need to be weighed against the gains in preserving bone health (Pietschmann et al., 2009). Interestingly, certain types of alcohol may be preventive for females. In a study of beer drinkers compared with those who drank no alcohol or other forms of alcohol, females who consumed beer had the lowest rates of osteoporosis, perhaps because beer contains dietary silicon, which can help promote bone regeneration (Rodella et al., 2014).

**Sleep.** The literature on sleep in adulthood clearly refutes a common myth about aging, namely that as people grow older they need less sleep. Regardless of age, everyone requires 7 to 9 hours of sleep a night (Ancoli-Israel & Cooke, 2005). However, sleeping 8 hours or more a night is associated with higher mortality risks and greater incidence of stroke in women (Chen et al., 2006). Unfortunately, sleep problems seem to affect up to one half of all older adults (Neikrug & Ancoli-Israel, 2009). In general, older adults have higher rates of sleep-wake disorders than do younger adults, and they are less able to adjust their sleep patterns to conditions such as jet lag and shift work (Duffy et al., 2015).

Older adults spend more time in bed relative to time spent asleep. They take longer to fall asleep, awaken more often during the night, lie in bed longer before rising, and have sleep that is shallower, more fragmented, and less efficient (Fetveit, 2009). Sleep patterns on an electroencephalogram (EEG) that measures electrical activity in the brain show some corresponding age alterations, including a rise in stage 1 sleep and a large decrease in both stage 4 and REM (rapid-eye movement) sleep (Kamel & Gammack, 2006). These changes occur even for people who are in excellent health.

Would you consider yourself an "early bird" or a "night owl"? Interestingly, it may be associated with the age group you fall into. At some point during middle to late adulthood, many people start to prefer working morning rather than later hours of the day and night. Adults over the age of 65 tend to classify themselves as "morning" people, whereas the large majority of younger adults classify themselves as "evening" people (Hasher et al., 2005). The circadian rhythms of older adults are shifted so they are slightly earlier than are those of young adults relative to clock time. This shift presumably occurs gradually throughout adulthood, along with changes in hormones that contribute to sleep-wake patterns.

# Psychological Functioning

Much of mainstream Western culture emphasizes loss and deficits when it comes to aging, not only physically, but psychologically as well. People can become preoccupied with the potential for memory loss and certain neurocognitive disorders that have the potential to accompany aging for some. We often fail to see that aging can coincide with increases in positivity and be affected by how we view ourselves and our identities across the life span.

**LO 11-4** **Describe the differences between Alzheimer's disease and other neurocognitive disorders.**

**LO 11-5** **Describe the link between identity processes and how we view aging during later life.**

**LO 11-6** **Identify some benefits of the use of positivity in later life.**

## Cognitive Perspective and Neurocognitive Disorders

**Memory and health-related behaviors.** There are several health-related behaviors, such as diet and exercise, related to the functioning of the central nervous system. Therefore, it should come as no surprise that memory in later adulthood is also related to health-related behaviors. For example, cigarette smoking is known to cause deleterious changes in the brain. One longitudinal study conducted in Scotland provided impressive data showing that people tested as children who eventually became smokers had significantly lower memory and information processing scores when followed up at age 64 and 66, controlling for early life intelligence (Starr et al., 2007).

**Neurocognitive disorders.** Neurocognitive disorders are present when a person experiences a loss of cognitive function severe enough to interfere with normal daily activities and social relationships. You may be familiar with the term **dementia**, which is a general term that refers to a loss of cognitive abilities and can include Alzheimer's disease. Major neurocognitive disorders can be distinguished from mild neurocognitive disorders. Mild cognitive disorders, such as mild cognitive impairment (MCI), refer to a form of neurocognitive disorder that signifies the individual may be at risk for developing Alzheimer's disease. The distinction between Alzheimer's disease and other forms of neurocognitive disorder is an important one. Other forms of neurocognitive disorder are different in their cause, prognosis, and treatment.

**FIGURE 11-5**

The causes of dementia

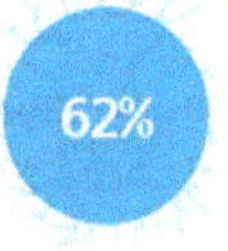


Alzheimer's disease
A physical disease caused by changes in the structure of the brain and a shortage of important chemicals that help with transmission of messages.

17%
Vascular dementia
Caused by problems in the supply of blood to the brain, commonly caused by a stroke or series of small strokes.

Mixed dementia
A type of dementia where a person has a diagnosis of both Alzheimer's disease and vascular dementia.

4%
Dementia with Lewy bodies
One of the less common forms of dementia, it is caused by irregularities in brain cells, leading to symptoms similar to Alzheimer's disease and Parkinson's disease.

3%
Rarer causes of dementia
There are many rarer diseases and syndromes that can lead to dementia or dementia-like symptoms, including corticobasal degeneration and Creutzfeldt–Jakob disease.

2%
Fronto-temporal dementia
Rare when all ages are taken into account but relatively common in people under 65, it is a physical disease that affects the brain.

*Source*: Copyright © Number 10 (CC BY-SA 2.0) at https://c1.staticflickr.com/8/7231/6871016212_be4fe7804b_b.jpg.

**Alzheimer's disease.** Alzheimer's disease is a neurocognitive disorder in which the individual suffers progressive and irreversible neuronal death. Over the years, Alzheimer's disease has been called by a variety of names, including senile dementia, pre-senile dementia, senile dementia of the Alzheimer's type, and organic brain disorder, but all of these terms refer to the same underlying disease.

**Prevalence of neurocognitive disorders and Alzheimer's disease.** The World Health Organization (2020) estimates a prevalence of all forms of neurocognitive disease (dementia) at 5 to 8%; with 60 to 70% due to Alzheimer's disease. Slightly more than half of these individuals (58%) live in low- to middle-income countries. U.S. sources cite a far higher prevalence rate of 5.3 million Americans (5.1 million of whom are age 65 and older), or the equivalent of 11% of the population according to the Alzheimer's Association (2015). Furthermore, according to the Alzheimer's Association, by 2050, the number of people 65 and older with Alzheimer's disease will nearly triple to 13.8 million.

Alzheimer's disease is one of a number of types of neurocognitive disorders. Perhaps as many as 20% of cases of neurocognitive disorder are due to vascular dementia (Knopman, 2007) and, as we will discuss, a number of other neurocognitive disorders share symptoms of Alzheimer's disease. In fact, one study of the autopsied brains of 533 individuals who, in life, had been diagnosed with Alzheimer's disease showed they instead had another neurocognitive disorder (Shim et al., 2013).

From a sociocultural point of view, what the public hears about the prevalence of Alzheimer's disease is also important because this information shapes people's attitudes about their own cognitive functioning. People who see these statistics may inaccurately conclude they are doomed to develop the disorder and there is nothing they can do to prevent it. In fact, not all neurocognitive disorders have the same inevitable progression as does Alzheimer's disease, and some can be prevented.

**Psychological symptoms.** The psychological symptoms of Alzheimer's disease evolve gradually over time. The earliest signs are occasional loss of memory for recent events or familiar tasks. Changes in personality and behavior eventually become evident as the disease progresses. By the time the disease has entered its most advanced stage, the individual has lost the ability to perform even the simplest and most basic of everyday functions. The rate of progression varies from person to person, but there is a fairly regular pattern of loss over the stages of the disease. The survival time following the diagnosis is 7 to 10 years for people diagnosed in their 60s and 70s, and drops to 3 years for people diagnosed in their 90s (Brookmeyer et al., 2002).

**Biological changes.** One of the most pervasive set of changes to occur in the brain of a person with Alzheimer's disease is the formation of abnormal deposits of protein fragments known as **amyloid plaques**. Amyloid is a generic name for protein fragments that collect together in a specific way to form insoluble deposits (meaning that they do not dissolve) that the body cannot dispose of or recycle.

The second major change to occur in the brain is an abundance of abnormally twisted fibers within the neurons themselves, known as **neurofibrillary tangles** (literally, tangled nerve fibers). It is now known that the neurofibrillary tangles are made up of a protein called tau, which seems to play a role in maintaining the stability of the microtubules that form the internal support structure of the axons. The **microtubules** are like train tracks that guide nutrients from the cell body down to the ends of the axon. The **tau proteins** are like the railroad ties or crosspieces of the microtubule train tracks. In Alzheimer's disease, the tau is changed chemically and loses its ability to separate and support the microtubules. With their support gone, the tubules begin to wind around each other and they can no longer perform their function. This collapse of the transport system within the neuron may first result in malfunctions in communication between neurons and may eventually lead to neuronal death.

**Proposed causes.** Most researchers believe genetic abnormalities are responsible for the neuronal death that is the hallmark of Alzheimer's. This hypothesis emerged after the discovery that certain families seemed more prone to develop a form of the disease, referred to as early-onset familial Alzheimer's disease, that strikes between age 40 and 50. Although certainly a difficult and painful situation for families, scientists learned a tremendous amount from studying the DNA of afflicted individuals. Since the discovery of early-onset Alzheimer's, genetic analyses have also uncovered a number of genes, as many as 21, that can individually or in combination increase a person's likelihood of developing the form of Alzheimer's disease that starts at a more conventional age between 60 and 65 years. This form of the disease is called late-onset Alzheimer's disease.

As inherited contributions to Alzheimer's disease were identified with the advent of new genetic testing methods, researchers also became interested in potential behavioral contributors. A unique longitudinal study was performed among the Sisters of Notre Dame, nuns who agreed to donate their brains upon their death. Researchers examined the women while alive and their cognitive performance, as well as their brains upon autopsy. One of the original findings showed that despite the appearance of plaques and tangles, many of the sisters did not show symptomatic deficits in cognitive performance. More recently, researchers found that higher mental activity in early adulthood seemed to protect the sisters from showing signs of cognitive decline in later life despite the presence of these changes in the brain (Iacono et al., 2009). Other research shows some people, who might be otherwise at risk for Alzheimer's disease, never have symptoms during their lifetimes. Exercise is one protective factor that seems to contribute to this. In one large study conducted in Japan, a group of highly active older individuals who exercised at least once a week had a lower rate of Alzheimer's disease than the nonactive participants (Kishimoto et al., 2016).

Predicting who will develop Alzheimer's disease, even in genetically at-risk individuals, is a challenging proposition given the many unknown processes that lead to its development. For example, Satizabal and colleagues (2016) suggested the improved health of the population may be playing a role in reducing the chances of even genetically susceptible individuals to avoid developing Alzheimer's disease.

**Diagnosis.** The diagnosis of a more general neurocognitive disorder is made when there is significant and progressive cognitive decline in one or more areas, including social cognition, memory, aphasia (loss of language ability), apraxia (loss of ability to carry out coordinated movement), agnosia (loss of ability to recognize familiar objects), and disturbance in executive functioning (loss of the ability to plan and organize) (American Psychiatric Association, 2013).

The diagnosis of Alzheimer's disease, specifically, is traditionally carried out through clinical methods using the process of exclusion, where other possible diagnoses are systematically ruled out. This is because no one specific test or clinical indicator can definitively identify the disorder. Though methods of diagnosis are improving considerably, only an autopsy will reveal the presence of neurofibrillary tangles and amyloid plaques that are the sure signs of the presence of Alzheimer's disease rather than another form of neurocognitive disorder. The National Institute of Neurological and Communicative Disorders and Stroke and Alzheimer's Disease and Related Diseases Association (NINCDS-ADRDA) criteria (McKhann et al., 1984) are considered the current "gold standard" for diagnosing Alzheimer's disease. These criteria are based on medical and neuropsychological screening tests, behavioral ratings, and mental status measures. The NINCDS-ADRDA criteria are said to be 85 to 90% accurate in the disease's later stages. The continued improvement of brain scanning provides the possibility for more reliable diagnoses in the early to moderate stages of the disorder (Panegyres et al., 2016).

**Treatments.** As researchers make advances in identifying the cause or causes of Alzheimer's disease, the hope is that medications will be found that can reverse its course. No current types of medications, either alone or in combination, have shown conclusive scientific evidence for their efficacy. At best, they can only treat symptoms, such as alleviating memory loss, and only for a limited time as they do not stop disease progression (Salloway, 2008; Stella et al., 2015). The side effects of medications used to treat neurocognitive disorders, including Alzheimer's disease, are considerable and can range as high as 37% of all patients (Kanagaratnam et al., 2016). These side effects include gastrointestinal effects; dizziness; drowsiness; fainting; frequent or painful urination; headache; joint pain, stiffness, or swelling; depression; unusual bleeding or bruising; weight loss; clumsiness or unsteadiness; confusion; changes in blood pressure; loss of bladder or bowel control; aggression; agitation; delusions; irritability; nervousness; restlessness; tremors; and respiratory difficulties.

Current research is aimed at identifying medications that will interfere with the disease progression rather than at treating its symptoms (Gauthier &

Scheltens, 2009). One approach targets beta-amyloids, and the second focuses on neuroprotective agents that will protect neurons from cell death. These agents would be most effective if used in the early stages of the disease, when it is possible to intervene most effectively (Salloway, 2008). Efforts to develop novel drugs for Alzheimer's have had limited success, and for the most part have been tested using animal models. Researchers believe a medical cure for Alzheimer's disease will eventually be found and may occur in your lifetime. However, it is unlikely that one "magic bullet" will serve this function. Instead, treatments will need target specific at-risk individuals based on genetic vulnerability, medical history, and exposure to environmental toxins (Roberson & Mucke, 2006).

A diet rich in antioxidants has been promoted as a way to prevent Alzheimer's. Antioxidants such as ginkgo biloba, melatonin, polyphenols, and vitamins E and C are thought to improve memory and thinking in those with Alzheimer's, although research has yet to support this. Research from a sample of Germans suggests that the serum concentration of vitamin C and beta-carotene are lower among patients with mild neurocognitive disorder compared with the control participants (von Arnim et al., 2012).

As intensively as research is progressing on treatments for Alzheimer's disease with the hope of someday soon finding a cure, the reality is no cure presently exists. Still, those affected by Alzheimer's must cope with the incapacitating cognitive and physical symptoms that accompany the deterioration of brain tissue. Clearly, until a cure is found, mental health workers will need to provide assistance in this difficult process so that the individual's functioning can be preserved for as long as possible. A critical step in providing conscientious symptom management is to recognize that Alzheimer's disease involves families as much as it does the patients. Family members, typically spouses and children, often provide care for the patient, particularly when the patient is no longer able to function independently.

**Parkinson's disease.** People who develop Parkinson's disease show a variety of motor disturbances, including tremors (shaking at rest), speech impediments, slowing of movement, muscular rigidity, shuffling gait, and postural instability or the inability to maintain balance. Neurocognitive disorder can develop during the later stages of the disease, and some people with Alzheimer's disease develop symptoms of Parkinson's disease. Patients typically survive 10 to 15 years after symptoms appear. There is no cure for Parkinson's disease, but medications can treat its symptoms. The primary drug used is Levadopa (L-dopa); however, over the years, this medication loses its effect and may even be toxic. Another, more radical, approach involves applying high-frequency deep brain stimulation (Sharma et al., 2016) of subcortical movement areas of the brain that in the past were removed surgically (Gradinaru et al., 2009). Research examining the activation of brain cells with flashes of light offers promising treatment for Parkinson's disease. This quickly emerging field of optogenetics presents exciting avenues to better understand the mechanisms involved in Parkinson's disease to advance and improve treatment (Guru et al., 2015).

**Lewy bodies** are tiny spherical structures of protein deposits found in dying nerve cells in damaged brain regions for those with Parkinson's disease. Neurocognitive disorder with Lewy bodies is similar to Alzheimer's disease in that it causes progressive loss of memory, language, calculation, and reasoning, as well as other higher mental functions. Estimates are that this form of neurocognitive disorder accounts for 10 to 15% of all cases of neurocognitive disorder (McKeith, 2006). Neurocognitive disorder with Lewy bodies can vary in severity, at least early on in the disease progression, and include episodes of confusion and hallucinations not typically found in Alzheimer's disease.

### Myths and Misconceptions

Neurocognitive disorders such as Alzheimer's disease and dementia afflict most older adults. **Myth**

Neurocognitive disorders such as Alzheimer's disease and dementia afflict a minority of older adults. **Fact**

Still, Alzheimer's disease and the variety of neurocognitive disorders described are major potential challenges that place limitations on the lives of older adults and their families. Nevertheless, breakthroughs in their treatment, along with contributions to understanding other major diseases, will be among the most significant achievements of science in the 21st century.

**Neuropsychological assessment.** Many specialized tests evaluate an individual's cognitive status, including the quality of their executive functioning. Neuropsychological assessment involves gathering information about a person's brain functioning from a series of standardized cognitive tests. In cases involving older adults with cognitive deficits, in particular, neuropsychologists may adapt their assessment to target the specific area in the brain they believe has suffered damage or decline.

Tests of executive functioning are typically part of a complete neuropsychological assessment. However, most neuropsychological assessments of older adults also include other measures of cognitive functioning. There are enough available neuropsychological tests within each category of cognitive functioning, so if a clinician wishes to investigate one area in depth for a particular client, then they will be able to probe into the individual's possible disorder by administering a variety tests from that category.

You might be surprised to learn there is no one standard procedure for conducting a neuropsychological assessment. In fact, neuropsychologists may have preferences for certain tests, especially if they tend to see the same type of client in their practice or area of research expertise. In clinical settings, though, neuropsychologists are expected to be trained in enough types of tests to adapt the assessment to the individual's symptoms. In working with older adults, neuropsychologists are also expected to be familiar with tests that are appropriate for people in this age group rather than those used in diagnosing a child or adolescent.

## Psychodynamic Theory

**Adult attachment theory.** Older adults are less likely to show anxious types of attachment in comparison with younger adults (Segal et al., 2009). Moreover, older adults who show secure attachment with their parents state they are currently happier on a daily basis than those who show less secure attachment (Consedine & Magai, 2003). Although attachment style might seem to be a stable feature of personality, there is evidence that it can change even in as short a period as a few years (Zhang & Labouvie-Vief, 2004).

Looking at attachment from a different perspective, Cicirelli (2010) examined the numbers of individuals older adults named as serving attachment-related functions in their lives. These functions include being protected from harm, providing emotional security, and serving as a "safe haven" during times of stress. Older adults may have fewer attachment figures in their social networks, according to this study, but those they have fit into a wider range of roles. Rather than seeing only their spouses or partners as serving these attachment functions, older adults turn to adult children, deceased spouses, in-laws, physicians, caregivers, clergy, and animals.

## Personality

**Five-factor model.** Studies based on the scales of the five-factor model and aging show a high degree of consistency over time throughout adulthood, with greater consistency among increasingly older groups of adults. However, the longer the time interval between measurements of personality, the less consistency there is between scores (Roberts & DelVecchio, 2000). People do maintain their relative positions along the traits in comparison with their age peers; the "highs" stay high and the "lows" stay low. If you had high neuroticism scores as a young adult, you would likely continue your high levels of worry, anxiety, and general malaise throughout adulthood.

Conscientiousness continues to play a role in mortality in later adulthood as well. Among a sample of more than 1,000 Medicare recipients ranging in age from 65 to 100 who were followed over a 3- to 5-year period, conscientiousness, particularly self-discipline (a facet of conscientiousness), predicted lower mortality risk over a 3-year period. As the study's authors point out, it is possible that high levels of self-discipline relate to a greater tendency to be proactive in engaging in behaviors that are protective of health and to avoid those behaviors that are damaging to health (Weiss & Costa, 2005). Reinforcing these findings, research from a large sample of Italian adults found that lower levels of conscientiousness (including impulsivity) were associated with lower levels of high-density lipoprotein (the "good" cholesterol) (Sutin et al., 2010) and interleukin-6, a protein important in bolstering immune function (Sutin et al., 2009).

Personality traits may be related to risk of developing cognitive disorders, including Alzheimer's disease. An investigation of nearly 1,000 Catholic nuns and priests indicated that high conscientiousness correlated with lower rates of Alzheimer's disease. Even among those whose brains showed a high degree of pathology upon autopsy, high levels of conscientiousness seemed to serve as a protective factor against cognitive symptoms associated with the disease (Wilson et al., 2007). High levels of neuroticism in midlife also appear to predict an earlier onset of the disease but only in women (Archer et al., 2009).

## Identity

Most people have fairly positive views of themselves, but as they get older, more and more experiences occur that can potentially erode self-esteem. We introduced you to the identity process model in earlier chapters and discussed identity accommodation, when a person changes themselves due to external or internal factors, and identity assimilation, when a person maintains a consistent sense of self over time. Research on identity processes shows that adults increasingly rely on identity assimilation, and this is how older people are able to maintain positive self-esteem. The edge that assimilation has over accommodation is theorized to be just enough to maintain this positive view without leading individuals into self-views that are so off-base that they are completely out of sync with experiences.

The **multiple threshold model** predicts individuals react to specific age-related changes in their physical and psychological functioning in terms of the identity processes. This model was tested out in a study of nearly 250 adults ranging in age from 40 to 95 years (Whitbourne & Collins, 1998). Individuals who used identity assimilation with regard to these specific changes (i.e., they did not think about these changes or integrate them into their identities) had higher self-esteem than people who used identity accommodation (i.e., they became preoccupied with these changes). A certain amount of denial, or at least minimization, seems to be important with regard to changes in the body and how they relate to identity. Others have examined the relation between identity and self-esteem more generally and found self-esteem to be higher in people who use identity assimilation (Sneed & Whitbourne, 2003). Identity accommodation, by contrast, is related to lower levels of self-esteem throughout adulthood. However, men and women differ in their use of identity processes in that women use identity accommodation more than men (Skultety & Whitbourne, 2004).

The potential advantage of identity assimilation in terms of health and mortality is supported by research on self-perceptions of aging and longevity (Levy et al., 2002). Older adults who managed to avoid adopting negative views of aging (which may be seen as a form of identity assimilation) lived 7.5 years longer than those individuals who did not develop a similar resistance to accommodating society's negative views about aging into their identities. The advantage of denial against negative self-evaluations associated with aging (a form of identity assimilation) was also demonstrated in a study in which people who used denial had better psychological health (Cramer & Jones, 2007). Conversely, relying primarily on identity accommodation is associated with the experience of depressive symptoms (Weinberger & Whitbourne, 2010).

Identity assimilation may also serve a protective function in other contexts in which older adults are faced with potentially negative information about their abilities. One group of researchers used a novel opportunity to study this process among older drivers referred to driver education classes due to a history of auto accidents. Those older drivers who overestimated their driving abilities became less depressed after receiving feedback about their actual driving abilities than older drivers who took a more pessimistic view of whether their driving abilities had changed (De Raedt & Ponjaert-Kristoffersen, 2006).

## Life Pathways

By studying the patterns of life changes, the first author identified five patterns of "life pathways" (Whitbourne, 2010). Others have used the pathways metaphor to capture the variations people's lives take as they develop and unfold over time (Friedman & Martin, 2011). The five pathways (see Table 11-1) have a connection to the identity process model. In identity assimilation, individuals try to maintain consistent views of themselves over time. Like those on the *straight and narrow* pathway, people who use identity assimilation fear change and prefer to think of themselves as stable even when situations might require that they change. Identity accommodation corresponds with the *meandering way* because this identity process involves excessively changing in response to experiences when it would be preferable to maintain some consistency. Identity balance is very much like the *authentic road*; people who use identity balance are able to change flexibly in response to experiences but still maintain consistency of their sense of self over time.

**TABLE 11-1** The Five Pathways of Development Identified in the Rochester Adult Longitudinal Study (Whitbourne, 2010)

| Pathway | Description |
|---|---|
| Authentic road | Achieves solid identity commitments through exploration and change |
| Triumphant trail | Overcomes challenges; is resilient |
| Straight and narrow way | Maintains consistent life pattern; is defensive about change |
| Meandering way | Fails to settle on a course in life; constantly searches for identity |
| Downward slope | Shows self-defeating behavior; makes poor decisions |

## Social Cognition

**Positivity.** Recall the socioemotional selectivity theory (SST) we discussed earlier. Related to aspects of motivation, people become more selective and set goals based on what's emotionally meaningful. Similarly, there is a cognitive preference for the positive over the negative. This idea was put to the test using eye-tracking instruments to examine the way in which older and younger adults approach stimuli varying in their positive emotional value. In one investigation (Isaacowitz et al., 2006), older and younger adults were compared in their eye movements when viewing faces conveying happy, sad, and neutral emotional expressions. Older adults were less likely than younger adults to look at parts of the face conveying anger and sadness and more likely to look at the parts conveying happiness. This study's findings imply that older adults would prefer, literally, to "accentuate the positive" when it comes to reading other people's facial expressions. Subsequent research has shown that older adults with higher levels of cognitive functioning are more likely to focus on positive images in an experimental manipulation that put them in a bad mood (Isaacowitz et al., 2009).

Findings on socioemotional selectivity are not consistent, however, in supporting the idea of a "positivity bias" among older adults. Murphy and Isaacowitz (2008) examined a large number of studies comparing younger and older adults and found that both older and younger adults show a preference for positive emotional stimuli, and older adults were more likely to avoid negative emotional stimuli. There may also be cultural factors involved in the relationship between age and a positivity bias. Among a Chinese sample, older adults looked away from, not toward, happy faces (Fung et al., 2008). It is also possible that older adults may display this positive-looking bias but not experience positive affect. Consequently, SST may not be able to explain entirely which factors account for the experience of positive emotional states in older adults (Isaacowitz, 2012).

It seems older adults have an advantage because they seem to react more slowly in emotionally provoking situations (Wieser et al., 2006). Rather than fly into a fit of rage when irked, an older adult may be more likely to think twice and maintain emotional control (Charles & Carstensen, 2010). This may be because older adults are better able to quickly regulate their emotions after being exposed to negative stimuli than are younger adults (Larcom & Isaacowitz, 2009). Most recently, Livingston and Isaacowitz (2015) found that older adults not only seemed to prefer avoiding situations that would provoke negative emotions but also to reduce as much as possible their exposure to such experiences, when given the opportunity.

Being less perturbed by emotional stimuli may also help older adults maintain their cognitive focus (Samanez-Larkin et al., 2009). If you are better able to think logically and maintain your "cool," you will be less likely to forget something or slip up and make a mistake. Perhaps older adults have learned the value of stepping back and not becoming highly aroused when something upsetting occurs (Magai et al., 2006).

**Coping.** The general pattern that emerges shows that older adults cope with anxiety, stress, or frustration by reacting in less self-destructive or emotional ways than they would have when they were younger. Rather than getting frustrated and giving up on a solution, older adults are more apt to try and understand the situation and figure out a way around it. They can suppress negative feelings or channel them into productive activities. By contrast, younger people (including adolescents and young adults) are more likely to react to psychologically demanding situations by acting out against others, projecting their anger onto others, or regressing to more primitive forms of behavior.

The objective nature of people's life circumstances may place constraints on their coping abilities, such as when people are unable to afford basic life necessities (Diener et al., 2003). However, coping can help individuals to withstand even very stressful life events such as personal illness and the death or illness of a friend or family member (Hardy et al., 2004). People who are characteristically able to cope with or show positive functioning in the face of particularly adverse life events are said to be high in **resilience**. This point was demonstrated among a sample of older adult widows and widowers followed intensively over a 6-week period while they rated their daily experiences of stressful events and emotional reactions (Ong et al., 2006). The measure of resilience used in this study tapped qualities such as the respondent's ability to overcome negative emotions and adapt to new situations. More resilient individuals were able to maintain a positive mood even on days when they experienced high degrees of stress.

The type of coping people use may reflect their own perceptions about their abilities to reduce stress. Older individuals with higher levels of self-efficacy are more likely to use problem-focused coping, compared with those who use emotion-focused coping, who are more likely to rate themselves high both in social support and in perceived stress (Trouillet et al., 2009).

Religion also plays a role in adapting to difficult life circumstances, serving as another important coping resource for many older adults (Van Ness & Larson, 2002). As we've discussed in earlier chapters, cultures and nations vary in their norms or expectations for experiencing emotions. For example, people in China have the lowest frequency and intensity of both positive and negative emotions compared with people living in the United States, Australia, and Taiwan (Eid & Diener, 2001).

Although some discussions of coping in later life regard older adults as passive rather than active copers, it is not necessarily a given that as people get older they adopt a fatalistic approach to managing their fortunes or that they become ineffective copers. A study of the victims of the 2005 Hurricane Katrina that devastated New Orleans showed older and younger adults were equally effective in engaging in coping strategies to manage their responses to the disaster (Cherry et al., 2009).

Thus, older adults can show initiative in managing their situations and making efforts to alter the course of events in their lives. People who show this type of initiative strongly wish to maintain a feeling of independence as they age, even if they have been forced to relinquish some of their actual independence due to functional changes in their abilities (Duner & Nordstrom, 2005). The ability to take charge of potentially stressful situations, before they become problems, is related to fewer health-related stressful situations for active older adults (Fiksenbaum et al., 2006).

Simply because many older adults tend to manage their emotions and demonstrate coping does not mean they don't feel stress. Researchers comparing the cardiovascular reactivity of older and younger adults during a stressful laboratory task found the blood pressure of older adults actually increased more in response to stress than the blood pressure of their younger counterparts. However, the older adults managed to keep their negative emotions in check, even when it was apparent that their bodies were registering heightened levels of stress (Uchino et al., 2006).

Social support is an important resource for people of any age when faced with stressful experiences. Everyone knows how important it is to be able to talk to someone who can if not help at least hear you out when you have had something bad happen to you. Loss of functional abilities is certainly one important stressful area for older adults. Close relationships among spouses is certainly a protective factor for psychological problems. Older adults with functional losses are able to maintain positive mood and self-regard if they are in marital relationships characterized by feeling loved, understood, and being able to communicate (Mancini & Bonanno, 2006).

# Social Contexts and Functioning

There are a number of social factors to consider when we examine later life. Financial resources may decrease when people retire, and age-related mobility and cognitive problems can make cooking a more difficult task for the older adult to manage. There are benefits to our social relationships and "what we do" when we retire that can affect our health and well-being as well as those around us.

**LO 11-7 Identify some benefits of the grandparenting role.**

**LO 11-8 Describe varying patterns of retirement.**

## Relationships and Social Support

Earlier we discussed successful coping, and research shows it is influenced by strong social networks (Brennan et al., 2006). It is not only the number of people in their social network but also the quality of social support that can help older people feel more satisfied with their lives (Berg et al., 2006). Think of how this process applies in your own life; by having others regard you positively, it is likely that you will develop an enhanced sense of self-esteem, which in turn has positive effects on your subjective health, which in turn enhances your well-being, and so on.

Social support and relationships with others have an influence on feelings of well-being by reinforcing the view that you are valued. At the same time, being concerned about family and having a sense of responsibility for children and other family members seem to have additional adaptive value. In one investigation of Australians ranging in age from 61 to 95, a sense of belonging and concern about family predicted high scores on a measure assessing reasons for living (Kissane & McLaren, 2006). Sense of mastery, particularly for men, also seems to play a key role in the relation between social support and perceived stress (Gadalla, 2009).

**Marriage.** Among people age 65 and older in the United States, an overall higher percentage of men (70%) are married and living with a spouse compared with women (45%) (U.S. Bureau of the Census, 2018). Consequently, women over the age of 65 are nearly twice as likely (35%) as men (19%) to be living alone. Therefore, older women are at greater risk for some of the disadvantages that come with single status, including fewer financial resources, access to care, and social support.

The percentage of older adults living with a spouse varies by age, sex, and race/ethnicity. Women are more likely than men not to live with a spouse, with the lowest percentage (12%) being Black women age 85 and older. The highest percentage of men living with a spouse is non-Hispanic Whites age 65 to 74. Because living with a spouse typically provides emotional and financial resources, these figures suggest Black women age 85 and older are at greatest risk for living without adequate support within the home.

**Cohabitation.** Most research on cohabitation involves younger adults, but older adults also enter into cohabiting relationships. As of the latest published data from 2012, 735,000 adults age 65 and older were living in a cohabitating relationship, with two thirds of these in the young-old category (Vespa et al., 2013). One study investigating cohabitation in older adults suggests the unions they form tend to persist longer than those formed by younger adults. Using data from the Health and Retirement Study, a longitudinal sample of more than 21,000 adults 50 and older followed from 1998 to 2006, Brown and colleagues (2012) reported that among the 4% who entered into cohabitation, only 18% ended in separation, and most people remained together either until one of them died or the study was over.

Compared with younger adults, older adults seem to be more likely, then, to view cohabitation as an alternative to marriage.

**FIGURE 11-6** Percent by age, sex, and race/ethnicity married with spouse present (2015).

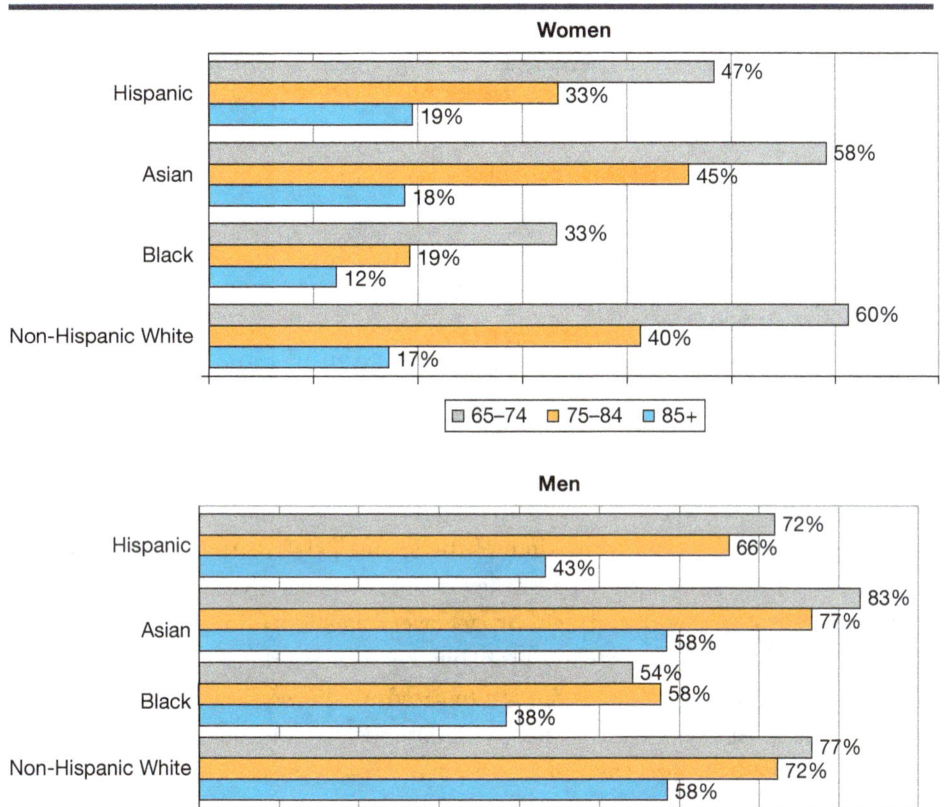


*Source:* United States Census Bureau, 2017.

Rather than sharing the same household, however, older adults may enter into an arrangement known as living apart together (LAT). This is a living arrangement increasingly adopted by unmarried older adults in intimate relationships who do not wish to share a residence. This arrangement may be prompted by concerns about finances (Lyssens-Danneboom & Mortelmans, 2014), caregiving (De Jong Gierveld, 2015), and simply a preference to remain in their separate households (Benson & Coleman, 2016).

**Widowhood.** The death of a spouse is one of the most stressful events of life, and for many older adults it can involve the loss of a relationship that may have lasted 50 years or more. As we shall see, however, the effect of widowhood on the bereaved individual varies greatly according to the circumstances surrounding the spouse's death and the nature of the couple's relationship (McNamara & Rosenwax, 2010).

In the United States, there are currently approximately 15 million widowed adults age 18 and older; 77% of these are 65 and older. The majority (77%) of widowed adults over the age of 65 are women. Another way to look at these statistics is in terms of what percentage of women and men age 65 and older are women; using this percentage, women are nearly three times as likely as men to be widowed. By age 85, 71% of women are widows compared with 34% of men (U.S. Bureau of the Census, 2018). Widows who experienced extensive caregiver burden at the end of their spouse's life no longer face these duties (Ferrario et al., 2004). Relief from the burdens of caregiving may alleviate some symptoms of depression and stress present during the spouse's dying months or years (Bonanno et al., 2004).

In general, men seem particularly vulnerable to depression after the death of their spouses (Bennett et al., 2005). Without remarriage, their levels of well-being may not return to preexisting levels even for as long as 8 years after the spouse has died (Lucas et al., 2003; Whitbourne & Bookwala, 2015). Among both men and women, anniversary reactions occur in which the bereaved experience a renewal of their feelings at or around the time of the spouse's death. These reactions may continue for 35 years or longer (Carnelley et al., 2006), signifying that people may not completely ever "work through" or "get over" their grief. In what is called the widowhood effect, there is a greater probability of death in those who have become widowed compared with those who are married. Widowed men have the highest mortality rates. This widowhood effect was demonstrated using data from a study involving nearly 6,000 older adults studied over an 11-year period (Williams et al., 2011). Even after controlling for health risks or causes of death, widowed individuals have a higher risk of mortality than the nonwidowed. Their higher mortality appears to be related to conditions such as depression, psychosocial stress, chronic economic hardship, and loss of social support and environmental resources. As a result, they suffer from physical and emotional declines that can lead to a relatively earlier death compared with their married counterparts. Based on a study of widows and widowers in Northern Ireland, it appears that widowers at highest risk are those living in urban areas (Wright et al., 2015).

Several studies support the notion that the widowed suffer more health problems than those still married, particularly in the period shortly after they lose their spouses. They may engage in riskier behaviors such as eating fewer fruits and vegetables and foods with higher fat content and engaging in less physical activity. They are more likely to drink alcohol (Stroebe et al., 2007) and more likely to smoke (Wilcox et al., 2003). Women who remarry after becoming widows have more favorable characteristics in a number of ways over women who remain widows. Women who remarry have fewer depressive symptoms, worry less about money, and have higher incomes than women who remain widowed (Moorman et al., 2006).

In a major prospective study of more than 200 widows, Bonanno and his collaborators (2004) followed women for 18 months after the death of their husbands. The majority showed relatively little distress following their loss, in a pattern called "resilient grief." However, some widows experienced chronic grief that did not subside during the study period, and some showed high levels of depression prior to and after the loss. Studies such as these underscore the notions that widowhood is a varied process and there are multiple factors influencing reactions to the loss of a spouse.

**Quality of late-life relationships.** Socioemotional selectivity theory, which we described earlier, implies that older adults would prefer to spend time with their marital partner (and other family members) rather than invest their energies in meeting new people. They may regard the long-term relationship as offering perhaps the most potential to serve emotional functions because their experiences together allow them to understand and respond to each other's needs. Indeed, research suggests that older adults are more likely to keep sight of the positive aspects of their relationships even when they have disagreements (Story et al., 2007). In addition, if older adults are better able to control their emotions, particularly negative ones, they should get along better with their partner because each is less likely to irritate the other. Finally, if older adults experience strong feelings, their affection for one another should not fade.

**Sexuality.** Sexuality remains an important component of happy relationships throughout adulthood. Although you may imagine older adults lose interest in sex, those who are in good physical health seem to maintain a virtually lifelong desire to engage in sexual relations (Lindau & Gavrilova, 2010). More than 40% of women and men in the 75–84 age range who are living with their partners engaged in intercourse at least once in the previous year. Even those older adults not living with a partner engage in at least yearly (if not more) sexual intercourse. Furthermore, a considerable number were engaged in some form of sexual activity on a much more frequent basis, with more than half of women and men (54%) in the 75–85 age bracket having sex two to three times a month, or more. Approximately one third in this age group also engaged in oral sex (Waite et al., 2009).

Thus, sexuality remains important to older adults in the context of their intimate relationships. We know that midlife, and particularly older adults, experience physical changes that could affect their ability to engage in some form of sexual activity. However, it appears that the majority of adults in their mid-50s and above find ways to incorporate sexuality into their lives on a regular basis, particularly if they are in an intimate relationship. Obviously more goes into the quality of long-term relationships than expressing sexuality. Alternative theories to marital satisfaction each have their own set of predictions about who will be happiest in a long-term relationship. Unfortunately, studies of marriage suffer from the obvious disadvantage of only including couples who remain married.

**Parent-adult child relationships.** As children move through their years of adulthood, many facets of their relationships with their own parents undergo change. For example, as children have their own families, they begin to gain greater insight into the role of being a parent. On the one hand, adult children may now appreciate what their parents did for them; on the other hand, they may resent their parents for not having done more. Another changing feature of the relationship stems from the child's increasing concern that parents will require help and support as they grow older. Adult children and their parents may also find they do not agree on various aspects of life, from an overall philosophy and set of values (such as in the area of politics) to specific habits and behaviors (such as methods of food preparation). Whether parents and their adult children live in the same geographic vicinity and actually see each other on a frequent basis must also be added into the equation.

FIGURE 11-7 Young adults living in their parents' home, 1960 to 2012: Census and CPS.

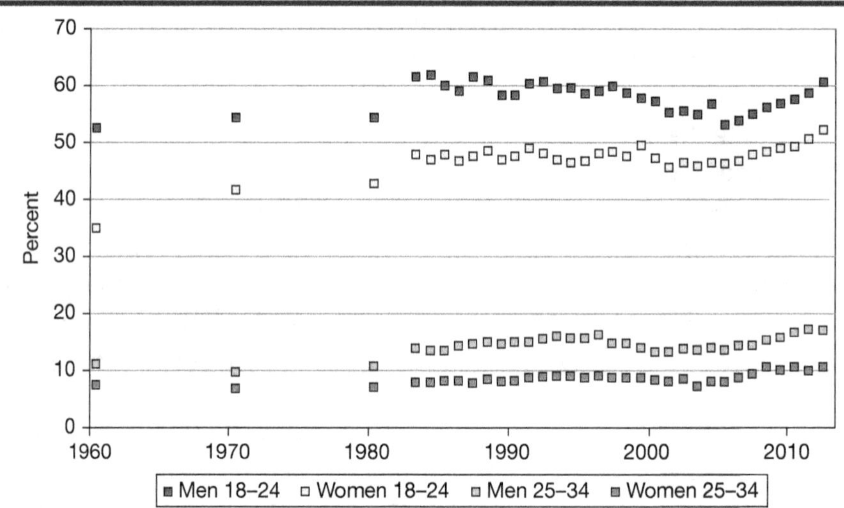


*Source*: Jonathan Vespa, Jamie M. Lewis, and Rose M. Kreider, America's Families and Living Arrangements: 2012, pp. 11, 2017.

Several concepts help us gain insight into parent-adult child relationships. Filial maturity occurs when children reach the age of relating to their parents as equals (Blenkner, 1963). Filial anxiety is the fear of having to take care of an aging, infirmed parent (Cicirelli, 1988). Filial obligation describes the cultural values that adult children are expected to care for their parents, including aging parents living in an adult child's home. Filial obligation is more likely to occur in African American (Wilson, 1986), Hispanic (Keefe et al., 1979), and Asian American families (Velkoff & Lawson, 1998) compared with White families of European descent. Filial obligation is also known as filial piety in China, represented by the character (*xiao*).

**Grandparents.** For many older adults, the rewards of family life begin to grow even richer when they reach the status of grandparents. At this point, many are in a position to be able to enjoy the benefits of expressing their generativity through interacting with the youngest generation, while avoiding some of the more difficult tasks of parenthood. Many people think of grandparents as the warm, generous, older adults portrayed in storybooks: kindly relatives who have ample time to spend with their families and want to do so. However, variations in patterns of grandparenting, along with a rapidly increasing growth in the number of grandparents in the population, may require a change in this image.

There may be as many as 70 million grandparents in the United States according to popular estimates as there are no official data in the U.S. Census on the grandparent status of an individual. We do know that more and more grandparents are involved in some form of caregiving of their grandchildren, with an estimated 22% in the United States (Fuller-Thomson & Minkler, 2001) and slightly more in Europe (33% of grandmothers and 26% of grandfathers) (Hank & Buber, 2009). Approximately 4.6% of all U.S. households are multigenerational (3.7 million households). Among these, the majority are three generational, but there are 62,000 households that qualify as four generational. Within most of these multigenerational families, more family members, other than the head of the household, are foreign born (Vespa et al., 2013).

There are also a substantial number of children who are raised entirely by their grandparents, with an estimated 1.6 million living in the homes of grandparents without the presence of their own parents (U.S. Bureau of the Census, 2019). The term "skip generation" family refers to the family living situation in which grandchildren live with their grandparents and not their parents. The skip generation family may occur when there is substance abuse by parents, child abuse or neglect by parents, teenage pregnancy or failure of parents to handle children, parental employment issues, divorce, health issues, or incarceration. African American and Hispanic children are more likely to grow up in a skip generation family or to be part of a multigenerational household headed by their grandparent (Luo et al., 2012).

Although only a small percentage (14%) of grandparents in skip generation households are over the age of 60, a substantial number of them live in poverty and many have a disability. However, on the positive side, their role as surrogate parent can contribute positively to the grandparents' sense of identity, particularly for African American grandmothers (Pruchno & McKenney, 2002). Feeling that others are supportive can help alleviate the negative effects of the stress and strain of caring for a grandchild (Musil et al., 2009).

Grandparents vary in the extent to which they become involved in the lives of their grandchildren. The classic study of grandparenting conducted by Neugarten and Weinstein (1964) identified five types of grandparents. The first type, the *formal grandparent*, follows what are believed to be the appropriate guidelines for the grandparenting role. Formal grandparents provide occasional services and maintain an interest in the grandchild but do not become overly involved. By contrast, the second type, the *fun seeker*, prefers the leisure aspects of the role and primarily provides entertainment for the grandchild. The *surrogate parent* is the third type; as the name implies, this type of grandparent takes over the caretaking role with the child. Fourth, the *reservoir of family wisdom*, typically a grandfather, is the head of the family who dispenses advice and resources but also controls the parent generation. Finally, the *distant figure* is the fifth type of grandparent; they have infrequent contact with the grandchildren, appearing only on holidays and special occasions. Other attempts to characterize or delineate styles or categories of grandparenting have followed a similar pattern, with distinctions typically made among the highly involved, friendly, and remote or formal types of grandparents (Mueller et al., 2002).

Although these variations may exist in patterns of grandparenting, it is safe to say that the role of grandparent is an important one for the older adult (Harwood et al., 2000) and that grandparent identity is an important contributor to well-being (Reitzes & Mutran, 2004). There is evidence that the role of grandparent is more central in the lives of grandmothers than grandfathers (Pollet et al., 2009). Grandparents feel a strong sense of connection to the younger generation (Crosnoe & Elder, 2002) and may play an important role in mediating conflicts between parents and grandchildren (Werner et al., 2005). Spending some time watching grandchildren may also help improve an older adult's executive functioning, as long as demands for caregiving do not invade the grandparent's time attending to their other needs (Burn & Szoeke, 2015).

Contact with grandchildren declines steadily through the grandchildren's early adulthood, particularly when they leave the home of their parents and start an independent life of their own (Geurts et al., 2015). Those grandparents who get along with their own children are more likely to maintain contact with their grandchildren throughout this period (Dunifon & Bajracharya, 2012). Research shows that such contact may be important to the mental health of the older generation. Grandparents who are unable to maintain contact with their grandchildren due to parental divorce or family disagreements are likely to suffer a variety of ill consequences, including poor mental and physical health, depression, feelings of grief, and poorer quality of life (Drew & Smith, 2002). However, as their grandchildren get older, many grandparents are able to stay in touch and even to consider their grandchildren as part of their social network (Geurts et al., 2012).

**Age stereotypes and social relationships.** Age stereotypes about the abilities of older adults can lead to others treating them in problematic ways and their own loss of self-efficacy. The communication predicament model shows that patronizing speech is often used with older adults as a result of these stereotypes. Infantilization, in which the older person loses the incentive to attempt to regain self-sufficiency in the basic activities of daily life, can also occur (Whitbourne et al., 1995; Whitbourne & Wills, 1993). When older adults in environments such as residential facilities are treated by younger staff in a patronizing manner, they lose the desire to socialize with each other, potentially leading to social isolation (Salari & Rich, 2001). The self-fulfilling nature of infantilization can also increase the older person's awareness of age stereotypes, causing negative self-beliefs to spread across multiple areas of functioning. If you think you are unable to carry out a task because you are too old, infirm, or feeble, then the chances are you will eventually lose the ability to carry out that task.

According to one analysis, infantilization may even produce symptoms of dementia, particularly in institutional settings where residents may feel they have no escape from the control of their caregivers (Marson & Powell, 2014). Because infantilization results in a loss of independence, researchers believe it is important to sensitize those who work with older adults so they avoid falling into this pattern. These programs have been implemented within assisted living facilities (Williams & Warren, 2009), but clearly more work in this area will have wide-ranging benefits.

## Work and Retirement

The share of the labor force that adults age 55 and older comprise is on the rise (see Figure 11-8). There are changes in work and leisure activities for many. Some look toward retirement on the horizon, whereas others continue to work, volunteer, and, as we've seen, contribute toward their adult children's needs.

**FIGURE 11-8** Labor force by age.

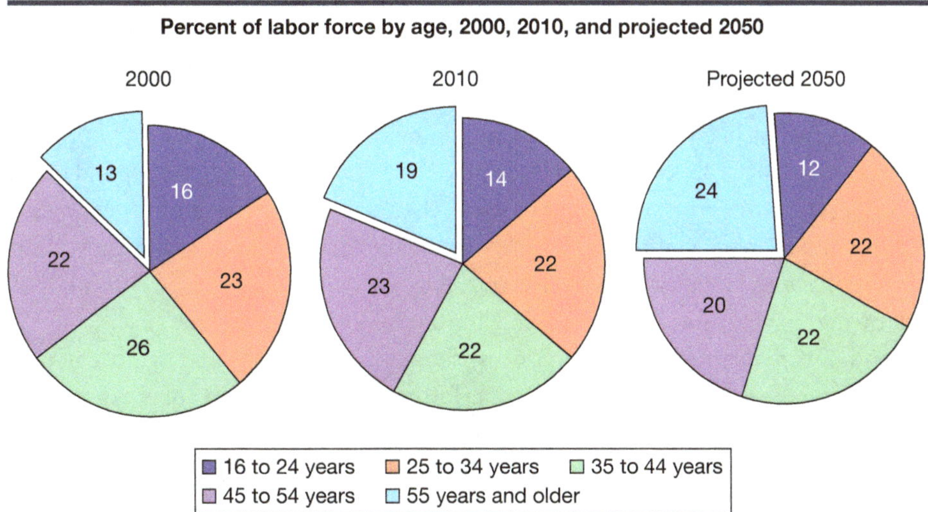


*Source:* U.S. Bureau of Labor Statistics, https://www.bls.gov/opub/ted/2012/ted_20121203.htm.

**Vocational performance.** Older workers have slightly lower core work performance, although the effect of age on work performance varies with the nature of the task (Warr, 1994). For example, those in jobs that require crystallized intelligence (which does not decrease until well past retirement) and depend on experience should theoretically show improved performance in later adulthood. They should be strongly motivated to put in the effort needed to perform well on the job because they realize their efforts will most likely meet with success. By contrast, if the job is highly dependent on strength, speed, or working memory, older workers may be less able to perform well and at the same time be less motivated to put in effort that, they believe, may not pay off (Kanfer & Ackerman, 2004). One area in which older adults may perform more poorly involves shift work, in which the individual's work hours change from daytime hours to evenings or nights. Although these schedules present a challenge for workers of all ages, they are particularly difficult for older workers (Bonnefond et al., 2006).

On the positive side, older workers show fewer counterproductive work behaviors, such as voluntary absenteeism. They are also more likely to engage in good "citizenship," meaning they participate in more voluntary activities. They also tend to be safer as they tend to take fewer risks on the job. Of course, some of these factors relate to survival effects in that the unhealthy, uncooperative, and risky workers tend to be the ones who do not last as long on the job.

Some older workers focus on maintaining their current employment status and plan how to end their careers without jeopardizing this. Others may experience some disability and attempt to compensate for their losses while still maintaining their position at work. Many older workers, however, do not experience a loss in work functioning and maintain high levels of performance until retirement (Ng & Feldman, 2012).

Injuries are also important in understanding the association between age and job performance. Overall, workers over the age of 55 are nearly half as likely to suffer a nonfatal injury as those who are 35 years and younger, and similarly older workers are about half as likely to suffer death due to a work-related injury. However, when older workers (ages 55–64) must miss work due to injury or illness, they spend twice as many days away from work (12) per year than do younger workers (ages 25–34) (U.S. Bureau of Labor Statistics, n.d.). Driving-related accidents in the transportation industry have the highest fatality rate of all U.S. industries, and it is in this job that older workers have the highest rate of dying as well (Pegula et al., 2007).

With regard to overall physical fitness, decreases in strength and agility can certainly have a negative influence on job performance in some areas of employment, particularly when physical exertion is involved (Sluiter, 2006). However, workers of any age can suffer from conditions that impair their performance, such as a cold or a muscle ache. Furthermore, as pointed out by Warr (1994), every worker has restrictions in the kind of work they can perform. The fact that older workers may have some limitations due to physical changes does not mean they cannot achieve adequate performance on all types of jobs. People learn to cope with their limitations and gravitate toward jobs they are able to perform (Daly & Bound, 1996). If they become disabled enough, they will leave the job market altogether.

**Retirement.** Retirement may be the furthest thing from your mind if you are a college student in your late teens or early 20s. You are most likely concentrating on finding a job rather than retiring from one. Ideally, you will find a job you enjoy that will give you a solid foundation for spending 10 or 20 years (or more!) enjoying your retirement years.

Many people think of retirement as an event marked by a ceremony such as the proverbial "gold watch" given to the retiree as thanks for years of loyal service. This traditional image of retirement was never really true, however. Even when careers had more predictable trajectories, people often continued to maintain some type of employment after they retired from their primary job. The definition of retirement is becoming even murkier with current changes in labor force participation by individuals in their middle and later years, as you will soon learn.

The economy's health affects not only the financial security of the employed, but also the financial security of the retired. Interest rates, tax policies, inflation, and the overall growth of the economy are some of the factors that determine the amount of money retired individuals receive from their various sources of income. Policies being decided on now by governments around the world will affect billions of older individuals in the decades to come. You may feel as though you are years away from retirement and therefore are not affected by these debates, but they are affecting your current paycheck now and will continue to have an impact on your financial stability throughout the rest of your life.

Retirement is defined as the withdrawal of an individual in later life from the labor force. However, for most workers, retirement occurs in a series of vocational phases through which they progress at least once, if not several, times throughout their lives. Because retirement is not simply an event with a defined start and end point, it is best conceptualized in terms of a period of adjustment (Wang, 2007).

The retirement process occurs over five phases (Sterns & Gray, 1999). People experience an anticipatory period that may last for decades. Eventually, they make the decision to retire. After their last day of work in the particular job (the act of retirement), workers go through an initial adjustment period followed, ultimately, by a more or less final restructuring of their activity patterns. Complicating this picture is the fact that fewer and fewer workers are showing the crisp retirement pattern, in which they leave the labor force in a single, unreversed, clear-cut exit. More typically, retirees show the blurred retirement pattern, in which they exit and reenter the labor force several times. Some accept bridge employment, which is when retirees work in a completely different occupation than they had during most of their adult life. For example, an insurance agent may retire from the insurance business but work as a crossing guard or server at a fast-food restaurant. Other workers may retire from one job in a company and accept another role in the same company. In general, involvement in bridge employment is strongly related to financial need. Workers who have a long, continuous history of employment in private sector jobs tend not to seek bridge employment because they typically have sufficient financial resources (Davis, 2003). Ultimately, the criteria for retirement are met when a person in later life with a cohesive past work pattern has not worked for a sustained period of time and is not psychologically invested in work any longer (Beehr et al., 2000).

**The effects of retirement on the individual.** Until the 1960s, most American workers resisted the idea of retiring because they believed retirement would place their financial security at risk. However, succeeding generations of workers are viewing retirement more positively. In part, this is true because their retirement earnings are higher than they were for past older Americans. Now that mandatory retirement is a thing of the past for most jobs, older workers no longer feel forced out of the labor market. Furthermore, retired individuals no longer necessarily experience the poor health, low income, and loss of status that was associated with exit from the labor force earlier in the 1900s. Many older individuals can also look forward to a healthy period of retirement in which they can continue to pursue part-time work as desired, travel, spend time with family, and move to more comfortable climates or housing situations.

The increasingly outdated view of retirement as an unwanted life change fits most closely with the role theory of retirement, which proposes that retirement has deleterious effects because the loss of the work role loosens the ties between the individual and society. The continuity theory of retirement proposes that retired individuals maintain their self-concept and identity over the retirement transition. For example, even though they no longer report to work on a daily basis, they can engage in many of the same activities they did when they were working. In addition, a retired person remains a retired accountant, plumber, or teacher in their community. These two theories focus on retirement as an isolated event. The life course perspective on retirement, on the other hand, proposes that changes in work roles in later life are best seen as logical outgrowths of earlier life events. The factors that shaped the individual's prior vocational development will have a persisting influence throughout retirement.

According to the resource model of retirement, the individual's adjustment to retirement reflects their physical, cognitive, motivational, financial, social, and emotional resources; the more resources, the more favorable the individual's adjustment will be at any one point through the retirement transition (Wang, 2007). The resource model fits well with the biopsychosocial perspective. In general, supporting the resource model, having a diverse set of physical, psychological, and social resources seems to ease the transition to retirement, even among individuals who initially experience poor adjustment (Wang et al., 2011). Additionally, easing the transition to retirement can be helped by invoking a sense of mastery, or the belief in one's ability to adapt successfully (Muratore & Earl, 2015).

People also adjust better to retirement if they retire in an "on-time" rather than "off-time" manner (Gill et al., 2006). Voluntarily retiring, instead of being forced to retire through downsizing, also promotes better adaptation (Clarke et al., 2012) The amount of time allowed for retiring is another related factor. A minimum planning time of 2 years prior to retirement is related to a positive retirement experience compared with a decision made 6 months or less prior to retirement (Hardy & Quadagno, 1995). As important as length of time, however, is the quality of retirement planning, which should include not only financial planning but also adequate discussion with the individual's spouse or partner (Noone et al., 2009).

Socioeconomic status (SES) is another influence on retirement adjustment. People at the high end of this scale are less likely to retire than people at the lower end, and higher-SES individuals tend to retire at a later age. When they do retire, those high in SES tend to be in better health than those at lower socioeconomic levels. Those high in SES also have a longer life expectancy (Majer et al., 2011). Their advantaged economic security means they are better able to take advantage of the opportunities retirement offers to engage in productive and enjoyable leisure activities, such as retirement learning communities and travel. Individuals with higher levels of education and previous experience in managerial or professional positions may be better able to find part-time employment after retirement if they desire it. Past experience in community organizations and activities may also make it easier for such individuals to find rewarding opportunities for unpaid volunteer work and participation in clubs, organizations, and informal networks.

**Retirement and marriage.** There has been some debate in the literature regarding the effect of retirement on a married couple's relationship. One school of thought describes the "spouse underfoot syndrome," whereby partners are more likely to experience conflict now that they are in each other's presence for most of the daytime and nighttime hours (the spouse who is underfoot is typically the husband). However, there is a contrasting view of retirement as a second honeymoon, in which couples are now free to enjoy each other's company on a full-time basis, without the constraints presented by having to leave home for 8 or more hours a day. As with much of the data on retirement, there is no simple answer. The transition itself from work to retirement seems to take its toll on marital satisfaction when partners have high levels of conflict. The greatest conflict is observed when one partner is working and the other has retired. Eventually, however, these problems seem to subside; after about 2 years of retirement for both partners, levels of marital satisfaction once again rise (Moen et al., 2001). Perhaps, relatedly, there is evidence that men and women engage in more equitable division of household tasks than they did prior to retirement. The convergence of the gender gap in everyday chores after retirement may be one of the factors that helps to promote a couple's feelings of satisfaction with their relationship as a whole (Leopold & Skopek, 2015).

**Gender differences in retirement.** The factors that influence retirement adjustment do appear to differ between women and men. Men operate according to the "usual" mode of retirement view, in which decisions regarding retirement do not involve the family. According to the new mode of retirement perspective, the characteristics of the person's spouse and lifelong family responsibilities play a role in retirement decisions and adjustment. Current cohorts of older women are more likely to operate according to the new modes of retirement; they are more likely than men to be influenced by the health, financial security, and work status of their spouses. However, among couples raised with more egalitarian values, both are likely to be influenced increasingly by the work status of their spouses (Pienta, 2003).

As we can see, work and retirement are broad and fascinating areas of study in the field of adult development and aging (Whitbourne & Bookwala, 2015). Research from a developmental perspective has been somewhat slow to get off the ground. However, increasing information on the topics of vocational satisfaction and retirement adjustment, and their interaction with personality and social structural factors, are providing greater clarification about this component of adult life.

**Leisure pursuits in later adulthood.** Throughout adulthood, people express themselves not only through their work but also through their hobbies and interests. Occupational psychologists and academics studying the association between job characteristics and satisfaction often neglect the fact that, for many adults, it is the off-duty hours rather than the on-duty hours that contribute the most to identity and personal satisfaction. In contrast, marketers recognize the value of developing promotional campaigns that appeal to these adults who potentially have resources to spend on leisure pursuits (Ferguson & Brohaugh, 2010).

As people move through adulthood and into retirement, it becomes more crucial for them to develop leisure interests so they will have activities to engage in during the day to provide focus and meaning to their lives. In addition, leisure pursuits can serve important functions by helping older adults maintain their health through physical activity and their cognitive functioning through intellectual stimulation. The social functions of leisure are also of potential significance, particularly for people who have become widowed or who have had to relocate because of a desire for more comfortable climates or poor health.

Researchers who study leisure time activities in later adulthood find strong evidence linking leisure participation to improvement in feelings of well-being, particularly among older adults who are trying to overcome deficits in physical functioning or in their social networks (Silverstein & Parker, 2002). Furthermore, cognitively challenging leisure activities can be at least as if not more beneficial than physical exercise to help individuals maintain their intellectual functioning, including lowering the risk for vascular dementia (Verghese et al., 2009).

Regular leisure-time physical activity can have important health consequences. A longitudinal study in Sweden followed men over five time points (Byberg et al., 2009). Participants were asked about their level of physical activity with questions such as, "Do you often go walking or cycling for pleasure?" People who engaged in physical activity in their leisure time died at later ages than those who did not over the 35-year period of the study. As people can be counseled to seek a person-environment fit for vocations, they might also be advised to find the leisure pursuit that will keep them motivated and, hence, active in a pursuit that will ultimately have value in maximizing their functional abilities (Kerby & Ragan, 2002).

Older adults are less likely than younger people to engage in physical activities as leisure-time pursuits. They may also not be aware of the potential benefits that mental and physical activity can provide. Not only can engaging in active leisure pursuits help preserve cognitive function and maintain cardiovascular health, but individuals can also benefit from the stress-reducing effects of engaging in enjoyable leisure-time pursuits (Lin et al., 2012). Maintaining an active social life in retirement also seems to have a variety of benefits in promoting retirement adjustment. Among a sample of Australian retirees, those who participated in a wider variety of social activities had higher levels of positive affect and, importantly, were higher in their self-efficacy and feelings of mastery (Earl et al., 2015).

# CHAPTER 12 Successful Aging

Many assume that as we get toward the end of life there is a quick drop in well-being and adjustment. However, as you probably have recognized, survival into the later years of adulthood requires individuals to negotiate the threats to living a long life that emerge along the way. To get old you have to not die, but to age successfully requires additional adaptive qualities. Because older adults have managed to avoid so many threats that could have ended their lives at younger ages, there may be some special quality about increasingly older individuals that have helped them reach this point in their lives.

We'll now explore the topics of psychological growth in the later adult years. Successful agers don't just "survive." They achieve greater levels of personal expression and happiness. We hope these inspirational qualities guide and sustain your optimism and hope about your own future.

# An Overview of Successful Aging

Who might you nominate as successful, or optimal, agers? Do you have a grandfather who can chop wood in his barn for hours on end? Can your grandmother beat everyone in the family at card games? How about your great aunt and uncle, who backpack around the world for 3 or 4 weeks a year? Perhaps your 80-year-old neighbor is outside every morning tending to her lawn and garden. Maybe you know someone in your town who is long past the traditional age of retirement but continues to work Monday through Friday at the hardware store. Think about some well-known older adults who have become cultural icons, in part due to their longevity, such as Betty White, the American television comedian. White had a resurgence in popularity in 2010 when a Facebook-inspired movement led the producers of *Saturday Night Live* to invite the then 88-year-old to host the show, a performance that garnered her an Emmy award.

**FIGURE 12-1** A camel ride across the desert is a leisure activity not many older adults partake in.

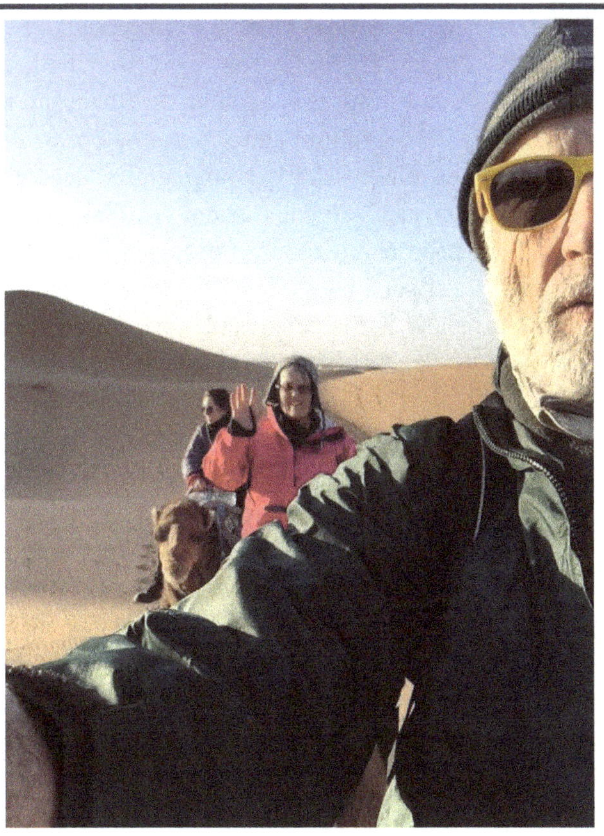

*Source*: Cynthia R. Davis

Unfortunately, many younger people tend to view the happy and productive older person as an anomaly. Cultural icons such as Betty White and fitness enthusiast Jack LaLanne, who kept physically fit and active well into his 80s before his death in 2011, have historically been admired by younger generations in part because they seem so atypical of their age group. Many assume aging inevitably brings about depression and hopelessness, so when people do not show these qualities, they must be truly special. However, most older people don't become depressed, and personality development in middle and later adulthood appears to be in the positive direction of greater adaptive ability.

# Definitions of Successful Aging

**LO 12-1 Compare some of the popular definitions of successful aging.**

The most widely researched theoretical model of optimal aging is that of Rowe and Kahn (1998) and is the foundation of the MacArthur Foundation Study of Aging in America and. Different from "usual" aging, the Rowe and Kahn definition of successful aging regards the optimum state to be the absence of disease and disability, high cognitive and physical functioning, and engagement with life as we age. Other researchers on successful aging have critiqued the Rowe and Kahn definition, stating it is unclear, overly focused on physical and cognitive health, and lacks psychological traits such as spirituality and well-being (Whitbourne & Bookwala, 2015). And a review of the successful aging literature shows that the majority of studies do not use all three criteria in their definitions of successful aging (Depp & Jeste, 2006).

Even when you think of the successful agers you know or see in the media, some may have one or more age-related limitations. That sharp grandmother may have a few memory lapses now and then, or perhaps she has had cataract surgery. That backpacking uncle may have just had cardiac surgery and need a walking stick from time to time as he navigates his way around the world. You may also know other individuals who have an age-related physical disability that severely limits their mobility but whose sense of optimism and hope rivals yours, even on your best days.

The Rowe and Kahn definition of successful aging has also been criticized because it does not take into account the individual's social context, including cultural norms or constraints on educational and occupational opportunities over the course of one's life. In some studies, successful agers are more heavily represented among Whites and among those with a college education or higher

(McLaughlin et al., 2010). Research has also found important contributors to successful aging that include early childhood conditions, such as parental social class and income (Brandt et al., 2012). Thus, successful aging is best viewed as a lifelong process reflecting the influence of multiple factors, including certain childhood conditions.

A model that focuses on a broader range of influences is the World Health Organization's (WHO, 2002a) definition of active aging, which includes "the process of optimizing opportunities for health, participation, and security to enhance quality of life as people age." The WHO model of active aging specifies a role for social, health care, and economic factors, and emphasizes the importance of the physical environment. WHO also makes the roles of autonomy and independence clear, placing more emphasis on an individual's ability to get around in the environment rather than on whether they need physical accommodations because of disability.

University of California at San Diego researchers attempted to overcome the limitations they identified in the Rowe and Kahn model (Vahia et al., 2012). They measured a range of qualities they thought were related to successful aging, including self-efficacy, optimism, attitudes toward aging in general, attitudes toward one's own aging, resilience, the endorsement of physical and emotional symptoms, depression, and a test of cognitive functioning (orientation, crystallized knowledge, and spatial skills). In their sample that used only women, they found that those highest in subjectively rated successful aging had high scores in self-efficacy, and optimism (what they called psychological protective factors of resilience); they were high in positive emotional functioning (low in depression and self-rated emotional symptoms); and they rated themselves low in physical symptoms, although physical symptoms were not as strongly related to successful aging as the resilience and emotional factors. Interestingly, performance on the cognitive tests did not predict self-rated successful aging in these women (Whitbourne & Bookwala, 2015). This study's findings support the argument that the Rowe and Kahn definition of successful aging is too narrow, and that psychological resilience and optimism are more important contributors to the older individual's own sense of successful aging than objective determinants. Building on these strengths, older adults may employ a range of active coping methods to help them achieve their desired goals that, as they think toward their future, can include preparing for potential stressors. Through proactive coping, successfully aging older adults can anticipate events they believe represent threats to their well-being and engage in mental preparation to reduce the impact of stress when it occurs. When the stressful event does occur, it will drain fewer coping resources (Ouwehand et al., 2007).

# Physical Health and Successful Aging

**LO 12-2 Describe how older adults come to their judgments on self-rated physical health.**

When it comes to successful aging, actual physical health appears to be less important than health behaviors, which appear vital to longevity. Examining the role of disability in the process of successful aging, researchers in Australia found that health behaviors, particularly physical exercise, predicted successful aging to an even greater extent than did social support or social contact (Parslow et al., 2011). These findings further reinforce what we've been saying about exercise and physical activity over the course of this book: Exercise is key for survival. It is an important predictor of overall well-being, especially as we get older. Despite the fact that even those highest on the successful aging factor reported several chronic health conditions, it appears those chronic diseases can still enjoy high levels of quality of life.

**FIGURE 12-2** Determinants of active aging.

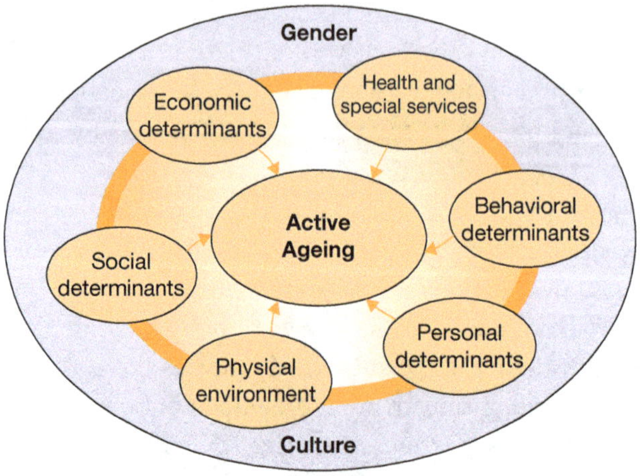

*Source:* World Health Organization, Global Age-Friendly Cities: A Guide, pp. 5, 2007, http://www.who.int/ageing/publications/Global_age_friendly_cities_Guide_English.pdf.

Satisfaction with health was one of the domains to show an accelerated decline in the oldest groups studied by McAdams et al. (2012). However, as we just noted, individuals may be in poor health objectively but still feel that they are aging successfully. As a result, self-rated physical health may differ from a more objective measure of physical functioning. Researchers believe older adults derive their self-rated health ratings through social comparison, the process that occurs when people rate themselves relative to their primary reference group.

If people in the older adult's reference group are in poorer health, the individual's self-rated health will be higher than if the reference group is in better health.

Yin et al. (2011) found that physical functioning had an inverse relation to self-rated health as individuals grew older. However, there were differences within the older groups in the physical functioning health ratings relation. Whites were more likely to have their actual physical functioning affect their self-rated health, as were older adults with advanced educational degrees. Thus, older adults from non-White racial/ethnic groups with less education whose health is disadvantaged may be more likely to compare themselves with members of a group that, like them, is in poor health. As a result, they may not show decreases in ratings of their own health.

Sexuality is another component of successful aging, known to play a role in overall health and well-being in the midlife and later years (Lindau & Gavrilova, 2010). Although sexual activity and functioning are negatively correlated with age (in other words, as we get older, our sexual activity and functioning lessen), there is no relation between age and sexual *satisfaction* for women. In fact, when it comes to successful aging, it has been linked to sexual satisfaction but not necessarily sexual activity.

# Social Support and Successful Aging

Having high levels of social support is generally recognized as beneficial to health throughout life, but particularly in the later years, and so social support often becomes part of the formula for achieving successful aging. Older adults with social support, particularly support from family, are most likely to have high ratings of successful aging (Bowling et al., 2002; Kissane & McLaren, 2006; Reichstadt et al., 2007). However, in addition to receiving, it seems important for older adults to be able to offer social support. Data from the Taiwanese Longitudinal Survey of Aging showed that in addition to the typical factors influencing health in later life, older adults who provided support to others seemed to benefit in terms of reduced rates of illness, disability, and mortality (Hsu & Chang, 2015).

# Successful Cognitive Aging

**LO 12-3** **What are some characteristics that set successful cognitive agers apart?**

Many believe successful cognitive aging is an important topic in its own right. An individual's cognitive functioning plays an important role in the ability to adapt to the demands of everyday life. As we know from earlier chapters, there are large interindividual differences in cognitive functioning. Some people maintain higher levels of cognitive performance in general, whereas others do not. Many older adults also regard cognitive functioning as central to their identities. This is one reason why some fear developing Alzheimer's disease and other neurocognitive disorders.

Most older adults preserve their cognitive abilities to a large degree. Studies of centenarians (Motta et al., 2005) and supercentenarians (those over age 110) show us that those who live to advanced ages are not only sturdy physiologically, but cognitively as well (Schoenhofen et al., 2006). Successful cognitive aging is cognitive performance above the average for an individual's age group, not based on standards for young adults (Fiocco & Yaffe, 2010; Negash et al., 2011). A sample of "superagers," defined as those 80 and older with superior episodic memory (i.e., comparable with that of middle-aged adults), were found by Harrison and colleagues (2012) on MRIs to have thicker cerebral cortex volume, and they showed greater volume of the cingulate cortex, an area that may be involved in preventing episodic memory loss (Whitbourne, 2015).

C-reactive protein (CRP), a known risk factor for cardiovascular disease in midlife, seems to serve a protective function against neurocognitive disorder for older adults. In a longitudinal study of male veterans and age-matched community volunteers, the individuals with the highest CRP levels were least likely to develop neurocognitive disorders over the 6-year period of the study (Silverman et al., 2012).

Successful cognitive aging in which an older individual is able to maintain superior memory performance may also reflect greater ability to engage in the compensatory activities involved in neuroplasticity that we discussed in the previous chapter. In comparing high- versus low-performing older adults on cognitive abilities, one team of researchers found that high-performing elders maintained their cognitive superiority by better encoding information while learning, which ultimately benefited their ability to retrieve the information when tested (Dockree et al., 2015).

# Life Satisfaction, Well-Being, and Successful Aging

**LO12-4** **Identify factors that affect life satisfaction and well-being as we age.**

Interest in successful aging fits more generally within the larger field of positive psychology, which seeks to provide a greater understanding of the strengths and virtues that enable individuals and communities to thrive. Within this positive psychology is the study of life satisfaction, the overall assessment of an individual's feelings and attitudes about their life at a particular point in time, and subjective well-being, the individual's overall sense of happiness. These two terms clearly are related; however, somewhat separate research traditions have developed around their use, so it is helpful to treat them as distinct. One difference is that life satisfaction may be more of a cognitive evaluation, but subjective well-being is more affective or emotional. Together, they represent a complete picture of a person's well-being (Diener, 1999). Therefore, unless we state otherwise, we will focus on subjective well-being as a way to understand the paths people take toward successful aging in adulthood.

One of the great puzzles for researchers who study successful aging is knowing exactly why so many adults are able to remain positive in their approach to life despite their accumulating chronic health conditions, normal age-related changes, and alterations in their social roles and financial security. The paradox of well-being refers to the well-established finding that older adults maintain high subjective well-being despite facing challenges from their objective circumstances. In support of this, subjective ratings of successful aging among old-old adults were found to be higher than the ratings made by young-old adults and to have a weaker association with actual physical and mental functioning (Martin et al., 2015).

As we mentioned earlier, some consider successful agers to be miraculous exceptions to the rule on aging. One reason why is that many theorists, researchers, and laypeople believe in the social indicator model (Mroczek & Kolarz, 1998), which suggests demographic and social structural variables, such as age, gender, marital status, and income, account for individual differences in levels of well-being. Because by demographic standards older individuals are in disadvantaged positions on these indices, they should therefore be less happy than the young. When an older adult maintains a high level of functioning despite potentially disturbing circumstances such as poor health, widowhood, and low income, then that person seems deserving of some kind of special recognition. There are connections between objective social indicators and subjective well-being. Studies of older adults show positive associations between feelings of well-being and personal resources, including physical functioning and adequacy of financial support (Katz, 2009). Not only physical functioning, but participation in physical activity also contributes to the subjective well-being of older adults (Mhaoláin et al., 2012). Education level then predicts high levels of physical and cognitive functioning, which predict high levels of subjective well-being (Jang et al., 2009).

If judged only by the standard of avoiding the despair brought about by lower status on important social indicators, there would be many successful agers. A national survey by the Pew Research Center of almost 3,000 Americans showed most older adults manage to enjoy relatively high subjective well-being on a variety of indices. Among respondents 75 and older, 81% said they were "very" or "pretty" happy, and only 19% rated themselves as "not too happy." Interestingly, most older adults rate their own experience of aging more favorably than younger adults would expect along a variety of dimensions from extent of memory loss to the feeling of being a burden on others.

The question then is whether some older adults have developed a set of coping skills over their lifetimes that allow them to frame events that younger adults would consider detrimental to their own well-being or even that the older adults would have found challenging when they themselves were younger. It is also possible that cohort effects lead current generations of older adults to feel higher levels of subjective well-being because they grew up with different expectations about what their lives would be like compared with current cohorts of young adults. Another possibility is that the paradox of well-being reflects a survival effect and that older adults who are still alive and available to be tested are hardier and more optimistic than those who are either no longer in the population or unwilling to participate in research studies. Perhaps these individuals were always inclined to view the world in a positive way, and the fact that they are the ones left standing at the end of life reflects their particular optimistic bias.

Some research has shown that the course of life satisfaction across adulthood is relatively stable until the very oldest ages, dropping slightly after the age of 70 and then more steadily in the 80s (Baird et al., 2010). However, subsequent research has shown different life patterns with life satisfaction decreasing in early in adulthood, increasing from mid- to late adulthood, and then decreasing again at the very end of life. In both cases, however, the results seemed to contradict predictions from the socioemotional selectivity theory we've discussed in previous chapters of a general upturn in satisfaction among the oldest-old. It appears that at the very end of life individuals may be influenced by objective life circumstances and, on average, show a gradual decline in their overall well-being.

It is still possible that those who remain happier longer are the ones who view the world in an optimistic manner, which, in turn, allows them to remain high in life satisfaction when their age peers are not. The set point perspective proposes that people's personalities influence their level of well-being throughout life. And it appears that personality traits may change in tandem with changes in well-being throughout adulthood. Using MIDUS data, Hill and colleagues (2012) found that people who scored higher on the traits of the five-factor model (see Chapter 9) had higher levels of well-being. Over time, positive changes in these traits correlated with further increases in well-being. This suggests personality acts as more than a set "point" in that its relation to changes in well-being continues to evolve.

Subjective well-being in later life also seems related to the tendency people have across adulthood to create and embellish their life story or narrative view of the past, in which they express their identities over the course of time (Whitbourne, 1985). Although individuals may differ in their narrative styles (Goodson, 2013), the process of constructing a life story continues throughout life and can serve a variety of adaptive functions (McAdams, 2011). Older adults seem to benefit from a life story that emphasizes their achievements and experiences that reflect favorably on their identity, altering the way they interpret events that might otherwise detract from their self-esteem (Whitbourne et al., 2002). Emerging adults seem to benefit from exploring alternatives as they arrive at identity commitments as long as this exploration does not involve a high degree of rumination and self-criticism (Ritchie et al., 2013). For older adults, identity processes may provide a means of maintaining high levels of well-being in the face of less than satisfactory circumstances. Identity assimilation allows them to place a positive interpretation on what might otherwise cause them to feel they are not accomplishing their desired objectives. Eventually, however, they may come to experience declines that they can no longer minimize, and at that point identity balance can bring their life story closer in line with the realities of their situation.

The ways individuals talk about their aging could influence the way they feel about aging and, ultimately, their actual ability to age successfully, according to the communicative ecology model of successful aging (CEMSA) (Fowler et al., 2015). According to CEMSA, people have great uncertainty about aging, which influences the way they talk about their own aging. The communication strategies they use in response to this uncertainty can alter their levels of self-efficacy about aging. The higher their self-efficacy, the more likely they will, as predicted by CEMSA, be able to age successfully. The communication strategies specific to CEMSA include expressing optimism about the aging process, not using age as a reason for general problems or limitations (i.e., not using the term "senior moment"), avoiding use of age stereotypes when referring to or thinking about other older adults, planning for the future with the assumption one will be there to enjoy it, and not giving up on trying to use new technology strategies such as social media and mobile phones. Older adults can also change the context in which they age by effectively managing ageist treatment by others to let them know that this sort of language is not acceptable. Finally, CEMSA advocates that older adults not allow themselves to be swayed by "peddlers of anti-aging products ... to recognize and resist the images propagated by an industry whose profitability rests on inducing their self-loathing" (Fowler et al., 2015, p. 437).

Successful aging is a complex process involving many moving parts. Older adults can develop a sense of high subjective well-being even in the face of many challenges. Although researchers are beginning to view subjective well-being as susceptible to potential threats very late in life, the majority of older adults avoid becoming depressed or even dissatisfied with their life situations.

# References

## A

Abar, C. C., Jackson, K. M., Colby, S. M., & Barnett, N. P. (2015). Parent-child discrepancies in reports of parental monitoring and their relationship to adolescent alcohol-related behaviors. *Journal of Youth and Adolescence, 44*(9), 1688–1701.

Abdou, C. M., Dunkel Schetter, C., Campos, B., Hilmert, C. J., Dominguez, T. P., Hobel, C. J., Glynn, L. M., & Sandman, C. (2010). Communalism predicts prenatal affect, stress, and physiology better than ethnicity and socioeconomic status. *Cultural Diversity and Ethnic Minority Psychology, 16*(3), 395–403. https://doi.org/10.1037/a0019808

Abrahin, O., Rodrigues, R. P., Nascimento, V. C., Da Silva-Grigoletto, M. E., Sousa, E. C., & Marcal, A. C. (2014). Single- and multiple-set resistance training improves skeletal and respiratory muscle strength in elderly women. *Clinical Interventions in Aging, 2014*(9), 1775–1782. https://doi.org/10.2147/CIA.S68529

Abrams, B., Altman, S. L., & Pickett, K. E. (2000). Pregnancy weight gain: Still controversial. *American Journal of Clinical Nutrition, 71*(5), 1233S–1241S.

Achem, S. R., & Devault, K. R. (2005). Dysphagia in aging. *Journal of Clinical Gastroenterology, 39*(5), 357–371.

Adachi, D., Nishiguchi, S., Fukutani, N., Kayama, H., Tanigawa, T., Yukutake, T., Hotta, T., Tashiro, Y., Morino, S., Yamata, M., & Aoyama, T. (2015). Factors associating with shuttle walking test results in community-dwelling elderly people. *Aging Clinical and Experimental Research, 27*(6), 829–834. https://doi.org/10.1007/s40520-015-0342-3

Adams, R. G., & Blieszner, R. (1994). An integrative conceptual framework for friendship research. *Journal of Social and Personal Relationships, 11*(2), 163–184.

Ades, P. A., & Toth, M. J. (2005). Accelerated decline of aerobic fitness with healthy aging: What is the good news? *Circulation, 112*(5), 624–626. doi:10.1161/CIRCULATIONAHA.105.553321

Ainsworth, M., Wittig, B., & Foss, B. (1969). Attachment and exploratory behavior of 1-year-olds in a strange situation. *Determinants of Infant Behavior*, Vol. 4 (pp. 11–136). Methuen.

Ainsworth, M. D. S. (1967). *Infancy in Uganda: Infant care and the growth of love.* Johns Hopkins University Press.

Alameel, T., Andrew, M. K., & Macknight, C. (2010). The association of fecal incontinence with institutionalization and mortality in older adults. *American Journal of Gastroenterology*. http://www.ncbi.nlm.nih.gov/entrez/query.fcgi?cmd=Retrieve&db=PubMed&dopt=Citation&list_uids=20216537doi:10.1038/ajg.2010.77

Aldwin, C. M., & Gilmer, D. F. (1999). Health and optimal aging. In J. C. Cavanaugh & S. K. Whitbourne (Eds.), *Gerontology: Interdisciplinary perspectives* (pp. 123–154). Oxford University Press.

Alkatan, M., Baker, J. R., Machin, D. R., Park, W., Akkari, A. S., Pasha, E. P., & Tanaka, H. (2016). Improved function and reduced pain after swimming and cycling training in patients with osteoarthritis. *Journal of Rheumatology, 43*(3), 666–672. https://doi.org/10.3899/jrheum.151110

Allely, C. S., & Wilson, P. (2011). Diagnosing autism spectrum disorder in primary care. *Practitioner, 255*(1745), 27–30, 3.

Allen, E. S., & Atkins, D. C. (2012). The association of divorce and extramarital sex in a representative U.S. sample. *Journal of Family Issues, 33*(11), 1477–1493. https://doi.org/10.1177/0192513x12439692

Allen, P. D., & Eddins, D. A. (2010). Presbycusis phenotypes form a heterogeneous continuum when ordered by degree and configuration of hearing loss. *Hearing Research, 264*(1–2), 10–20.

Almquist, Y. B., & Brännström, L. (2014). Childhood peer status and the clustering of social, economic, and health-related circumstances in adulthood. *Social Science & Medicine, 105*, 67–75.

Alonso-Fernandez, P., Puerto, M., Mate, I., Ribera, J. M., & de la Fuente, M. (2008). Neutrophils of centenarians show function levels similar to those of young adults. *Journal of the American Geriatrics Society, 56*(12), 2244–2251. https://doi.org/10.1111/j.1532-5415.2008.02018.x

Alvik, A., Torgersen, A. M., Aalen, O. O., & Lindemann, R. (2011). Binge alcohol exposure once a week in early pregnancy predicts temperament and sleeping problems in the infant. *Early Human Development, 87*(12), 827–833. https://doi.org/10.1016/j.earlhumdev.2011.06.009

Alzheimer's Association. (2015). 2015 Alzheimer's disease facts and figures. *Alzheimer's & dementia: the journal of the Alzheimer's Association, 11*(3), 332.

Amato, P. R. (2000). The consequences of divorce for adults and children. *Journal of Marriage and the Family, 62*(4), 511–521.

Amato, P. R., & Afifi, T. D. (2006). Feeling caught between parents: Adult children's relations with parents and subjective well-being. *Journal of Marriage and Family, 68*(1), 222–235.

American Academy of Pediatrics. (2019a). *Nutrition and exercise during pregnancy*. http://www.healthychildren.org/English/ages-stages/prenatal/pages/Nutrition-and-Exercise-During-Pregnancy.aspx

American Academy of Pediatrics. (2019b). *Where we stand: Smoking during pregnancy*. http://www.healthychildren.org/English/ages-stages/prenatal/pages/Where-We-Stand-Smoking-During-Pregnancy.aspx

American College of Obstetricians and Gynecologists. (2013). Definition of term pregnancy. *Obstetrics & Gynecology, 122*(5), 1139–1140.

American Psychiatric Association. (2013). *DSM-5 Diagnostic and Statistical Manual of Mental Disorders 5*. Author.

Ancoli-Israel, S., & Cooke, J. R. (2005). Prevalence and comorbidity of insomnia and effect on functioning in elderly populations. *Journal of the American Geriatrics Society, 53*(7), S264–S271.

Anestis, S. F. (2010). Hormones and social behavior in primates. *Evolutionary Anthropology: Issues, News, and Reviews, 19*(2), 66–78.

Angelucci, L. (2000). The glucocorticoid hormone: From pedestal to dust and back. *European Journal of Pharmacology, 405*(1–3), 139–147. https://doi.org/10.1016/S0014-2999(00)00547-1

Anger, J. T., Saigal, C. S., & Litwin, M. S. (2006). The prevalence of urinary incontinence among community dwelling adult women: Results from the National Health and Nutrition Examination Survey. *Journal of Urology, 175*(2), 601–604. https://doi.org/10.1016/S0022-5347(05)00242-9

Aoi, W. (2009). Exercise and food factors. *Forum in Nutrition, 61*, 147–155. https://doi.org/10.1159/000212747

Arabin, B. (2009). OP05.09: The development of senses—a concept for future trials. *Ultrasound in Obstetrics & Gynecology, 34*(S1), 78–78. https://doi.org/10.1002/uog.6696

Arabin, B., Bos, R., Rijlaarsdam, R., Mohnhaupt, A., & van Eyck, J. (1996). The onset of inter-human contacts: Longitudinal ultrasound observations in early twin pregnancies. *Ultrasound Obstetrics and Gynecology, 8*(3), 166–173.

Archer, N., Brown, R. G., Reeves, S., Boothby, H., Lovestone, S., & Nicholas, H. (2009). Midlife neuroticism and the age of onset of Alzheimer's disease. *Psychological Medicine, 39*(4), 665–673.

Arias, C., & Chotro, M. G. (2005). Increased preference for ethanol in the infant rat after prenatal ethanol exposure, expressed on intake and taste reactivity tests. *Alcoholism: Clinical and Experimental Research, 29*(3), 337–346. https://doi.org/10.1097/01.alc.0000156115.35817.21

Armstrong, P. I., & Anthoney, S. F. (2009). Personality facets and RIASEC interests: An integrated model. *Journal of Vocational Behavior, 75*(3), 346–359.

Armstrong-Stassen, M., & Ursel, N. D. (2009). Perceived organizational support, career satisfaction, and the retention of older workers. *Journal of Occupational and Organizational Psychology, 82*(1), 201–220.

Arnett, J. J. (2000). Emerging adulthood: A theory of development from the late teens through the twenties. *American Psychologist, 55*(5), 469–480.

Atladóttir, H. Ó., Henriksen, T. B., Schendel, D. E., & Parner, E. T. (2012). Autism after infection, febrile episodes, and antibiotic use during pregnancy: An exploratory study. *Pediatrics, 130*(6), e1447–e1454. https://doi.org/10.1542/peds.2012-1107

Aviles, A., & Neri, N. (2001). Hematological malignancies and pregnancy: A final report of 84 children who received chemotherapy in utero. *Clinical Lymphoma, 2*(3), 173–177.

Aykan, N. F. (2015). Red meat and colorectal cancer. *Oncology Reviews, 9*(1), 288. https://doi.org/10.4081/oncol.2015.288


# B


Baan, R., Grosse, Y., Straif, K., Secretan, B., El Ghissassi, F., Bouvard, V., Benbrahim-Talla, L., Guha, N., Freeman, C., Galichet, L., & Cogliano, V. (2009). A review of human carcinogens—Part F: Chemical agents and related occupations. *Lancet Oncology, 10*(12), 1143–1144.

Baird, B. M., Lucas, R. E., & Donnellan, M. B. (2010). Life satisfaction across the lifespan: Findings from two nationally representative panel studies. *Social Indicators Research, 99*, 183–203. https://doi.org/10.1007/s11205-010-9584-9

Baliunas, D. O., Taylor, B. J., Irving, H., Roerecke, M., Patra, J., Mohapatra, S., & Rehm, J. (2009). Alcohol as a risk factor for type 2 diabetes: A systematic review and meta-analysis. *Diabetes Care, 32*(11), 2123–2132. https://doi.org/10.2337/dc09-0227

Ball, H. L. (2009). Bed-sharing and co-sleeping: Research overview. *National Childbirth Trust New Digest, 48*, 22–27.

Baltes, P. B. (1979). Life-span developmental psychology: Some converging observations on history and theory. In P. B. Baltes & J. O. G. Brim (Eds.), *Life-span development and behavior*, Vol. 2 (pp. 255–279). Academic Press.

Baltes, P. B., & Graf, P. (1997). *Psychological aspects of aging: Facts and frontiers*. Cambridge University Press.

Bandura, A. (1989). Social cognitive theory. *Annals of Child Development, 6*, 1–60.

Bandura, A. (2002). Social foundations of thought and action. *The health psychology reader*, 94–106.

Barker, D. H., Quittner, A. L., Fink, N. E., Eisenberg, L. S., Tobey, E. A., & Niparko, J. K. (2009). Predicting behavior problems in deaf and hearing children: The influences of language, attention, and parent–child communication. *Development and Psychopathology, 21*(2), 373–392. https://doi.org/10.1017/S0954579409000212

Barth, F. D. (2015). Social media and adolescent development: Hazards, pitfalls and opportunities for growth. *Clinical Social Work Journal, 43*, 201–208.

Barwegen, L. M., Falciani, N. K., Putnam, S. J., Reamer, M. B., & Stair, E. E. (2004). Academic achievement of homeschool and public school students and student perception of parent involvement. *School Community Journal, 14*(1), 39–58.

Bauer, P. J., Larkina, M., & Deocampo, J. (2011). Early memory development. In U. Goswami (Ed.), *The Wiley-Blackwell handbook of childhood cognitive development* (2nd ed.) (153–179). Wiley-Blackwell.

Baumeister, R. F. (1996). Self-regulation and ego threat: Motivated cognition, self deception, and destructive goal setting. In P. M. Gollwitzer & J. A. Bargh (Eds.), *The psychology of action: Linking cognition and motivation to behavior* (pp. 27–47). Guilford.

Baumeister, R. F. (1997). Identity, self-concept, and self-esteem: The self lost and found. In R. Hogan, J. A. Johnson, & S. R. Briggs (Eds.), *Handbook of personality psychology* (pp. 681–710). Academic Press.

Baumeister, R. F., Bratslavsky, E., Finkenauer, C., & Vohs, K. D. (2001). Bad is stronger than good. *Review of General Psychology, 54*(4), 323–370.

Baumrind, D. (1991). The influence of parenting style on adolescent competence and substance use. *Journal of Early Adolescence, 11*(1), 56–95.

Beehr, T. A., Glazer, S., Nielson, N. L., & Farmer, S. J. (2000). Work and nonwork predictors of employees' retirement ages. *Journal of Vocational Behavior, 57*(2), 206–225.

Bellipanni, G., Bianchi, P., Pierpaoli, W., Bulian, D., & Ilyia, E. (2001). Effects of melatonin in perimenopausal and menopausal women: A randomized and placebo controlled study. *Experimental Gerontology, 36*(2), 297–310.

Beltrand, J., Soboleva, T. K., Shorten, P. R., Derraik, J. G., Hofman, P., Albertsson-Wikland, K., Hockberg, Z., & Cutfield, W. S. (2012). Post-term birth is associated with greater risk of obesity in adolescent males. *Journal of Pediatrics, 160*(5), 769–773. https://doi.org/10.1016/j.jpeds.2011.10.030

Benasich, A. A., Choudhury, N., Friedman, J. T., Realpe-Bonilla, T., Chojnowska, C., & Gou, Z. (2006). The infant as a prelinguistic model for language learning impairments: Predicting from event-related potentials to behavior. *Neuropsychologia, 44*(3), 396–411. https://doi.org/10.1016/j.neuropsychologia.2005.06.004

Benes, F. M. (1998). Brain development, VII: Human brain growth spans decades. *American Journal of Psychiatry, 155*(11), 1489–1489.

Benjamin, E. J., Blaha, M. J., Chiuve, S. E., Cushman, M., Das, S. R., Deo, R., de Ferranti, S. D., Floyd, J., Fornage, M., Gillespie, C., Isasi, C. R., Jiménez, M. C., Jordan, L. C., Judd, S. E., Lackland, D., Lichtman, J. H., Lisabeth, L., Liu, S., Longenecker, C. T., ... & Muntner, P. (2017). Heart disease and stroke statistics—2017 update: A report from the American Heart Association. *Circulation, 135*(10), e145–e603.

Benloucif, S., Orbeta, L., Ortiz, R., Janssen, I., Finkel, S. I., Bleiberg, J., & Zee, P. C. (2004). Morning or evening activity improves neuropsychological performance and subjective sleep quality in older adults. *Sleep, 27*(8), 1542–1551.

Bennett, K. M., Smith, P. T., & Hughes, G. M. (2005). Coping, depressive feelings and gender differences in late life widowhood. *Aging and Mental Health, 9*(4), 348–353.

Benson, J. J., & Coleman, M. (2016). Older adults developing a preference for living apart together. *Journal of Marriage and Family, 78*(3), 797–812. https://doi.org/10.1111/jomf.12292

Benson, L. A., McGinn, M. M., & Christensen, A. (2012). Common principles of couple therapy. *Behavior Therapy, 43*(1), 25–35. https://doi.org/10.1016/j.beth.2010.12.009

Berg, A. I., Hassing, L. B., McClearn, G. E., & Johansson, B. (2006). What matters for life satisfaction in the oldest-old? *Aging and Mental Health, 10*(3), 257–264.

Bernardes, S. F., Marques, S., & Matos, M. (2015). Old and in pain: Enduring and situational effects of cultural aging stereotypes on older people's pain experiences. *European Journal of Pain, 19*(7), 994–1001. https://doi.org/10.1002/ejp.626

Bernstein, H. H., Spino, C., Lalama, C. M., Finch, S. A., Wasserman, R. C., & McCormick, M. C. (2013). Unreadiness for postpartum discharge following healthy term pregnancy: Impact on health care use and outcomes. *Academic Pediatrics, 13*(1), 27–39. https://doi.org/10.1016/j.acap.2012.08.005

Best, P., Manktelow, R., & Taylor, B. (2014). Online communication, social media and adolescent wellbeing: A systematic narrative review. *Children and Youth Services Review, 41*, 27–36.

Bharucha, A. E., & Camilleri, M. (2001). Functional abdominal pain in the elderly. *Gastroenterology Clinics of North America, 30*(2), 517–529.

Bhave, D. P., Kramer, A., & Glomb, T. M. (2010). Work-family conflict in work groups: Social information processing, support, and demographic dissimilarity. *Journal of Applied Psychology, 95*(1), 145–158.

Biblarz, T. J., & Stacey, J. (2010). How does the gender of parents matter? *Journal of Marriage and Family, 72*(1), 3–22. https://doi.org/10.1111/j.1741-3737.2009.00678.x

Birditt, K. S., Fingerman, K. L., & Almeida, D. M. (2005). Age differences in exposure and reactions to interpersonal tensions: A daily diary study. *Psychology and Aging, 20*(2), 330–340. https://doi.org/10.1037/0882-7974.20.2.330

Birditt, K. S., Tighe, L. A., Fingerman, K. L., & Zarit, S. H. (2012). Intergenerational relationship quality across three generations. *Journals of Gerontology: Series B: Psychological Sciences And Social Sciences, 67*(5), 627–638. https://doi.org/10.1093/geronb/gbs050

Bischoff-Ferrari, H. A., Kiel, D. P., Dawson-Hughes, B., Orav, J. E., Li, R., Spiegelman, D., Dietrich, T., & Willett, W. C. (2009). Dietary calcium and serum 25-hydroxyvitamin D status in relation to BMD among U.S. adults. *Journal of Bone and Mineral Research, 24*(5), 935–942. https://doi.org/10.1359/jbmr.081242

Bleich, S. N., Barry, C. L., Gary-Webb, T. L., & Herring, B. J. (2014). Reducing sugar-sweetened beverage consumption by providing caloric information: How Black adolescents alter their purchases and whether the effects persist. *American Journal of Public Health, 104*(12), 2417–2424.

Blenkner, M. (1963). Social work and family relations in later life with some thoughts on filial maturity. In E. Shanas & G. F. Streib (Eds.), *Social structure and the family: Generational relations* (pp. 46–59). Prentice-Hall.

Bloom, H. G., Ahmed, I., Alessi, C. A., Ancoli-Israel, S., Buysse, D. J., Kryger, M. H., Phillips, B. A., Thorpy, M. J., Vitiello, M. V., & Zee, P. C. (2009). Evidence-based recommendations for the assessment and management of sleep disorders in older persons. *Journal of the American Geriatrics Society, 57*(11), 761–789.

Boaz, N. T., & Almquist, A. J. (1999). *Essentials of biological anthropology.* Prentice Hall.

Boling, M. C., Bolgla, L. A., Mattacola, C. G., Uhl, T. L., & Hosey, R. G. (2006). Outcomes of a weight-bearing rehabilitation program for patients diagnosed with patellofemoral pain syndrome. *Archives of Physical Medicine and Rehabilitation, 87*(11), 1428–1435.

Bonanno, G. A., Wortman, C. B., Lehman, D. R., Tweed, R. G., Haring, M., Sonnega, J., Carr, D., & Nesse, R. M. (2002). Resilience to loss and chronic grief: A prospective study from preloss to 18-months postloss. *Journal of Personality & Social Psychology, 83*(5), 1150–1164.

Bonanno, G. A., Wortman, C. B., & Nesse, R. M. (2004). Prospective patterns of resilience and maladjustment during widowhood. *Psychology and Aging, 19*(2), 260–271.

Bonnefond, A., Härmä, M., Hakola, T., Sallinen, M., Kandolin, I., & Virkkala, J. (2006). Interaction of age with shift-related sleep-wakefulness, sleepiness, performance, and social life. *Experimental Aging Research, 32*(2), 185–208.

Boron, W., & Boulpaep, E. (2004). *Medical physiology: A cellular and molecular approach.* Elsevier.

Bortz, W. M. (2005). Biological basis of determinants of health. *American Journal of Public Health, 95*, 389–392.

Botwinick, J. (1977). Intellectual abilities. In J. E. Birren & K. W. Schaie (Eds.), *Handbook of the psychology of aging* (pp. 580–605). Van Nostrand Reinhold.

Bouchard, T. J. J. (2004). Genetic influence on human psychological traits: A survey. *Current Directions in Psychological Science, 13*(4), 148–151.

Bowlby, J. (1969). *Attachment and loss, Vol 1: Attachment.* Basic Books.

Bowlby, J. (1973). *Attachment and Loss: Vol. 2. Separation.* Basic Books.

Bowlby, J. (1980). Attachment and loss: Loss, sadness and depression (Vol. 3): Basic Books.

Bowling, A., Banister, D., Sutton, S., Evans, O., & Windsor, J. (2002). A multidimensional model of the quality of life in older age. *Aging and Mental Health, 6*(4), 355–371.

Boylan, S., Welch, A., Pikhart, H., Malyutina, S., Pajak, A., Kubinova, R., Bragina, O., Simonova, G., Stepaniak, U., Gilis-Januszewska, A., Milla, L., Peasey, A., Marmot, M., & Bobak, M. (2009). Dietary habits in three Central and Eastern European countries: The HAPIEE study. *BMC Public Health, 9*, 439. https://doi.org/10.1186/1471-2458-9-439

Boyle, J. (2011). Speech and language delays in preschool children. *BMJ, 343*. https://doi.org/10.1136/bmj.d5181

Boyle, S. H., Jackson, W. G., & Suarez, E. C. (2007). Hostility, anger, and depression predict increases in C3 over a 10-year period. *Brain, Behavior, and Immunity*. http://www.ncbi.nlm.nih.gov/entrez/query.fcgi?cmd=Retrieve&db=PubMed&dopt=Citation&list_uids=17321106

Bramlett, M. D., & Mosher, W. D. (2002). Cohabitation, marriage, divorce, and remarriage in the United States. National Center for Health Statistics. *Vital and Health Statistics, 23*(22), 1–93.

Brand, E., Kothari, C., & Stark, M. A. (2011). Factors related to breastfeeding discontinuation between hospital discharge and 2 weeks postpartum. *Journal of Perinatal Education, 20*(1), 36–44. https://doi.org/10.1891/1058-1243.20.1.36

Brandt, M., Deindl, C., & Hank, K. (2012). Tracing the origins of successful aging: The role of childhood conditions and social inequality in explaining later life health. *Social Science & Medicine, 74*(9), 1418–1425. https://doi.org/10.1016/j.socscimed.2012.01.004

Breborowicz, G. H. (2001). Limits of fetal viability and its enhancement. *Early Pregnancy, 5*(1), 49–50.

Brechwald, W. A., & Prinstein, M. J. (2011). Beyond homophily: A decade of advances in understanding peer influence processes. *Journal of Research on Adolescence, 21*(1), 166–179. https://doi.org/10.1111/j.1532-7795.2010.00721.x

Brendgen, M., Dishion, T. J., & Tremblay, R. E. (2010). Transactional analysis of the reciprocal links between peer experiences and academic achievement from middle childhood to early adolescence. *Developmental Psychology, 46*(4), 773.

Brennan, P. L., Schutte, K. K., & Moos, R. H. (2006). Long-term patterns and predictors of successful stressor resolution in later life. *International Journal of Stress Management, 13*(3), 253–272.

Brim, D., Townsend, D. B., DeQuinzio, J. A., & Poulson, C. L. (2009). Analysis of social referencing skills among children with autism. *Research in Autism spectrum disorder, 3*(4), 942–958. https://doi.org/10.1016/j.rasd.2009.04.004

Broesch, T. L., & Bryant, G. A. (2013). Prosody in infant-directed speech is similar across western and traditional cultures. *Journal of Cognition and Development, 16*(1), 31–43. https://doi.org/10.1080/15248372.2013.833923

Bromley, R. L., Baker, G. A., & Meador, K. J. (2009). Cognitive abilities and behaviour of children exposed to antiepileptic drugs in utero. *Current Opinion in Neurology, 22*(2), 162–166. https://doi.org/10.1097/WCO.0b013e3283292401

Brookmeyer, R., Corrada, M. M., Curriero, F. C., & Kawas, C. (2002). Survival following a diagnosis of Alzheimer disease. *Archives Neurology, 59*(11), 1764–1767.

Brooks-Gunn, J., & Warren, M. P. (1989). Biological and social contributions to negative affect in young adolescent girls. *Child Development, 60*(1), 40–55.

Brotherson, S. (2009). *Understanding brain development in young children*. http://www.ag.ndsu.edu/pubs/yf/famsci/fs609.pdf

Brown, S. L., Bulanda, J. R., & Lee, G. R. (2012). Transitions into and out of cohabitation in later life. *Journal of Marriage and Family, 74*(4), 774–793.

Brummett, B. H., Babyak, M. A., Williams, R. B., Barefoot, J. C., Costa, P. T., & Siegler, I. C. (2006). NEO personality domains and gender predict levels and trends in body mass index over 14 years during midlife. *Journal of Research in Personality, 40*(3), 222–236.

Bryant, G. A., Liénard, P., & Clark Barrett, H. (2012). Recognizing infant-directed speech across distant cultures: Evidence from Africa. *Journal of Evolutionary Psychology, 10*(2), 47–59.

Buckner, R. L., Andrews-Hanna, J. R., & Schacter, D. L. (2008). The brain's default network: Anatomy, function, and relevance to disease. *Annals of the New York Academy of Science, 1124*(1), 1–38. https://doi.org/10.1196/annals.1440.011

Burgmans, S., van Boxtel, M. P., Gronenschild, E. H., Vuurman, E. F., Hofman, P., Uylings, H. B., Jolles, J., & Raz, N. (2010). Multiple indicators of age-related differences in cerebral white matter and the modifying effects of hypertension. *Neuroimage, 49*(3), 2083–2093. https://doi.org/10.1016/j.neuroimage.2009.10.035

Burke, K. E., & Wei, H. (2009). Synergistic damage by UVA radiation and pollutants. *Toxicology and Industrial Health, 25*(4–5), 219–224. https://doi.org/10.1177/0748233709106067

Burn, K., & Szoeke, C. (2016). Boomerang families and failure-to-launch: Commentary on adult children living at home. *Maturitas, 83*, 9–12.

Byberg, L., Melhus, H. K., Gedeborg, R., Sundstrom, J., Ahlbom, A., Zethelius, B., … Michaelsson, K. (2009). Total mortality after changes in leisure time physical activity in 50 year old men: 35 year follow-up of population based cohort. *BMJ: British Medical Journal, 338*. https://doi.org/10.1136/bmj.b688

Byrne, C. M., Solomon, M. J., Young, J. M., Rex, J., & Merlino, C. L. (2007). Biofeedback for fecal incontinence: Short-term outcomes of 513 consecutive patients and predictors of successful treatment. *Diseases of the Colon and Rectum, 50*(4), 417–427. https://doi.org/10.1007/s10350-006-0846-1

Bystrova, K., Widstrom, A. M., Matthiesen, A. S., Ransjo-Arvidson, A. B., Welles-Nystrom, B., Wassberg, C., Vorontsov, I., & Uvnas-Moberg, K. (2003). Skin-to-skin contact may reduce negative consequences of "the stress of being born": A study on temperature in newborn infants, subjected to different ward routines in St. Petersburg. *Acta Paediatrica, 92*(3), 320–326.

# C

Callahan, C. M., Boustani, M. A., Unverzagt, F. W., Austrom, M. G., Damush, T. M., Perkins, A. J., Fultz, B. A., Hui, S. L., Counsell, S. R., & Hendrie, H. C. (2006). Effectiveness of collaborative care for older adults with Alzheimer disease in primary care: A randomized controlled trial. *Journal of the American Medical Association, 295*(18), 2148–2157.

Calle, E. E., Rodriguez, C., Walker-Thurmond, K., & Thun, M. J. (2003). Overweight, obesity, and mortality from cancer in a prospectively studied cohort of U.S. adults. *New England Journal of Medicine, 348*(17), 1625–1638. https://doi.org/10.1056/NEJMoa021423

Callister, L. C., Khalaf, I., Semenic, S., Kartchner, R., & Vehvilainen-Julkunen, K. (2003). The pain of childbirth: Perceptions of culturally diverse women. *Pain Management Nursing, 4*(4), 145–154.

Campbell, B. (2011a). Adrenarche and middle childhood. *Human Nature, 22*(9), 327–349. https://doi.org/10.1007/s12110-011-9120-x

Campbell, B. (2011b). An introduction to the special issue on middle childhood. *Human Nature, 22*, 247–248. https://doi.org/10.1007/s12110-011-9118-4

Cao, J. J., Wronski, T. J., Iwaniec, U., Phleger, L., Kurimoto, P., Boudignon, B., & Halloran, B. P. (2005). Aging increases stromal/osteoblastic cell-induced osteoclastogenesis and alters the osteoclast precursor pool in the mouse. *Journal of Bone and Mineral Research, 20*(9), 1659–1668.

Card, N. A., Stucky, B. D., Sawalani, G. M., & Little, T. D. (2008). Direct and indirect aggression during childhood and adolescence: A meta-analytic review of gender differences, intercorrelations, and relations to maladjustment. *Child Development, 79*(5), 1185–1229.

Carlson, S. M. (2003). Executive function in context: Development, measurement, theory, and experience. *Monographs of the Society for Research in Child Development, 68*(3), 138–151.

Carlson, S. M., & Wang, T. S. (2007). Inhibitory control and emotion regulation in preschool children. *Cognitive Development, 22*(4), 489–510. https://doi.org/10.1016/j.cogdev.2007.08.002

Carnelley, K. B., Wortman, C. B., Bolger, N., & Burke, C. T. (2006). The time course of grief reactions to spousal loss: Evidence from a national probability sample. *Journal of Personality and Social Psychology, 91*(3), 476–492.

Carroll, C. C., Dickinson, J. M., Haus, J. M., Lee, G. A., Hollon, C. J., Aagaard, P., Magnusson, S. P., & Trappe, T. A. (2008). Influence of aging on the in vivo properties of human patellar tendon. *Journal of Applied Physiology, 105*(6), 1907–1915. https://doi.org/10.1152/japplphysiol.00059.2008

Cates, C. B., Dreyer, B. P., Berkule, S. B., White, L. J., Arevalo, J. A., & Mendelsohn, A. L. (2012). Infant communication and subsequent language development in children from low-income families: The role of early cognitive stimulation. *Journal of Developmental & Behavioral Pediatrics, 33*(7), 577–585.

Cattell, R. B. (1963). Theory of fluid and crystallized intelligence: A critical experiment. *Journal of Educational Psychology, 54*(1), 1–22.

Cattell, R. B. (1971). *Abilities: Their structure, growth, and action.* Houghton Mifflin.

Cauley, J. A., Lui, L. Y., Barnes, D., Ensrud, K. E., Zmuda, J. M., Hillier, T. A., Hochberg, M. C., Schwartz, A. V., Yaffe, K., Cummings, S. R., & Newman, A. B. (2009). Successful skeletal aging: A marker of low fracture risk and longevity. The Study of Osteoporotic Fractures (SOF). *Journal of Bone Mineral Research, 24*(1), 134–143. https://doi.org/10.1359/jbmr.080813

Cauley, J. A., Palermo, L., Vogt, M., Ensrud, K. E., Ewing, S., Hochberg, M., Schwartz, A. V., Yaffe, K., Cummings, S. R., & Black, D. M. (2008). Prevalent vertebral fractures in black women and white women. *Journal of Bone Mineral Research, 23*, 1458–1467. https://doi.org/10.1359/jbmr.080411

Caviness, V., Kennedy, D., Richelme, C., Rademacher, J., & Filipek, P. (1996). The human brain age 7–11 years: A volumetric analysis based on magnetic resonance images. *Cerebral Cortex, 6*(5), 726–736.

Center on the Developing Child. *Child development fact sheet.* Harvard University.

Centers for Disease Control and Prevention. (2010b). *Defining overweight and obesity.* http://www.cdc.gov/obesity/defining.html

Centers for Disease Control and Prevention. (2011a). *Assisted reproductive technology success rates: National summary and fertility clinic reports.* American Society for Reproductive Medicine, Society for Assisted Reproductive Technology.

Centers for Disease Control and Prevention. (2011b). *Child development.* http://www.cdc.gov/ncbddd/childdevelopment/positiveparenting/index.html

Centers for Disease Control and Prevention. (2013d). *Preventing shaken baby syndrome: A guide for health departments and community-based organizations. Head's up.* http://www.cdc.gov/concussion/pdf/preventing_sbs_508-a.pdf

Centers for Disease Control and Prevention. (2013e). *What is premature birth.* http://www.cdc.gov/features/prematurebirth/

Centers for Disease Control and Prevention. (2013f). *School connectedness: Strategies for increasing protective factors among youth.* U.S. Department of Health and Human Services.

Centers for Disease Control and Prevention. (2017a). *Health United States.* https://www.cdc.gov/nchs/data/hus/2016/057.pdf

Centers for Disease Control and Prevention. (2018). *Obesity.* http://www.cdc.gov/healthyyouth/obesity/facts.htm

Centers for Disease Control and Prevention. (2019). *Facts about birth. Birth defects.* http://www.cdc.gov/NCBDDD/birthdefects/facts.html

Centers for Disease Control and Prevention. (2020). *ADHD.* http://www.cdc.gov/ncbddd/adhd/facts.html

Centers for Disease Control and Prevention. (2020). *Infant health.* http://www.cdc.gov/nchs/fastats/infant_health.htm

Centers for Disease Control and Prevention. (2020). *National diabetes statistics report, 2017.* https://www.cdc.gov/diabetes/pdfs/data/statistics/national-diabetes-statistics-report.pdf

Centers for Disease Control and Prevention. (2020). *Marriage and divorce.* https://www.cdc.gov/nchs/fastats/marriage-divorce.htm

Centers for Disease Control and Prevention. (2020). *Burden of tobacco use in the U.S.* https://www.cdc.gov/tobacco/campaign/tips/resources/data/cigarette-smoking-in-united-states.html

Chamberlain, D. B. (2013). *The fetal senses: A classical view.* http://birthpsychology.com/free-article/fetal-senses-classical-view

Chandola, T., Brunner, E., & Marmot, M. (2006). Chronic stress at work and the metabolic syndrome: Prospective study. *BMJ: British Medical Journal, 332*(7540), 521–525.

Chang, Y.-K., & Etnier, J. L. (2009). Exploring the dose-response relationship between resistance exercise intensity and cognitive function. *Journal of Sport and Exercise Psychology, 31*(5), 640–656.

Charles, S. T., & Carstensen, L. L. (2010). Social and emotional aging. *Annual Review of Psychology, 61*(1), 383–409.

Charlton, R. A., Barrick, T. R., Markus, H. S., & Morris, R. G. (2009). The relationship between episodic long-term memory and white matter integrity in normal aging. *Neuropsychologia, 48*(1), 114–122. https://doi.org/10.1016/j.neuropsychologia.2009.08.018

Chase, P. A., Hilliard, L. J., Geldhof, G. J., Warren, D. J., & Lerner, R. M. (2014). Academic achievement in the high school years: The changing role of school engagement. *Journal of Youth and Adolescence, 43*(6), 884–896.

Chedraui, P., Perez-Lopez, F. R., Mendoza, M., Leimberg, M. L., Martinez, M. A., Vallarino, V., & Hidalgo, L. (2010). Factors related to increased daytime sleepiness during the menopausal transition as evaluated by the Epworth sleepiness scale. *Maturitas, 65*(1), 75–80. https://doi.org/10.1016/j.maturitas.2009.11.003

Chen, H., Cohen, P., Kasen, S., Johnson, J. G., Ehrensaft, M., & Gordon, K. (2006). Predicting conflict within romantic relationships during the transition to adulthood. *Personal Relationships, 13*(4), 411–427.

Cherry, K. E., Silva, J. L., & Galea, S. (2009). Natural disasters and the oldest-old: A psychological perspective on coping and health in late life. In *Life span perspectives on natural disasters: Coping with Katrina, Rita, and other storms* (pp. 171–193). Springer.

Chess, S., & Thomas, A. (1999). *Goodness of fit: Clinical applications from infancy through adult life.* Psychology Press.

Child Welfare Information Gateway. (2010). *Impact of adoption on adoptive parents. Factsheets for families.* https://www.childwelfare.gov/pubs/factsheets/impact_parent/index.cfm

Chiriaco, G., Cauci, S., Mazzon, G., & Trombetta, C. (2016). An observational retrospective evaluation of 79 young men with long-term adverse effects after use of finasteride against androgenetic alopecia. *Andrology, 4*(2), 245–250. https://doi.org/10.1111/andr.12147

Chodzko-Zajko, W. J., Proctor, D. N., Fiatarone Singh, M. A., Minson, C. T., Nigg, C. R., Salem, G. J., & Skinner, J. S. (2009). American College of Sports Medicine position stand. Exercise and physical activity for older adults. *Medicine and Science in Sports and Exercise, 41*(7), 1510–1530. https://doi.org/10.1249/MSS.0b013e3181a0c95c

Choudhury, S., Blakemore, S.-J., & Charman, T. (2006). Social cognitive development during adolescence. *Social Cognitive and Affective Neuroscience, 1*(3), 165–174. https://doi.org/10.1093/scan/nsl024

Christiansen, S. L., & Palkovitz, R. (2001). Why the "good provider" role still matters: Providing as a form of paternal involvement. *Journal of Family Issues, 22*(1), 84–106.

Chung, C.-S., Lee, Y.-C., & Wu, M.-S. (2015). Prevention strategies for esophageal cancer: Perspectives of the East vs. West. *Best Practice & Research Clinical Gastroenterology, 29*(6), 869–883.

Cicirelli, V. G. (1988). A measure of filial anxiety regarding anticipated care of elderly parents. *Gerontologist, 28*(4), 478–482.

Cicirelli, V. G. (2010). Attachment relationships in old age. *Journal of Social and Personal Relationships, 27*(2), 191–199. https://doi.org/10.1177/0265407509360984

Ciechanowski, P., Sullivan, M., Jensen, M., Romano, J., & Summers, H. (2003). The relationship of attachment style to depression, catastrophizing and health care utilization in patients with chronic pain. *Pain, 104*(3), 627–637.

Clarke, P., Marshall, V. W., & Weir, D. (2012). Unexpected retirement from full time work after age 62: Consequences for life satisfaction in older Americans. *European Journal of Ageing, 9*(3), 207–219. https://doi.org/10.1007/s10433-012-0229-5

Coelho, S. G., Choi, W., Brenner, M., Miyamura, Y., Yamaguchi, Y., Wolber, R., Smuda, C., Batzer, J., Kolbe, L., Ito, S., Wakamatsu, K., Zmudzka, B. Z., Beer, J. Z., Miller, S. A., & Hearing, V. J. (2009). Short- and long-term effects of UV radiation on the pigmentation of human skin. *Journal of Investigative Dermatology Symposium Proceedings, 14*(1), 32–35. https://doi.org/10.1038/jidsymp.2009.10

Cohan, C. L., & Kleinbaum, S. (2002). Toward a greater understanding of the cohabitation effect: Premarital cohabitation and marital communication. *Journal of Marriage and Family, 64*(1), 180–192.

Coie, J. D., & Dodge, K. A. (1983). Continuities and changes in children's social status: A five-year longitudinal study. *Merrill-Palmer Quarterly, 29*(3), 261–282.

Coie, J. D., Dodge, K. A., & Coppotelli, H. (1982). Dimensions and types of social status: A cross-age perspective. *Developmental Psychology, 18*(4), 557–570.

Colombo, J., & Fagen, J. (2014). *Individual differences in infancy: Reliability, stability, and prediction*: Psychology Press.

Coltrane, S. (2000). Research on household labor: Modeling and measuring the social embeddedness of routine family work. *Journal of Marriage and Family, 62*(4), 1208–1233.

Combs, J. L., Pearson, C. M., & Smith, G. T. (2011). A risk model for preadolescent disordered eating. *International Journal of Eating Disorders, 44*(7), 596–604. https://doi.org/10.1002/eat.20851

Comijs, H. C., Gerritsen, L., Penninx, B. W., Bremmer, M. A., Deeg, D. J., & Geerlings, M. I. (2010). The association between serum cortisol and cognitive decline in older persons. *American Journal of Geriatric Psychiatry, 18*(1), 42–50. https://doi.org/10.1097/JGP.0b013e3181b970ae

Committee on Child Abuse and Neglect. (2001). Shaken baby syndrome: Rotational cranial injuries—Technical report. *Pediatrics, 108*(1), 206–210. https://doi.org/10.1542/peds.108.1.206

Committee on Fetus and Newborn. (2004). Hospital stay for healthy term newborns. *Pediatrics, 113*(5), 1434–1436.

Common Sense Media. (2012). Children, teens, and entertainment media: The view from the classroom. https://www.commonsensemedia.org/research/children-teens-and-entertainment-media-the-view-from-the-classroom

Common Sense Media. (2013, February 13). Media and violence: An analysis of current research. https://www.commonsensemedia.org/research/media-and-violence-an-analysis-of-current-research

Conde-Agudelo, A., Diaz-Rossello, J. L., & Belizan, J. M. (2003). Kangaroo mother care to reduce morbidity and mortality in low birthweight infants. *Cochrane Database of Systematic Reviews*, CD002771. https://doi.org/10.1002/14651858.CD002771

Connolly, J., McIsaac, C., Shulman, S., Wincentak, K., Joly, L., Heifetz, M., & Bravo, V. (2014). Development of romantic relationships in adolescence and emerging adulthood: Implications for community mental health. *Canadian Journal of Community Mental Health, 33*(1), 7–19.

Conroy, K., Sandel, M., & Zuckerman, B. (2010). Poverty grown up: How childhood socioeconomic status impacts adult health. *Journal of Developmental and Behavioral Pediatrics, 31*(2), 154–160. https://doi.org/10.1097/DBP.0b013e3181c21a1b

Consedine, N. S., & Magai, C. (2003). Attachment and emotion experience in later life: The view from emotions theory. *Attachment and Human Development, 5*(2), 165–187. https://doi.org/10.1080/1461673031000108496

Conway, A., & Stifter, C. A. (2012). Longitudinal antecedents of executive function in preschoolers. *Child Development, 83*(3), 1022–1036. https://doi.org/10.1111/j.1467-8624.2012.01756.x

Cooper, B. S., & Sureau, J. (2007). The politics of homeschooling: New developments, new challenges. *Educational Policy, 21*(1), 110–131.

Copeland, W. E., Wolke, D., Angold, A., & Costello, E. J. (2013). Adult psychiatric outcomes of bullying and being bullied by peers in childhood and adolescence. *JAMA Psychiatry, 70*(4), 419–426.

Copen, C. E., Daniels, K., Vespa, J., & Mosher, W. D. (2012, March 22). First marriages in the United States: Data from the 2006–2010 National Survey of Family Growth. *National Health Statistics Reports* (no. 49). http://www.cdc.gov/nchs/data/nhsr/nhsr049.pdf

Coplan, R. J., & Weeks, M. (2010). Unsociability in middle childhood: Conceptualization, assessment, and associations with socioemotional functioning. *Merrill-Palmer Quarterly, 56*(2), 105–130.

Cornwell, B. (2012). Spousal network overlap as a basis for spousal support. *Journal of Marriage and Family, 74*(2), 229–238. https://doi.org/10.1111/j.1741-3737.2012.00959.x

Costa, P. T., Jr., & McCrae, R. R. (1992). *NEO-PI-R manual.* Psychological Assessment Resources.

Covay, E., & Carbonaro, W. (2010). After the bell: Participation in extracurricular activities, classroom behavior, and academic achievement. *Sociology of Education, 83*(1), 20–45. https://doi.org/10.1177/0038040709356565

Covinsky, K. E., Lindquist, K., Dunlop, D. D., & Yelin, E. (2009). Pain, functional limitations, and aging. *Journal of the American Geriatrics Society, 57*(9), 1556–1561. https://doi.org/10.1111/j.1532-5415.2009.02388.x

Cramer, P., & Jones, C. J. (2007). Defense mechanisms predict differential lifespan change in self-control and self-acceptance. *Journal of Research in Personality, 41*(4), 841–855.

Cranley, M. S. (1981). Development of a tool for the measurement of maternal attachment during pregnancy. *Nursing Research, 30*(5), 281–284.

Criss, M. M., Lee, T. K., Morris, A. S., Cui, L., Bosler, C. D., Shreffler, K. M., & Silk, J. S. (2015). Link between monitoring behavior and adolescent adjustment: An analysis of direct and indirect effects. *Journal of Child and Family Studies, 24*(3), 668–678.

Crockett, L. J. (1997). Cultural, historical, and subcultural contexts of adolescence: Implications for health and development. *Health Risks and Developmental Transitions During Adolescence*, 23–53.

Crosnoe, R., & Elder, G. H., Jr. (2002). Life course transitions, the generational stake, and grandparent-grandchild relationships. *Journal of Marriage and Family, 64*(4), 1089–1096.

Crowe, F., Roddam, A., Key, T., Appleby, P., Overvad, K., Jakobsen, M., Tjønneland, A., Hansen, L., Boeing, H.,

Weikert, C., Linseisen, J., Kaaks, R., Trichopoulou, R., Misirli, G., Lagiou, P., Sacerdote, C., Pala, V., Palli, D., Tumino. R., ... & Riboli, E. (2011). Fruit and vegetable intake and mortality from ischaemic heart disease: Results from the European Prospective Investigation into Cancer and Nutrition (EPIC)-Heart Study. *European Heart Journal, 32*(10), 1235–1243.

Crowe, L. M., Catroppa, C., Babl, F. E., Rosenfeld, J. V., & Anderson, V. (2012). Timing of traumatic brain injury in childhood and intellectual outcome. *Journal of Pediatric Psychology, 37*, 745–754. https://doi.org/10.1093/jpepsy/jss070

Crowell, J. A., Dearing, E., Davis, C. R., Miranda-Julian, C., Barkai, A. R., Usher, N., Trifiletti, S., & Mantzoros, C. (2014). Partnership and extended family relationship quality moderate associations between lifetime psychiatric diagnoses and current depressive symptoms in midlife. *Journal of Social and Clinical Psychology, 33*(7), 612–629. https://doi.org/10.1521/jscp.2014.33.7.612

Crowell, J. A., & Feldman, S. S. (1988). Mothers' internal models of relationships and children's behavioral and developmental status: A study of mother-child interaction. *Child Development, 59*(5), 1273–1285. https://doi.org/10.2307/1130490

Crowell, J. A., Treboux, D., Gao, Y., Fyffe, C., Pan, H., & Waters, E. (2002). Assessing secure base behavior in adulthood: Development of a measure, links to adult attachment representations and relations to couples' communication and reports of relationships. *Developmental Psychology, 38*(5), 679–693. https://doi.org/10.1037/0012-1649.38.5.679

Cyr, C., Euser, E. M., Bakermans-Kranenburg, M. J., & Van Ijzendoorn, M. H. (2010). Attachment security and disorganization in maltreating and high-risk families: A series of meta-analyses. *Development and Psychopathology, 22*(1), 87–108. https://doi.org/10.1017/S0954579409990289

# D

Dahl, R. E. (2001). Affect regulation, brain development, and behavioral/emotional health in adolescence. *CNS Spectrums, 6*(1), 60–72.

Daly, M. C., & Bound, J. (1996). Worker adaptation and employer accommodation following the onset of a health impairment. *Journal of Gerontology: Social Sciences, 51*(2), S53–S60.

da Silva Lara, L. A., Useche, B., Rosa, E. S. J. C., Ferriani, R. A., Reis, R. M., de Sa, M. F., de Carvalho, B. R., Carvalho, M. A., C., R., & de Sa Rosa, E. S. A. C. (2009). Sexuality during the climacteric period. *Maturitas, 62*(2), 127–133. https://doi.org/10.1016/j.maturitas.2008.12.014

Davies, L. N., Croft, M. A., Papas, E., & Charman, W. N. (2016). Presbyopia: Physiology, prevention and pathways to correction. *Ophthalmic and Physiological Optics, 36*(1), 1–4. https://doi.org/10.1111/opo.12272

Davis, C. R., Dearing, E., Usher, N., Trifiletti, S., Zaichenko, L., Ollen, E., Brinkoetter, M. T., Crowell-Doom, C., Joung, K., Park, K. H., Mantzoros, C. S., & Crowell, J. A. (2014). Detailed assessments of childhood adversity enhance prediction of central obesity independent of gender, race, adult psychosocial risk and health behaviors. *Metabolism-Clinical and Experimental, 63*(2), 199–206.

Davis, C. R., Dearing, E., Weber, E. R., Brinkoetter, M. T., Crowell-Doom, C., Joung, K., Park, K. H., Mantzoros, C. S., Crowell, J. A. (under review). Beyond 'modifiable' risks: Enhanced prediction of central obesity using detailed assessments of childhood adversities, adult psychosocial risk, and health behaviors.

Davis, C. R., Usher, N., Dearing E., Barkai, A.R., Crowell-Doom, C., Neupert, S. D, Mantzoros, C. S., & Crowell, J. A. (2014). Attachment and the metabolic syndrome in midlife: The role of interview-based discourse patterns. *Psychosomatic Medicine, 76*(8), 611–621. http://europepmc.org/abstract/med/25264975

Davis, E. P., & Sandman, C. A. (2010). The timing of prenatal exposure to maternal cortisol and psychosocial stress is associated with human infant cognitive development. *Child Development, 81*(1), 131–148. https://doi.org/10.1111/j.1467-8624.2009.01385.x

Davis, M. A. (2003). Factors related to bridge employment participation among private sector early retirees. *Journal of Vocational Behavior, 63*(1), 55–71.

Davis, S. D., Lebow, J. L., & Sprenkle, D. H. (2012). Common factors of change in couple therapy. *Behavior Therapy, 43*(1), 36–48. https://doi.org/10.1016/j.beth.2011.01.009

Dawson-Hughes, B., & Bischoff-Ferrari, H. A. (2007). Therapy of osteoporosis with calcium and vitamin D. *Journal of Bone and Mineral Research, 22*(2), V59–V63. https://doi.org/10.1359/jbmr.07s209

de Alencar, A. E., Arraes, L. C., de Albuquerque, E. C., & Alves, J. G. (2009). Effect of kangaroo mother care on postpartum depression. *Journal of Tropical Pediatrics, 55*(1), 36–38. https://doi.org/10.1093/tropej/fmn083

De Jong Gierveld, J. (2015). Intra-couple caregiving of older adults living apart together: Commitment and independence. *Canadian Journal on Aging, 34*(3), 356–365. https://doi.org/10.1017/S0714980815000264

De Luca, C. R., & Leventer, R. J. (2008). Developmental trajectories of executive functions across the lifespan. *Executive functions and the frontal lobes: A lifespan perspective*, 23–56.

Delbaere, I., Cammu, H., Martens, E., Tency, I., Martens, G., & Temmerman, M. (2012). Limiting the caesarean section rate in low risk pregnancies is key to lowering the trend of increased abdominal deliveries: An observational study. *BMC Pregnancy Childbirth, 12*(3). https://doi.org/10.1186/1471-2393-12-3

De Raedt, R., & Ponjaert-Kristoffersen, I. (2006). Self-serving appraisal as a cognitive coping strategy to deal with age-related limitations: An empirical study with elderly adults in a real-life stressful situation. *Aging and Mental Health, 10*(2), 195–203.

De Souza, Z., & Dick, G. N. (2009). Disclosure of information by children in social networking—Not just a case of "you show me yours and I'll show you mine." *International Journal of Information Management, 29*(4), 255–261.

de Vries, B., & Megathlin, D. (2009). The meaning of friendships for gay men and lesbians in the second half of life. *Journal of GLBT Family Studies, 5*(1–2), 82–98.

Deng, C.-P., Armstrong, P. I., & Rounds, J. (2007). The fit of Holland's RIASEC model to US occupations. *Journal of Vocational Behavior, 71*(1), 1–22. https://doi.org/10.1016/j.jvb.2007.04.002

Deng, H., Miao, D., Liu, J., Meng, S., & Wu, Y. (2009). The regeneration of gingiva: Its potential value for the recession of healthy gingiva. *Medical Hypotheses, 74*(1), 76–77. https://doi.org/10.1016/j.mehy.2009.07.051

Dennerstein, L., Dudley, E., & Guthrie, J. (2002). Empty nest or revolving door? A prospective study of women's quality of life in midlife during the phase of children leaving and re-entering the home. *Psychological Medicine, 32*(3), 545–550.

Depp, C. A., & Jeste, D. V. (2006). Definitions and predictors of successful aging: A comprehensive review of larger quantitative studies. *American Journal of Geriatric Psychiatry, 14*(1), 6–20.

Derauf, C., LaGasse, L., Smith, L., Newman, E., Shah, R., Arria, A., Huestis, M., Haning, W., Strauss, A., Grotta, S., Dansereau, L., Lin, H., & Lester, B. (2011). Infant temperament and high-risk environment relate to behavior problems and language in toddlers. *Journal of Developmental and Behavioral Pediatrics, 32*(2), 125–135. https://doi.org/10.1097/DBP.0b013e31820839d7

Desai, S., Upadhyay, M., & Nanda, R. (2009). Dynamic smile analysis: Changes with age. *American Journal of Orthodontic and Dentofacial Orthopathy, 136*(3), e311–e310. https://doi.org/10.1016/j.ajodo.2009.01.021

Devine, A., Dick, I. M., Islam, A. F., Dhaliwal, S. S., & Prince, R. L. (2005). Protein consumption is an important predictor of lower limb bone mass in elderly women. *American Journal of Clinical Nutrition, 81*(6), 1423–1428.

Diab, T., Condon, K. W., Burr, D. B., & Vashishth, D. (2006). Age-related change in the damage morphology of human cortical bone and its role in bone fragility. *Bone, 38*(3), 427–431.

Diallo, Y., Hagemann, F., Etienne, A., Gurbuzer, Y., & Mehran, F. (2010). *Global child labour developments: Measuring trends from 2004 to 2008.* International Labour Organization.

Diamond, A. (2002). Normal development of prefrontal cortex from birth to young adulthood: Cognitive functions, anatomy, and biochemistry. In D. T. Stuss, & R. T. Knight (Ed.), *Principles of frontal lobe function.* Oxford University Press.

Dich, N., Hansen, Å. M., Avlund, K., Lund, R., Mortensen, E. L., Bruunsgaard, H., & Rod, N. H. (2015). Early life adversity potentiates the effects of later life stress on cumulative physiological dysregulation. *Anxiety, Stress, & Coping, 28*(4), 372–390. https://doi.org/10.1080/10615806.2014.969720

Diehl, M., Coyle, N., & Labouvie-Vief, G. (1996). Age and sex differences in coping and defense across the lifespan. *Psychology and Aging, 11*(1), 127–139.

Diener, E. (1999). Subjective well-being: Three decades of progress. *Psychological Bulletin, 125*(2), 276–302.

Diener, E., Oishi, S., & Lucas, R. E. (2003). Personality, culture, and subjective well-being: Emotional and cognitive evaluations of life. *Annual Review of Psychology, 54*(1), 403–425.

Diez, J. J., & Iglesias, P. (2004). Spontaneous subclinical hypothyroidism in patients older than 55 years: An analysis of natural course and risk factors for the development of overt thyroid failure. *Journal of Clinical Endocrinology and Metabolism, 89*(10), 4890–4897.

Dik, B. J., & Duffy, R. D. (2015). Strategies for discerning and living a calling. In P. J. Hartung, M. L. Savickas, & W. B. Walsh (Eds.), *APA handbook of career intervention: Vol. 2. Applications* (pp. 305–317). American Psychological Association.

Ding, C., Cicuttini, F., Blizzard, L., Scott, F., & Jones, G. (2007). A longitudinal study of the effect of sex and age on rate of change in knee cartilage volume in adults. *Rheumatology (Oxford), 46*(2), 273-290. https://doi.org/10.1093/rheumatology/kel243

Dobrow, S. R., & Tosti-Kharas, J. (2011). Calling: The development of a scale measure. *Personnel Psychology, 64*(4), 1001–1049. https://doi.org/10.1111/j.1744-6570.2011.01234.x

Dockree, P. M., Brennan, S., O'Sullivan, M., Robertson, I. H., & O'Connell, R. G. (2015). Characterising neural signatures of successful aging: Electrophysiological correlates of preserved episodic memory in older age. *Brain and Cognition, 97,* 40–50. https://doi.org/10.1016/j.bandc.2015.04.002

Domar, A. D., Moragianni, V. A., Ryley, D. A., & Urato, A. C. (2012). The risks of selective serotonin reuptake inhibitor use in infertile women: A review of the impact on fertility, pregnancy, neonatal health and beyond. *Human Reproduction, 28*(1), 160–171 https://doi.org/10.1093/humrep/des383

Donoho, C. J., Crimmins, E. M., & Seeman, T. E. (2013). Marital quality, gender, and markers of inflammation in the MIDUS cohort. *Journal of Marriage and Family, 75*(1), 127–141. https://doi.org/10.1111/j.1741-3737.2012.01023.x

Donohue, R. (2006). Person-environment congruence in relation to career change and career persistence. *Journal of Vocational Behavior, 68*(3), 504–515.

Doss, B. D., Rhoades, G. K., Stanley, S. M., & Markman, H. J. (2009). The effect of the transition to parenthood on relationship quality: An 8-year prospective study. *Journal of Personality and Social Psychology, 96*(3), 601–619. https://doi.org/10.1037/a0013969

Drew, L. M., & Smith, P. K. (2002). Implications for grandparents when they lose contact with their grandchildren: Divorce, family feud, and geographical separation. *Journal of Mental Health & Aging, 8*(2), 95–119.

Drozdowski, L., & Thomson, A. B. (2006). Aging and the intestine. *World Journal of Gastroenterology, 12*(47), 7578–7584.

Duffy, J. F., Zitting, K. M., & Chinoy, E. D. (2015). Aging and circadian rhythms. *Sleep Medicine Clinics, 10*(4), 423–434. https://doi.org/10.1016/j.jsmc.2015.08.002

Duffy, R. D., Allan, B. A., Autin, K. L., & Bott, E. M. (2013). Calling and life satisfaction: It's not about having it, it's about living it. *Journal of Counseling Psychology, 60*(1), 42–52. https://doi.org/10.1037/a0030635

Duffy, R. D., Bott, E. M., Allan, B. A., Torrey, C. L., & Dik, B. J. (2012). Perceiving a calling, living a calling, and job satisfaction: Testing a moderated, multiple mediator model. *Journal of Counseling Psychology, 59*(1), 50–59. https://doi.org/10.1037/a0026129

Duffy, R. D., & Dik, B. J. (2013). Research on calling: What have we learned and where are we going? *Journal of Vocational Behavior, 83*(3), 428–436. https://doi.org/10.1016/j.jvb.2013.06.006

Dufour, A., & Candas, V. (2007). Ageing and thermal responses during passive heat exposure: Sweating and sensory aspects. *European Journal of Applied Physiology, 100*(1), 19–26. https://doi.org/10.1007/s00421-007-0396-9

Dufour, A. B., Broe, K. E., Nguyen, U. S., Gagnon, D. R., Hillstrom, H. J., Walker, A. H., Kivell, E., & Hannan, M. T. (2009). Foot pain: Is current or past shoewear a factor? *Arthritis & Rheumatism, 61*(10), 1352–1358. https://doi.org/10.1002/art.24733

Duner, A., & Nordstrom, M. (2005). Intentions and strategies among elderly people: Coping in everyday life. *Journal of Aging Studies, 19*(4), 437–451.

Dunifon, R., & Bajracharya, A. (2012). The role of grandparents in the lives of youth. *Journal of Family Issues, 33*(9), 1168–1194. https://doi.org/10.1177/0192513x12444271

Dunst, C. J., Gorman, E., & Hamby, D. W. (2012). Child-directed motionese with infants and toddlers with and without hearing impairments. *Center for Early Literacy Learning, 5*(8).

Dykas, M. J., & Cassidy, J. (2011). Attachment and the processing of social information across the lifespan: Theory and evidence. *Psychological Bulletin, 137*(1), 19–46.

# E

Earl, J. K., Gerrans, P., & Halim, V. A. (2015). Active and adjusted: Investigating the contribution of leisure, health and psychosocial factors to retirement adjustment. *Leisure Sciences, 37*(4), 354–372. https://doi.org/10.1080/01490400.2015.1021881

Eaton, D. K., Kann, L., Kinchen, S., Shanklin, S., Ross, J., Hawkins, J., ... Chyen, D. (2010). Youth risk behavior surveillance—United States, 2009. *MMWR Surveillance Summaries, 59*, 1–142.

Edwards, J. R., & Rothbard, N. P. (2000). Mechanisms linking work and family: Clarifying the relationship between work and family constructs. *Academy of Management Review, 25*(1), 178–199. https://doi.org/10.2307/259269

Eggum, N. D., Eisenberg, N., Reiser, M., Spinrad, T. L., Valiente, C., Liew, J., & Sallquist, J. (2012). Relations over time among children's shyness, emotionality, and internalizing problems. *Social Development, 21*(1), 109–129.

Eid, M., & Diener, E. (2001). Norms for experiencing emotions in different cultures: Inter- and intranational differences. *Journal of Personality & Social Psychology, 81*(5), 869–885.

Eisenach, J. C., Pan, P., Smiley, R. M., Lavand'homme, P., Landau, R., & Houle, T. T. (2013). Resolution of pain after childbirth. *Anesthesiology, 118*(1), 143–151. https://doi.org/10.1097/ALN.0b013e318278ccfd

Ekman, P., Sorenson, E. R., & Friesen, W. V. (1969). Pan-cultural elements in facial displays of emotion. *Science, 164*(3875), 86–88.

Elder, G. H., Jr., Shanahan, M., & Clipp, E. C. (1994). When war comes to men's lives: Life course patterns in family, work, and health. *Psychology and Aging, 9*(1), 5–16.

El Marroun, H., Zeegers, M., Steegers, E. A., van der Ende, J., Schenk, J. J., Hofman, A., Jaddoe, V. W. V., Verhulst, F. C., & Tiemeier, H. (2012). Post-term birth and the risk of behavioural and emotional problems in early childhood. *International Journal of Epidemiology*, 41*(3)*, 773–781 https://doi.org/10.1093/ije/dys043

Eliasson, L., Birkhed, D., Osterberg, T., & Carlen, A. (2006). Minor salivary gland secretion rates and immunoglobulin A in adults and the elderly. *European Journal of Oral Sciences, 114*(6), 494–499.

Elkind, D. (1967). Egocentrism in adolescence. *Child Development, 38*(4), 1025–1034.

Elliot, S. J., Karl, M., Berho, M., Xia, X., Pereria-Simon, S., Espinosa-Heidmann, D., & Striker, G. E. (2006). Smoking induces glomerulosclerosis in aging estrogen-deficient mice through cross-talk between TGF-beta1 and IGF-I signaling pathways. *Journal of the American Society Nephrology, 17*(12), 3315–3324. https://doi.org/10.1681/ASN.2006070799

Emaus, N., Berntsen, G. K., Joakimsen, R., & Fonnebo, V. (2006). Longitudinal changes in forearm bone mineral density in women and men aged 45–84 years: The Tromso Study, a population-based study. *American Journal of Epidemiology, 163*(5), 441–449.

Endowment for Human Development. (2013). Interactive prenatal development timeline. http://www.ehd.org/science_main.php

Ericsson, K. A., Krampe, R. T., & Tesch-Römer, C. (1993). The role of deliberate practice in the acquisition of expert performance. *Psychological Review, 100*(3), 363–406.

Erikson, E. H. (1968). The life cycle: Epigenesis of identity. *Identity, youth and crisis*, 91–141.

Escott, D., Slade, P., & Spiby, H. (2009). Preparation for pain management during childbirth: The psychological aspects of coping strategy development in antenatal education. *Clinical Psychology Review, 29*(7), 617–622. https://doi.org/10.1016/j.cpr.2009.07.002

Espiritu, J. R. (2008). Aging-related sleep changes. *Clinics in Geriatric Medicine, 24*(1), 1–14, v. https://doi.org/10.1016/j.cger.2007.08.007

Espy, K. A., Sheffield, T. D., Wiebe, S. A., Clark, C. A. C., & Moehr, M. J. (2011). Executive control and dimensions of problem behaviors in preschool children. *Journal of Child Psychology and Psychiatry, 52*(1), 33–46. https://doi.org/10.1111/j.1469-7610.2010.02265.x

Evans, E. H., Tovée, M. J., Boothroyd, L. G., & Drewett, R. F. (2013). Body dissatisfaction and disordered eating attitudes in 7- to 11-year-old girls: Testing a sociocultural model. *Body Image, 10*(1), 8–15. https://doi.org/10.1016/j.bodyim.2012.10.001

# F

Faith, M. S. (2010). Development of child taste and food preferences: The role of exposure. In W. S. Agras (Ed.), *The Oxford handbook of eating disorders* (pp. 137–147). Oxford University Press.

Farley, C., Alimi, Y., Espinosa, L. R., Perez, S., Knechtle, W., Hestley, A., Carlson, G. W., Russell, M. C., Delman, K. A., & Rizzo, M. (2015). Tanning beds: A call to action for further educational and legislative efforts. *Journal of Surgical Oncology, 112*(2), 183–187.

Féart, C., Samieri, C., Allès, B., & Barberger-Gateau, P. (2013). Potential benefits of adherence to the Mediterranean diet on cognitive health. *Proceedings of the Nutrition Society, 72*(1), 140–152.

Feeney, J. A., & Ryan, S. M. (1994). Attachment style and affect regulation: Relationships with health behavior and family experiences of illness in a student sample. *Health Psychology, 13*(4), 334–345. https://doi.org/10.1037/0278-6133.13.4.334

Feldman, H. A., Longcope, C., Derby, C. A., Johannes, C. B., Araujo, A. B., Coviello, A. D., Bremner, W. J., & McKinlay, J. B. (2002). Age trends in the level of serum testosterone and other hormones in middle-aged men: Longitudinal results from the Massachusetts male aging study. *Journal of Clinical Endocrinology and Metabolism, 87*(2), 589–598.

Feldman, R., & Eidelman, A. I. (2003). Skin-to-skin contact (kangaroo care) accelerates autonomic and neurobehavioural maturation in preterm infants. *Developmental Medicine and Child Neurology, 45*(4), 274–281.

Feldt, K., Raikkonen, K., Eriksson, J. G., Andersson, S., Osmond, C., Barker, D. J., Phillips, D. I. W., & Kajantie, E. (2007). Cardiovascular reactivity to psychological stressors in late adulthood is predicted by gestational age at birth. *Journal of Human Hypertension, 21*, 401–410. https://doi.org/10.1038/sj.jhh.1002176

Ferguson, R., & Brohaugh, B. (2010). The aging of Aquarius. *Journal of Consumer Marketing, 27*(1), 76–81.

Fergusson, D. M., Boden, J. M., & Horwood, L. J. (2013). Bullying in childhood, externalizing behaviors, and adult offending: Evidence from a 30-year study. *Journal of School Violence, 13*(1), 136–164.

Fernald, A. (1985). Four-month-old infants prefer to listen to motherese. *Infant Behavior and Development, 8*(2), 181–195. https://doi.org/10.1016/S0163-6383(85)80005-9

Ferrari, S. L., & Rizzoli, R. (2005). Gene variants for osteoporosis and their pleiotropic effects in aging. *Molecular Aspects of Medicine, 26*(3), 145–167.

Ferrario, S. R., Cardillo, V., Vicario, F., Balzarini, E., & Zotti, A. M. (2004). Advanced cancer at home: Caregiving and bereavement. *Palliative Medicine, 18*(2), 129–136.

Ferri, R., Gschliesser, V., Frauscher, B., Poewe, W., & Hogl, B. (2009). Periodic leg movements during sleep and periodic limb movement disorder in patients presenting with unexplained insomnia. *Clinics in Neurophysiology, 120*(2), 257–263. https://doi.org/10.1016/j.clinph.2008.11.006

Ferrucci, L., Baroni, M., Ranchelli, A., Lauretani, F., Maggio, M., Mecocci, P., & Ruggiero, C. (2014). Interaction between bone and muscle in older persons with mobility limitations. *Current Pharmaceutical Design, 20*(19), 3178–3197.

Fetto, J. (2002). Friends forever *Ad Age*. http://adage.com/article/american-demographics/friends-forever/44657/

Fetveit, A. (2009). Late-life insomnia: A review. *Geriatrics and Gerontology International, 9*(3), 220–234. https://doi.org/10.1111/j.1447-0594.2009.00537.x

Field, T. (2010). Postpartum depression effects on early interactions, parenting, and safety practices: A review. *Infant Behavioral Development, 33*(1), 1–6. https://doi.org/10.1016/j.infbeh.2009.10.005

Figlio, D. N., & Stone, J. A. (2000). Are private schools really better? *Research in labor economics* (pp. 115–140): Emerald Group.

Fiksenbaum, L. M., Greenglass, E. R., & Eaton, J. (2006). Perceived social support, hassles, and coping among the elderly. *Journal of Applied Gerontology, 25*(1), 17–30.

Fingerman, K. L., & Griffiths, P. C. (1999). Seasons greetings: Adults' social contacts at the holiday season. *Psychology and Aging, 14*(2), 192–205.

Fingerman, K. L., Hay, E. L., & Birditt, K. S. (2004). The best of ties, the worst of ties: Close, problematic, and ambivalent social relationships. *Journal of Marriage and Family, 66*(3), 792–808.

Finkel, E. J., Cheung, E. O., Emery, L. F., Carswell, K. L., & Larson, G. M. (2015). The suffocation model: Why marriage in America is becoming an all-or-nothing institution. *Current Directions in Psychological Science, 24*(3), 238–244. https://doi.org/10.1177/0963721415569274

Fiocco, A. J., & Yaffe, K. (2010). Defining successful aging: The importance of including cognitive function over time. *Archives of Neurology, 67*(7), 876–880. https://doi.org/10.1001/archneurol.2010.130

Fitzpatrick, C., & Pagani, L. S. (2012). Toddler working memory skills predict kindergarten school readiness. *Intelligence, 40*(2), 205–212. https://doi.org/10.1016/j.intell.2011.11.007

Fitzpatrick, S., & Bussey, K. (2014). The role of perceived friendship self-efficacy as a protective factor against the negative effects of social victimization. *Social Development, 23*(1), 41–60.

Fjell, A. M., Walhovd, K. B., Fennema-Notestine, C., McEvoy, L. K., Hagler, D. J., Holland, D., Brewer, J. B., & Dale, A. M. (2009). One-year brain atrophy evident in healthy aging. *Journal of Neuroscience, 29*(48), 15223–15231. https://doi.org/10.1523/JNEUROSCI.3252-09.2009

Fleischman, A. R., Oinuma, M., & Clark, S. L. (2010). Rethinking the definition of "term pregnancy." *Obstetrics and Gynecology, 116*(1), 136–139.

Flora, C. (2013). *Friendfluence: The surprising ways friends make us who we are.* Random House.

Foley, D. J., Vitiello, M. V., Bliwise, D. L., Ancoli-Israel, S., Monjan, A. A., & Walsh, J. K. (2007). Frequent napping is associated with excessive daytime sleepiness, depression, pain, and nocturia in older adults: Findings from the National Sleep Foundation '2003 Sleep in America' Poll. *American Journal of Geriatric Psychiatry, 15*(4), 344–350.

Foley, P. F., & Lytle, M. C. (2015). Social cognitive career theory, the theory of work adjustment, and work satisfaction of retirement-age adults. *Journal of Career Development, 42*(3), 199–214. https://doi.org/10.1177/0894845314553270

Fomon, S. (2001). Infant feeding in the 20th century: Formula and beikost. *Journal of Nutrition, 131*(2), 409S–420S.

Ford, D. H., & Lerner, R. M. (1992). *Developmental systems theory: An integrative approach.* SAGE.

Forsmo, S., Langhammer, A., Forsen, L., & Schei, B. (2005). Forearm bone mineral density in an unselected population of 2,779 men and women—the HUNT Study, Norway. *Osteoporos International, 16*(5), 562–567.

Fowler, C., Gasiorek, J., & Giles, H. (2015). The role of communication in aging well: Introducing the communicative ecology model of successful aging. *Communication Monographs, 82*(4), 431–457. https://doi.org/10.1080/03637751.2015.1024701

Fox, K. (2009). *The smell report.* http://www.sirc.org/publik/smell.pdf

Frankenberger, K. D. (2000). Adolescent egocentrism: A comparison among adolescents and adults. *Journal of Adolescence, 23*, 343–354.

Fraser, J., Maticka-Tyndale, E., & Smylie, L. (2004). Sexuality of Canadian women at midlife. *Canadian Journal of Human Sexuality, 13*(3), 171–188.

Fricchione, G. (2011). *Compassion and healing in medicine and society. On the nature and uses of attachment solutions to separation challenges.* Johns Hopkins University Press.

Friedman, H. S., & Martin, L. R. (2011). *The longevity project: Surprising discoveries for health and long life from the landmark eight-decade study.* Hudson Street Press/Penguin.

Friedman, H. S., Tucker, J. S., Schwartz, J. E., Martin, L. R., Tomlinson-Keasey, C., Wingard, D. L., & Criqui, M. H. (1995). Childhood conscientiousness and longevity: Health behaviors and cause of death. *Journal of Personality and Social Psychology, 68*(4), 696–703.

Friedman, M., & Rosenman, R. H. (1974). *Type A behavior and your heart.* Knopf.

Frisby, B. N., Booth-Butterfield, M., Dillow, M. R., Martin, M. M., & Weber, K. D. (2012). Face and resilience in divorce: The impact on emotions, stress, and post-divorce relationships. *Journal of Social and Personal Relationships, 29*(6), 715–735. https://doi.org/10.1177/0265407512443452

Fuiano, G., Sund, S., Mazza, G., Rosa, M., Caglioti, A., Gallo, G., Natale, G., Andreucci, M., Memoli, B., De Nicola, L., & Conte, G. (2001). Renal hemodynamic response to maximal vasodilating stimulus in healthy older subjects. *Kidney International, 59*(3), 1052–1058.

Fuller-Thomson, E., & Minkler, M. (2001). American grandparents providing extensive childcare to their grandchildren: Prevalence and profile. *Gerontologist, 41*(2), 201–209.

Fung, H. H., Lu, A. Y., Goren, D., Isaacowitz, D. M., Wadlinger, H. A., & Wilson, H. R. (2008). Age-related positivity enhancement is not universal: Older Chinese look away from positive stimuli. *Psychology and Aging, 23*(2), 440–446.

Furnham, A., Eracleous, A., & Chamorro-Premuzic, T. (2009). Personality, motivation and job satisfaction: Hertzberg meets the big five. *Journal of Managerial Psychology, 24*(8), 765–779.


# G


Gabelle, A., & Dauvilliers, Y. (2010). Editorial: Sleep and dementia. *Journal of Nutrition Health and Aging, 14*(3), 201–202.

Gadalla, T. M. (2009). Sense of mastery, social support, and health in elderly Canadians. *Journal of Aging and Health, 21*(4), 581–595.

Gagnon, M., Hersen, M., Kabacoff, R. L., & Van Hasselt, V. B. (1999). Interpersonal and psychological correlates of marital dissatisfaction in late life: A review. *Clinical Psychology Review, 19*(3), 359–378.

Gallese, V., Rochat, M. J., & Berchio, C. (2013). The mirror mechanism and its potential role in autism spectrum disorder. *Developmental Medicine and Child Neurology, 55*(1), 15–22. https://doi.org/10.1111/j.1469-8749.2012.04398.x

Gardner, H. (1993). *Multiple intelligences: The theory in practice.* Basic Books.

Garg, S. K., Maurer, H., Reed, K., & Selagamsetty, R. (2014). Diabetes and cancer: Two diseases with obesity as a common risk factor. *Diabetes, Obesity and Metabolism, 16*(2), 97–110. https://doi.org/10.1111/dom.12124

Gaunt, R. (2006). Couple similarity and marital satisfaction: Are similar spouses happier? *Journal of Personality, 74*(5), 1401–1420.

Gauthier, S., & Scheltens, P. (2009). Can we do better in developing new drugs for Alzheimer's disease? *Alzheimers and Dementia, 5*(6), 489–491. https://doi.org/10.1016/j.jalz.2009.09.002

Geoffroy, M.-C., Côté, S. M., Giguère, C.-É., Dionne, G., Zelazo, P. D., Tremblay, R. E., Boivin, M., & Séguin, J. R. (2010). Closing the gap in academic readiness and achievement: The role of early childcare. *Journal of Child Psychology and Psychiatry, 51*(12), 1359–1367. https://doi.org/10.1111/j.1469-7610.2010.02316.x

George, C., & Solomon, J. (1996). Representational models of relationships: Links between caregiving and attachment. *Infant Mental Health Journal, 17*(3), 198–216.

George, C., & Solomon, J. (1999). The development of caregiving: A comparison of attachment theory and psychoanalytic approaches to mothering. *Psychoanalytic Inquiry, 19*(4), 618–646. https://doi.org/10.1080/07351699909534268

George, C., & Solomon, J. (2008). The caregiving system: A behavioral systems approach to parenting. In J. Cassidy & P. R. Shaver (Eds.), *Handbook of attachment: Theory, research, and clinical applications* (2nd ed.) (pp. 833–856). Guilford Press.

Gerber, R. J., Wilks, T., & Erdie-Lalena, C. (2010). Developmental milestones: Motor development. *Pediatrics in Review, 31*(7), 267–277. https://doi.org/10.1542/pir.31-7-267

Gerber, R. J., Wilks, T., & Erdie-Lalena, C. (2011). Developmental milestones 3: Social-emotional development. *Pediatrics in Review, 32*(12), 533–536. https://doi.org/10.1542/pir.32-12-533

Gerstorf, D., Ram, N., Lindenberger, U., & Smith, J. (2013). Age and time-to-death trajectories of change in indicators of cognitive, sensory, physical, health, social, and self-related functions. *Developmental Psychology, 49*(10), 1805–1821. https://doi.org/10.1037/a0031340

Gettler, L. T., McDade, T. W., Agustin, S. S., & Kuzawa, C. W. (2011). Short-term changes in fathers' hormones during father–child play: Impacts of paternal attitudes and experience. *Hormones and Behavior, 60*(5), 599–606.

Gettler, L. T., McDade, T. W., Feranil, A. B., & Kuzawa, C. W. (2011). Longitudinal evidence that fatherhood decreases testosterone in human males. *Proceedings of the National Academy of Sciences, 108*(39), 16194–16199.

Geurts, T., van Tilburg, T. G., & Poortman, A.-R. (2012). The grandparent–grandchild relationship in childhood and adulthood: A matter of continuation? *Personal Relationships, 19*(2), 267–278.

Geurts, T., van Tilburg, T., Poortman, A.-R., & Dykstra, P. A. (2015). Child care by grandparents: Changes between 1992 and 2006. *Ageing & Society, 35*(6), 1318–1334. https://doi.org/10.1017/S0144686X14000270

Ghetti, S., & Bunge, S. A. (2012). Neural changes underlying the development of episodic memory during middle childhood. *Developmental Cognitive Neuroscience, 2*(4), 381–395. https://doi.org/10.1016/j.dcn.2012.05.002

Giannotti, F., & Cortesi, F. (2009). Family and cultural influences on sleep development. *Child and Adolescent Psychiatric Clinics of North America, 18*(4), 849–861. https://doi.org/10.1016/j.chc.2009.04.003

Gibbons, L., Belizán, J. M., Lauer, J. A., Betrzán, A. P., Merialdi, M., & Althabe, F. (2010). The global numbers and costs of additionally needed and unnecessary caesarean sections performed per year: Overuse as a barrier to universal coverage [World Health Report Background Paper no. 30]. http://www.who.int/healthsystems/topics/financing/healthreport/30C-sectioncosts.pdf

Gill, S. C., Butterworth, P., Rodgers, B., Anstey, K. J., Villamil, E., & Melzer, D. (2006). Mental health and the timing of men's retirement. *Social Psychiatry and Psychiatric Epidemiology, 41*(7), 933–954.

Gimeno, D., Tabak, A. G., Ferrie, J. E., Shipley, M. J., De Vogli, R., Elovainio, M., Vahtera, J., Marmot, M., G., & Kivimaki, M. (2010). Justice at work and metabolic syndrome: The Whitehall II study. *Occupational and Environmental Medicine, 67,* 256–262. https://doi.org/10.1136/oem.2009.047324

Ginsburg, K. R., & Pediatrics, A. A. o. (2007). Committee on Communications, Committee on Psychosocial Aspects of Child and Family Health. The importance of play in promoting healthy child development and maintaining strong parent-child bonds. *Pediatrics, 119*(1), 182–191.

Gladwell, M. (2008). *Outliers: The story of success.* Penguin.

Glanz, K., & Schwartz, M. (2008). Stress, coping and health behavior. In K. Glanz, B. Rimer, & K. Viswanath (Eds.), *Health behavior and health education: Theory, research and practice* (pp. 211–236). Jossey-Bass.

Gluck, J., & Bluck, S. (2007). Looking back across the lifespan: A life story account of the reminiscence bump. *Memory and Cognition, 35*(8), 1928–1939.

Gogtay, N., Giedd, J. N., Lusk, L., Hayashi, K. M., Greenstein, D., Vaituzis, A. C., Nugent, T. F., III, Herman, D. S., Clasen. L. S., Toga, J. W., Rapaport, J. L., & Thompson, P. M. (2004). Dynamic mapping of human cortical development during childhood through early adulthood. *Proceedings of the National Academy of Sciences of the USA, 101*(21), 8174–8179.

Goh, J. O., & Park, D. C. (2009). Neuroplasticity and cognitive aging: The scaffolding theory of aging and cognition. *Restorative Neurology and Neuroscience, 27*(5), 391–403. https://doi.org/10.3233/RNN-2009-0493

Goldberg, A. E., & Sayer, A. (2006). Lesbian couples' relationship quality across the transition to parenthood. *Journal of Marriage and Family, 68*(1), 87–100.

Goldberg, A. E., & Smith, J. Z. (2011). Stigma, social context, and mental health: Lesbian and gay couples across the transition to adoptive parenthood. *Journal of Counseling Psychology, 58*, 139–150. doi:10.1037/a0021684

Goodson, I. F. (2013). *Developing narrative theory: Life histories and personal representation.* Routledge.

Goodwin, P. Y., Mosher, W. D., & Chandra, A. (2010). Marriage and cohabitation in the United States: A statistical portrait based on cycle 6 (2002) of the National Survey of Family Growth. *Vital Health and Statistics, 23*(26), 1–45.

Goodwin, R. D., Fergusson, D. M., & Horwood, L. J. (2004). Early anxious/withdrawn behaviours predict later internalising disorders. *Journal of Child Psychology and Psychiatry, 45*(4), 874–883.

Goossens, L., Beyers, W., Emmen, M., & Van Aken, M. A. (2002). The imaginary audience and personal fable: Factor analyses and concurrent validity of the "new look" measures. *Journal of Research on Adolescence, 12*(2), 193–215.

Gottfredson, G. D. (2002). Interests, aspirations, self-estimates, and the self-directed search. *Journal of Career Assessment, 10*(2), 200–208.

Gottman, J. M., & Driver, J. L. (2005). Dysfunctional marital conflict and everyday marital interaction. *Journal of Divorce and Remarriage, 43*(3–4), 63–78.

Gouin, J. P., Hantsoo, L., & Kiecolt-Glaser, J. K. (2008). Immune dysregulation and chronic stress among older adults: A review. *Neuroimmunomodulation, 15*, 251–259. https://doi.org/10.1159/000156468

Goyal, D., Gay, C., & Lee, K. (2009). Fragmented maternal sleep is more strongly correlated with depressive symptoms than infant temperament at three months postpartum. *Archives of Women's Mental Health, 12*(4), 229–237. https://doi.org/10.1007/s00737-009-0070-9

Goyal, D., Gay, C., & Lee, K. A. (2010). How much does low socioeconomic status increase the risk of prenatal and postpartum depressive symptoms in first-time mothers? *Women's Health Issues, 20*(2), 96–104. https://doi.org/10.1016/j.whi.2009.11.003

Gradinaru, V., Mogri, M., Thompson, K. R., Henderson, J. M., & Deisseroth, K. (2009). Optical deconstruction of Parkinsonian neural circuitry. *Science, 324*(5925), 354–359. https://doi.org/10.1126/science.1167093

Graziano, P. A., Calkins, S. D., & Keane, S. P. (2010). Toddler self-regulation skills predict risk for pediatric obesity. *International Journal of Obesity, 34*(4), 633–641.

Green, T. L., & Darity, W. A., Jr. (2010). Under the skin: Using theories from biology and the social sciences to explore the mechanisms behind the Black-White health gap. *American Journal of Public Health, 100*(1), S36–S40. https://doi.org/10.2105/AJPH.2009.171140

Greenhaus, J. H., Collins, K. M., & Shaw, J. D. (2003). The relation between work-family balance and quality of life. *Journal of Vocational Behavior, 63*(3), 510–531.

Greenhaus, J. H., & Powell, G. N. (2006). When work and family are allies: A theory of work-family enrichment. *Academy of Management Review, 31*, 72–92.

Greenwald, D. A. (2004). Aging, the gastrointestinal tract, and risk of acid-related disease. *American Journal of Medicine, 117*(5A), 8S–13S.

Greif, G. L., & Deal, K. H. (2012). Platonic couple love: How couples view their close couple friends. In M. A. Paludi (Ed.), *The psychology of love*, Vols. 1–4 (pp. 19–33). Praeger/ABC-CLIO.

Griffiths, L. J., Parsons, T. J., & Hill, A. J. (2010). Self-esteem and quality of life in obese children and adolescents: A systematic review. *International Journal of Pediatric Obesity, 5*(4), 282–304. https://doi.org/10.3109/17477160903473697

Grivell, R. M., Reilly, A. J., Oakey, H., Chan, A., & Dodd, J. M. (2012). Maternal and neonatal outcomes following induction of labor: A cohort study. *Acta Obstetricia et Gynecologica Scandinavica, 91*(2), 198–203. https://doi.org/10.1111/j.1600-0412.2011.01298.x

Groeneveld, M. G., Vermeer, H. J., van Ijzendoorn, M. H., & Linting, M. (2010). Children's wellbeing and cortisol levels in home-based and center-based childcare. *Early Childhood Research Quarterly, 25*(4), 502–514. https://doi.org/10.1016/j.ecresq.2009.12.004

Gross, J., Jack, F., Davis, N., & Hayne, H. (2013). Do children recall the birth of a younger sibling? Implications for the study of childhood amnesia. *Memory, 21*(3), 336–346.

Grote, N. K., Clark, M. S., & Moore, A. (2004). Perceptions of injustice in family work: The role of psychological distress. *Journal of Family Psychology, 18*(1), 480–492.

Grubeck-Loebenstein, B. (2010). Fading immune protection in old age: Vaccination in the elderly. *Journal of Comparative Physiology, 142*(1), S116–S119. https://doi.org/10.1016/j.jcpa.2009.10.002

Guadalupe-Grau, A., Fuentes, T., Guerra, B., & Calbet, J. A. (2009). Exercise and bone mass in adults. *Sports Medicine, 39*(6), 439–468.

Gubin, D. G., Gubin, G. D., Waterhouse, J., & Weinert, D. (2006). The circadian body temperature rhythm in the elderly: Effect of single daily melatonin dosing. *Chronobiology International, 23*(3), 639–658.

Guest, A. M. (2011). Cultures of play during middle childhood: Interpretive perspectives from two distinct marginalized communities. *Sport, Education and Society, 18*(2), 167–183. https://doi.org/10.1080/13573322.2011.555478

Guhn, M., Schonert-Reichl, K., Gadermann, A., Marriott, D., Pedrini, L., Hymel, S., & Hertzman, C. (2012). Well-being in middle childhood: An assets-based population-level research-to-action project. *Child Indicators Research, 5*, 393–418. https://doi.org/10.1007/s12187-012-9136-8

Gulmezoglu, A. M., Crowther, C. A., & Middleton, P. (2006). Induction of labour for improving birth outcomes for women at or beyond term. *Cochrane Database of Systematic Reviews*, CD004945. https://doi.org/10.1002/14651858.CD004945.pub2

Gulmezoglu, A. M., Crowther, C. A., Middleton, P., & Heatley, E. (2012). Induction of labour for improving birth outcomes for women at or beyond term. *Cochrane Database of Systematic Reviews, 6*, CD004945. https://doi.org/10.1002/14651858.CD004945.pub3

Guru, A., Post, R. J., Ho, Y. Y., & Warden, M. R. (2015). Making sense of optogenetics. *International Journal of Neuropsychopharmacology, 18*(11), pyv079. https://doi.org/10.1093/ijnp/pyv079

# H

Hackman, D. A., Farah, M. J., & Meaney, M. J. (2010). Socioeconomic status and the brain: Mechanistic insights from human and animal research. *Nature Reviews Neuroscience, 11*, 651–659. https://doi.org/10.1038/nrn2897

Hadders-Algra, M. (2004). General movements: A window for early identification of children at high risk for developmental disorders. *Journal of Pediatrics, 145*(2), S12–S18. https://doi.org/10.1016/j.jpeds.2004.05.017

Hadders-Algra, M., Heineman, K. R., Bos, A. F., & Middelburg, K. J. (2010). The assessment of minor neurological dysfunction in infancy using the Touwen Infant Neurological Examination: Strengths and limitations. *Developmental Medicine & Child Neurology, 52*(1), 87–92. https://doi.org/10.1111/j.1469-8749.2009.03305.x

Hall, D. T. (1993). *The new "career contract": Wrong on both counts.* Boston University Executive Development Roundtable Report.

Hall, D. T., & Chandler, D. E. (2005). Psychological success: When the career is a calling. *Journal of Organizational Behavior, 26*(2), 155–176. https://doi.org/10.1002/job.301

Hambrick, D. Z., Altmann, E. M., Oswald, F. L., Meinz, E. J., Gobet, F., & Campitelli, G. (2014). Accounting for expert performance: The devil is in the details. *Intelligence, 45*, 112–114. https://doi.org/10.1016/j.intell.2014.01.007

Hamilton, B. E., Martin, J. A., & Ventura, S. J. (2011). Births: Preliminary data for 2010. *National Vital Statistics Reports*, Vol. 60 Centers for Disease Control and Prevention.

Hank, K., & Buber, I. (2009). Grandparents caring for their grandchildren: Findings from the 2004 Survey of Health, Ageing, and Retirement in Europe. *Journal of Family Issues, 30*(1), 53–73. https://doi.org/10.1177/0192513x08322627

Hanke, T. A., & Tiberio, D. (2006). Lateral rhythmic unipedal stepping in younger, middle-aged, and older adults. *Journal of Geriatric Physical Therapy, 29*(1), 22–27.

Hanna, E. Z., Yi, H.-y., Dufour, M. C., & Whitmore, C. C. (2001). The relationship of early-onset regular smoking to alcohol use, depression, illicit drug use, and other risky behaviors during early adolescence: Results from the youth supplement to the third national health and nutrition examination survey. *Journal of Substance Abuse, 13*(3), 265–282.

Hanna, L. G. (2012). Homeschooling education: Longitudinal study of methods, materials, and curricula. *Education and Urban Society, 44*(5), 609–631. https://doi.org/10.1177/0013124511404886

Hanushek, E. A., Schwerdt, G., Woessmann, L., & Zhang, L. (2017). General education, vocational education, and labor-market outcomes over the lifecycle. *Journal of Human Resources, 52*(1), 48–87.

Harber, M. P., Konopka, A. R., Douglass, M. D., Minchev, K., Kaminsky, L. A., Trappe, T. A., & Trappe, S. (2009). Aerobic exercise training improves whole muscle and single myofiber size and function in older women. *American Journal of Physiology: Regulative, Integrative, and Comparative Physiology, 297*(5), R1452–R1459. https://doi.org/10.1152/ajpregu.00354.2009

Hardy, M. A., & Quadagno, J. (1995). Satisfaction with early retirement: Making choices in the auto industry. *Journals of Gerontology: Series B: Psychological Sciences and Social Sciences, 50B*(4), S217–S228. https://doi.org/10.1093/geronb/50B.4.S217

Hardy, S. E., Concato, J., & Gill, T. M. (2004). Resilience of community-dwelling older persons. *Journal of the American Geriatrics Society, 52*(2), 257–262.

Harmer, P. A., & Li, F. (2008). Tai chi and falls prevention in older people. *Medicine and Science in Sports and Exercise, 52*, 124–134. https://doi.org/10.1159/000134293

Harmon, L. W., Hansen, J. C., Borgen, F. H., & Hammer, A. L. (1994). *Strong Interest Inventory applications and technical guide.* Consulting Psychologists Press.

Harms, C. A. (2006). Does gender affect pulmonary function and exercise capacity? *Respiratory Physiology and Neurobiology, 151*(2–3), 124–131.

Harrington, J., & Lee-Chiong, T. (2009). Obesity and aging. *Clinics in Chest Medicine, 30*(3), 609–614. https://doi.org/10.1016/j.ccm.2009.05.011

Harris, G. (2008). Development of taste and food preferences in children. *Current Opinion in Clinical Nutrition & Metabolic Care, 11*(3), 315–319.

Harrison, T. M., Weintraub, S., Mesulam, M. M., & Rogalski, E. (2012). Superior memory and higher cortical volumes in unusually successful cognitive aging. *Journal of the International Neuropsychological Society, 18*(6), 1081–1085. https://doi.org/10.1017/s1355617712000847

Hart, H. M., McAdams, D. P., Hirsch, B. J., & Bauer, J. J. (2001). Generativity and social involvement among African Americans and White adults. *Journal of Research in Personality, 35*(2), 208–230. https://doi.org/10.1006/jrpe.2001.2318

Harwood, D. G., Sultzer, D. L., & Wheatley, M. V. (2000). Impaired insight in Alzheimer disease: Association with cognitive deficits, psychiatric symptoms, and behavioral disturbances. *Neuropsychiatry, Neuropsychology, and Behavioral Neurology, 13*(2), 83–88.

Hasher, L., Goldstein, F., & May, C. (2005). It's about time: Circadian rhythms, memory and aging. In C. Izawa & N. Ohta (Eds.), *Human learning and memory: Advances in theory and application,* Vol. 18 (pp. 179–186). Lawrence Erlbaum.

Haskell, W. L., Lee, I. M., Pate, R. R., Powell, K. E., Blair, S. N., Franklin, B. A., Macera, C. A., Heath, G. W., Thompson, P. D., & Bauman, A. (2007). Physical activity and public health: Updated recommendation for adults from the American College of Sports Medicine and the American Heart Association. *Medicine and Science in Sports and Exercise, 39*(8), 1423–1434. https://doi.org/10.1249/mss.0b013e3180616b27

Hatfield, E., & Rapson, R. L. (2012). Equity theory in close relationships. In P. A. M. Van Lange, A. W. Kruglanski, & E. T. Higgins (Eds.), *Handbook of theories of social psychology* (Vol. 2) (pp. 200–217). SAGE.

Hatfield, E., Rapson, R. L., & Aumer-Ryan, K. (2008). Social justice in love relationships: Recent developments. *Social Justice Research, 21*(4), 413–431.

Hawes, D., Dadds, M., Frost, A. J., & Russell, A. (2013). Parenting practices and prospective levels of hyperactivity/inattention across early- and middle-childhood. *Journal of Psychopathology and Behavioral Assessment, 35*(3), 273–282. https://doi.org/10.1007/s10862-013-9341-x

Hawkins, N., Richards, P. S., Granley, H. M., & Stein, D. M. (2004). The impact of exposure to the thin-ideal media image on women. *Eating Disorders, 12*(1), 35–50.

Hazan, C., & Shaver, P. R. (1994). Attachment as an organizational framework for research on close relationships. *Psychological Inquiry, 5*(1), 1–22.

Hebblethwaite, S., & Norris, J. (2011). Expressions of generativity through family leisure: Experiences of grandparents and adult grandchildren. *Family Relations: An Interdisciplinary Journal of Applied Family Studies, 60*(1), 121–133. https://doi.org/10.1111/j.1741-3729.2010.00637.x

Heilmann, S. G., Holt, D. T., & Rilovick, C. Y. (2008). Effects of career plateauing on turnover: A test of a model. *Journal of Leadership & Organizational Studies, 15*(1), 59–68.

Heinonen, K., Raikkonen, K., Pesonen, A. K., Kajantie, E., Andersson, S., Eriksson, J. G., Niemelä, A., Vartia, T., Peltola, J., & Lano, A. (2008). Prenatal and postnatal growth and cognitive abilities at 56 months of age: A longitudinal study of infants born at term. *Pediatrics, 121*(5), e1325–e1333. https://doi.org/10.1542/peds.2007-1172

Henry, D. E., Cheng, Y. W., Shaffer, B. L., Kaimal, A. J., Bianco, K., & Caughey, A. B. (2008). Perinatal outcomes in the setting of active phase arrest of labor. *Obstetrics & Gynecology, 112*(5), 1109–1115.

Henry, K. L., Knight, K. E., & Thornberry, T. P. (2012). School disengagement as a predictor of dropout, delinquency, and problem substance use during adolescence and early adulthood. *Journal of Youth and Adolescence, 41*(2), 156–166.

Heraclides, A. M., Chandola, T., Witte, D. R., & Brunner, E. J. (2009). Psychosocial stress at work doubles the risk of type 2 diabetes in middle-aged women: Evidence from the Whitehall II study. *Diabetes Care, 32*(12), 2230–2235. https://doi.org/10.2337/dc09-0132

Heraclides, A. M., Chandola, T., Witte, D. R., & Brunner, E. J. (2012). Work stress, obesity and the risk of type 2 diabetes: Gender-specific bidirectional effect in the Whitehall II Study. *Obesity, 20*(2), 428–433. https://doi.org/10.1038/oby.2011.95

Heron, M. (2016). Deaths: Leading causes for 2014. *National Vital Statistics Report, 65.*

Hetherington, E. M. (1989). Coping with family transitions: Winners, losers, and survivors. *Child Development, 60*(1), 1–14.

Heymsfield, S. B., Peterson, C. M., Thomas, D. M., Heo, M., & Schuna, J. M. (2016). Why are there race/ethnic differences in adult body mass index–adiposity relationships? A quantitative critical review. *Obesity Reviews, 17*(3), 262–275.

Hill, P. L., Turiano, N. A., Mroczek, D. K., & Roberts, B. W. (2012). Examining concurrent and longitudinal relations between personality traits and social well-being in adulthood. *Social Psychological and Personality Science, 3*(6), 698–705. https://doi.org/10.1177/1948550611433888

Hirschi, A. (2012). Callings and work engagement: Moderated mediation model of work meaningfulness, occupational identity, and occupational self-efficacy. *Journal of Counseling Psychology, 59*(3), 479–485. https://doi.org/10.1037/a0028949

Hirsh-Pasek, K. (2009). *A mandate for playful learning in preschool: Presenting the evidence.* Oxford University Press.

Hjelmstedt, A., Widstrom, A. M., & Collins, A. (2006). Psychological correlates of prenatal attachment in women who conceived after in vitro fertilization and women who conceived naturally. *Birth, 33*(4), 303–310. https://doi.org/10.1111/j.1523-536X.2006.00123.x

Hmelo-Silver, C. E., & Pfeffer, M. G. (2004). Comparing expert and novice understanding of a complex system from the perspective of structures, behaviors, and functions. *Cognitive Science, 28*(1), 127–138.

Hobfoll, S. E. (2002). Social and psychological resources and adaptation. *Review of General Psychology, 6*(4), 307–324. https://doi.org/10.1037/1089-2680.6.4.307

Hofferth, S. (2009). Media use vs. work and play in middle childhood. *Social Indicators Research, 93*(1), 127–129. https://doi.org/10.1007/s11205-008-9414-5

Hoffman, B. J., & Woehr, D. J. (2006). A quantitative review of the relationship between person-organization fit and behavioral outcomes. *Journal of Vocational Behavior, 68*(3), 389–399.

Hoffmann, J. P., & Bahr, S. J. (2014). Parenting style, religiosity, peer alcohol use, and adolescent heavy drinking. *Journal of Studies on Alcohol and Drugs, 75*(2), 222–227.

Hofvander, Y. (2003). Why women don't breastfeed: A national survey. *Acta Paediatr, 92*(11), 1243–1244.

Hogervorst, E., Huppert, F., Matthews, F. E., & Brayne, C. (2008). Thyroid function and cognitive decline in the MRC Cognitive Function and Ageing Study. *Psychoneuroendocrinology, 33*(7), 1013–1022. https://doi.org/10.1016/j.psyneuen.2008.05.008

Holland, J. L. (1997). *Making vocational choices: A theory of vocational personalities and work environments* (3rd ed.). Psychological Assessment Resources.

Home School Legal Defense Associaiton. (2013). *Am I homeschooling under the "home school" law or the "private school" law.* http://www.hslda.org/docs/news/201103100.asp

Hook, J. L., & Chalasani, S. (2008). Gendered expectations? Reconsidering single fathers' child-care time. *Journal of Marriage and Family, 70*(4), 978–990.

Hooker, K., & Kaus, C. R. (1994). Health-related possible selves in young and middle adulthood. *Psychology and Aging, 9*(1), 126–133.

Hooper, S. R., Roberts, J., Sideris, J., Burchinal, M., & Zeisel, S. (2010). Longitudinal predictors of reading and math trajectories through middle school for African American versus Caucasian students across two samples. *Developmental Psychology, 46*(5), 1018–1029.

Horn, J. L., & Cattell, R. B. (1966). Refinement and test of the theory of fluid and crystallized intelligence. *Journal of Educational Psychology, 57*(5), 253–270.

Hostinar, C. E., Stellern, S. A., Schaefer, C., Carlson, S. M., & Gunnar, M. R. (2012). Associations between early life adversity and executive function in children adopted internationally from orphanages. *Proceedings of the National Academy of Sciences, 109*(2), 17208–17212. https://doi.org/10.1073/pnas.1121246109

Houston, D. K., Nicklas, B. J., & Zizza, C. A. (2009). Weighty concerns: The growing prevalence of obesity among older adults. *Journal of the American Dietetic Association, 109*(11), 1886–1895. https://doi.org/10.1016/j.jada.2009.08.014

Howie, L. D., Lukacs, S. L., Pastor, P. N., Reuben, C. A., & Mendola, P. (2010). Participation in activities outside of school hours in relation to problem behavior and social skills in middle childhood. *Journal of School Health, 80*(3), 119–125. https://doi.org/10.1111/j.1746-1561.2009.00475.x

Hrdy, S. (1999). *Mother nature: A history of mothers, infants and natural selection.* Pantheon.

Hsu, H. C., & Chang, W. C. (2015). Social connections and happiness among the elder population of Taiwan. *Aging and Mental Health, 19*(12), 1131–1137. https://doi.org/10.1080/13607863.2015.1004160

*Huffington Post.* (2013, January 7). Hollister nurse-in: Breastfeeding advocates feud with shopping mall following protest. http://www.huffingtonpost.com/2013/01/07/hollister-nurse-in_n_2425541.html

Hughes, M. E., & Waite, L. J. (2009). Marital biography and health at mid-life. *Journal of Health and Social Behavior, 50*(3), 344–358.

Hunter, D. J., & Eckstein, F. (2009). Exercise and osteoarthritis. *Journal of Anatomy, 214*(2), 197–207. https://doi.org/10.1111/j.1469-7580.2008.01013.x

Huston, T. L. (2009). What's love got to do with it? Why some marriages succeed and others fail. *Personal Relationships, 16*(3), 301–327. https://doi.org/10.1111/j.1475-6811.2009.01225.x

## I

Iacono, D., Markesbery, W. R., Gross, M., Pletnikova, O., Rudow, G., Zandi, P., & Troncoso, J. C. (2009). The nun study: Clinically silent AD, neuronal hypertrophy, and linguistic skills in early life. *Neurology, 73*(9), 665–673. https://doi.org/10.1212/WNL.0b013e3181b01077

Ijzendoorn, M. H., Dijkstra, J., & Bus, A. G. (1995). Attachment, intelligence, and language: A meta-analysis. *Social development, 4*(2), 115–128.

Ilies, R., Johnson, M. D., Judge, T. A., & Keeney, J. (2011). A within-individual study of interpersonal conflict as a work stressor: Dispositional and situational moderators. *Journal of Organizational Behavior, 32*(1), 44–64. https://doi.org/10.1002/job.677

Imhoff-Kunsch, B., Stein, A. D., Martorell, R., Parra-Cabrera, S., Romieu, I., & Ramakrishnan, U. (2011). Prenatal docosahexaenoic acid supplementation and infant morbidity: Randomized controlled trial. *Pediatrics, 128*(3), e505–e512. https://doi.org/10.1542/peds.2010-1386

Isaacowitz, D. M. (2012). Mood regulation in real time: Age differences in the role of looking. *Current Directions in Psychological Science, 21*(4), 237–242. https://doi.org/10.1177/0963721412448651

Isaacowitz, D. M., Toner, K., & Neupert, S. D. (2009). Use of gaze for real-time mood regulation: Effects of age and attentional functioning. *Psychology and Aging, 24*(4), 989–994.

Isaacowitz, D. M., Wadlinger, H. A., Goren, D., & Wilson, H. R. (2006). Selective preference in visual fixation away from negative images in old age? An eye-tracking study. *Psychology and Aging, 21*(1), 40–48.

# J

Jackson, R. A., Vittinghoff, E., Kanaya, A. M., Miles, T. P., Resnick, H. E., Kritchevsky, S. B., ... Brown, J. S. (2004). Urinary incontinence in elderly women: Findings from the Health, Aging, and Body Composition Study. *Obstetrics and Gynecology, 104*(2), 301–307. https://doi.org/10.1097/01.AOG.0000133482.20685.d1

Jambon, M., & Smetana, J. G. (2014). Moral complexity in middle childhood: Children's evaluations of necessary harm. *Developmental Psychology, 50*(1), 22–33.

Janakiraman, V., Ecker, J., & Kaimal, A. J. (2010). Comparing the second stage in induced and spontaneous labor. *Obstetrics and Gynecology, 116*(3), 606–611. https://doi.org/10.1097/AOG.0b013e3181eeb968

Jang, S.-N., Choi, Y.-J., & Kim, D.-H. (2009). Association of socioeconomic status with successful ageing: Differences in the components of successful ageing. *Journal of Biosocial Science, 41*(2), 207–219.

Janse, E. (2009). Processing of fast speech by elderly listeners. *Journal of the Acoustical Society of America, 125*(4), 2361–2373. https://doi.org/10.1121/1.3082117

Jaunin, J., Bochud, M., Marques-Vidal, P., Vollenweider, P., Waeber, G., Mooser, V., & Paccaud, F. (2009). Smoking offsets the metabolic benefits of parental longevity in women: The CoLaus study. *Preventive Medicine, 48*(3), 224–231. https://doi.org/10.1016/j.ypmed.2008.12.007

Jerome, G. J., Ko, S. U., Kauffman, D., Studenski, S. A., Ferrucci, L., & Simonsick, E. M. (2015). Gait characteristics associated with walking speed decline in older adults: Results from the Baltimore Longitudinal Study of Aging. *Archives of Gerontology and Geriatrics, 60*(2), 239–243. https://doi.org/10.1016/j.archger.2015.01.007

Johnson, M. H. (1995). The inhibition of automatic saccades in early infancy. *Developmental Psychobiology, 28*(5), 281–291. https://doi.org/10.1002/dev.420280504

Johnson, S., Li, J., Kendall, G., Strazdins, L., & Jacoby, P. (2013). Mothers' and fathers' work hours, child gender, and behavior in middle childhood. *Journal of Marriage and Family, 75*(1), 56–74. https://doi.org/10.1111/j.1741-3737.2012.01030.x

Johnston, C. C., Stevens, B., Pinelli, J., Gibbins, S., Filion, F., Jack, A., Steele, S., Boyer, K., & Veilleux, A. (2003). Kangaroo care is effective in diminishing pain response in preterm neonates. *Archives of Pediatrics and Adolescent Medicine, 157*(11), 1084–1088. https://doi.org/10.1001/archpedi.157.11.1084

Jonassaint, C. R., Boyle, S. H., Williams, R. B., Mark, D. B., Siegler, I. C., & Barefoot, J. C. (2007). Facets of openness predict mortality in patients with cardiac disease. *Psychosomatic Medicine, 69*(4), 319–322. https://doi.org/10.1097/PSY.0b013e318052e27d

Jones, L. (2012). Pain management for women in labour: an overview of systematic reviews. *Journal of Evidence-Based Medicine, 5*(2), 101–102.

Joung, K. E., Park, K.-H., Zaichenko, L., Sahin-Efe, A., Thakkar, B., Brinkoetter, M., et al. (2014). Early life adversity is associated with elevated levels of circulating leptin, irisin, and decreased levels of adiponectin in midlife adults. *The Journal of Clinical Endocrinology & Metabolism, 99*(6), E1055–E1060.

# K

Kagan, J. (2005). Temperament. In *Encyclopedia on early child development.* Centre of Excellence for Early Child Development. http://www.excellence-earlychildhood.ca/documents/KaganANGxp.pdf

Kajantie, E., Hovi, P., Raikkonen, K., Pesonen, A. K., Heinonen, K., Jarvenpaa, A. L., Eriksson, J. G., Strang-Karlsson, S., & Andersson, S. (2008). Young adults with very low birth weight: Leaving the parental home and sexual relationships—Helsinki study of very low birth weight adults. *Pediatrics, 122*(1), e62–e72. https://doi.org/10.1542/peds.2007-3858

Kakinami, L., Barnett, T., & Paradis, G. (2014). Abstract MP34: In praise of demanding parenting: The effects of parenting style and poverty on obesity risk in children: Evidence from a nationally representative sample. *Circulation, 129*(1), AMP34.

Kalmijn, M. (2003). Shared friendship networks and the life course: An analysis of survey data on married and cohabiting couples. *Social Networks, 25*(3), 231–249.

Kamel, N. S., & Gammack, J. K. (2006). Insomnia in the elderly: Cause, approach, and treatment. *American Journal of Medicine, 119*(6), 463–469.

Kamijo, K., Khan, N. A., Pontifex, M. B., Scudder, M. R., Drollette, E. S., Raine, L. B., Evans, E. L., Castelli, D. M., & Hillman, C. H. (2012). The relation of adiposity to cognitive control and scholastic achievement in preadolescent children. *Obesity, 20*(12), 2406–2411.

Kanagaratnam, L., Drame, M., Trenque, T., Oubaya, N., Nazeyrollas, P., Novella, J. L., ... Mahmoudi, R. (2016). Adverse drug reactions in elderly patients with cognitive disorders: A systematic review. *Maturitas, 85*, 56–63. https://doi.org/10.1016/j.maturitas.2015.12.013

Kaneshiro, N. K. Z., & Zieve, D. (2010). Sudden Infant Death Syndrome. Retrieved February 15, 2018, from https://www.texashealth.org/allen/health-information/?productId=617&pid=1&gid=001566

Kanfer, R., & Ackerman, P. L. (2004). Aging, adult development, and work motivation. *Academy of Management Review, 29*(3), 440–458.

Kannus, P., Uusi-Rasi, K., Palvanen, M., & Parkkari, J. (2005). Non-pharmacological means to prevent fractures among older adults. *Annals of Medicine, 37*(4), 303–310.

Karney, B., & Bradbury, T. (1997). Neuroticism, marital interaction, and the trajectory of marital satisfaction. *Journal of Personality and Social Psychology, 72*(5), 1075–1092.

Kastorini, C.-M., Milionis, H. J., Esposito, K., Giugliano, D., Goudevenos, J. A., & Panagiotakos, D. B. (2011). The effect of Mediterranean diet on metabolic syndrome and its Components: A meta-analysis of 50 studies and 534,906 individuals. *Journal of the American College of Cardiology (JACC), 57*(11), 1299–1313.

Kato, K., Zwelq, R., Barzilai, N., & Atzmon, G. (2012). Positive attitude towards life and emotional expression as personality phenotypes for centenarians. *Aging, 4*(5), 359–367.

Katz, R. (2009). Intergenerational family relations and subjective well-being in old age: A cross-national study. *European Journal of Ageing, 6*(2), 79–90.

Keefe, S. E., Padilla, A. M., & Carlos, M. L. (1979). The Mexican-American extended family as an emotional support system. *Human Organization, 38*(2), 144–152.

Kelley-Quon, L. I., Tseng, C.-H., Janzen, C., & Shew, S. (2012). *Congenital malformations associated with assisted reproductive technology: A California statewide analysis* [Paper presentation, American Academy of Pediatrics, New Orleans, LA].

Kelley, P., Lockley, S. W., Foster, R. G., & Kelley, J. (2015). Synchronizing education to adolescent biology: "Let teens sleep, start school later." *Learning, Media and Technology, 40*(2), 210–226.

Kendler, K. S., Myers, J., Damaj, M. I., & Chen, X. (2013). Early smoking onset and risk for subsequent nicotine dependence: A monozygotic co-twin control study. *American Journal of Psychiatry, 170*(4), 408–413.

Kennedy, A. C., Bybee, D., Sullivan, C. M., & Greeson, M. (2009). The effects of community and family violence exposure on anxiety trajectories during middle childhood: The role of family social support as a moderator. *Journal of Clinical Child & Adolescent Psychology, 38*(3), 365–379. https://doi.org/10.1080/15374410902851713

Keown, L. (2012). Predictors of Boys' ADHD symptoms from early to middle childhood: The role of father–child and mother–child interactions. *Journal of Abnormal Child Psychology, 40*(4), 569–581. https://doi.org/10.1007/s10802-011-9586-3

Kerby, D. S., & Ragan, K. M. (2002). Activity interests and Holland's RIASEC system in older adults. *International Journal of Aging & Human Development, 55*(2), 117–139.

Kessel, L., Jorgensen, T., Glumer, C., & Larsen, M. (2006). Early lens aging is accelerated in subjects with a high risk of ischemic heart disease: An epidemiologic study. *BMC Ophthalmology, 18*(6), 16.

Khaddouma, A., Norona, J. C., & Whitton, S. W. (2015). Individual, couple, and contextual factors associated with same-sex relationship instability. *Couple and Family Psychology: Research and Practice, 4*(2), 106–125. https://doi.org/10.1037/cfp0000043

Kidd, T., & Sheffield, D. (2005). Attachment style and symptom reporting: Examining the mediating effects of anger and social support. *British Journal of Health Psychology, 10*(4), 531–541. https://doi.org/10.1348/135910705x43589

Kieffer, K. M., Schinka, J. A., & Curtiss, G. (2004). Person-environment congruence and personality domains in the prediction of job performance and work quality. *Journal of Counseling Psychology, 51*(2), 168–177.

Kikkert, H. K., Middelburg, K. J., & Hadders-Algra, M. (2010). Maternal anxiety is related to infant neurological condition, paternal anxiety is not. *Early Human Development, 86*(3), 171–177. https://doi.org/10.1016/j.earlhumdev.2010.02.004

Kim, G., Walden, T. A., & Knieps, L. J. (2010). Impact and characteristics of positive and fearful emotional messages during infant social referencing. *Infant Behavior and Development, 33*(2), 189–195. https://doi.org/10.1016/j.infbeh.2009.12.009

Kim, H., Yoshida, H., & Suzuki, T. (2010). The effects of multidimensional exercise on functional decline, urinary incontinence, and fear of falling in community-dwelling elderly women with multiple symptoms of geriatric syndrome: A randomized controlled and 6-month follow-up trial. *Archives of Gerontology and Geriatrics, 52*(1), 99–105. https://doi.org/10.1016/j.archger.2010.02.008

Kim, J.-M., Stewart, R., Kim, S.-W., Yang, S.-J., Shin, I., & Yoon, J.-S. (2009). Insomnia, depression, and physical disorders in late life: A 2-year longitudinal community study in Koreans. *Sleep, 32*(9), 1221–1228.

King, A. C., Atienza, A., Castro, C., & Collins, R. (2002). Physiological and affective responses to family caregiving in the natural setting in wives versus daughters. *International Journal of Behavioral Medicine, 9*(3), 176–194.

King, K. M., Lengua, L. J., & Monahan, K. C. (2013). Individual differences in the development of self-regulation during pre-adolescence: Connections to context and adjustment. *Journal of Abnormal Child Psychology, 41*(1), 57–69.

King, M., Ruggles, S., Alexander, J. T., Flood, S., Genadek, K., Schroeder, M. B., ... Vick, R. (2010). *Integrated public use microdata series, current population survey: Version 3.0.* University of Minnesota.

Kishimoto, H., Ohara, T., Hata, J., Ninomiya, T., Yoshida, D., Mukai, N., Nagat, M., Ikeda, F., Fukuhara, M., Kumagai, S., Kanba, S., Kitazano, T., & Kiyohara, Y. (2016). The long-term association between physical activity and risk of dementia in the community: The Hisayama Study. *European Journal of Epidemiology, 31*, 267–274. https://doi.org/10.1007/s10654-016-0125-y

Kisilevsky, B. S., Hains, S. M. J., Brown, C. A., Lee, C. T., Cowperthwaite, B., Stutzman, S. S., Swansburg, M. L., Lee, K., Huang, H., Ye, H.-H., Zhang, K., & Wang, Z. (2009). Fetal sensitivity to properties of maternal speech and language. *Infant Behavior and Development, 32*(1), 59–71.

Kissane, M., & McLaren, S. (2006). Sense of belonging as a predictor of reasons for living in older adults. *Death Studies, 30*(3), 243–258.

Klass, M., Baudry, S., & Duchateau, J. (2006). Voluntary activation during maximal contraction with advancing age: A brief review. *European Journal of Applied Physiology, 100*(5), 543–551.

Klemmack, D. L., Roff, L. L., Parker, M. W., Koenig, H. G., Sawyer, P., & Allman, R. M. (2007). A cluster analysis typology of religiousness/spirituality among older adults. *Research on Aging, 29*(2), 163–183.

Klerman, E. B., Duffy, J. F., Dijk, D. J., & Czeisler, C. A. (2001). Circadian phase resetting in older people by ocular bright light exposure. *Journal of Investigative Medicine, 49*(1), 30–40.

Klomek, A. B., Sourander, A., & Gould, M. (2010). The association of suicide and bullying in childhood to young adulthood: A review of cross-sectional and longitudinal research findings. *Canadian Journal of Psychiatry, 55*(5), 282–288.

Knoester, C., & Eggebeen, D. J. (2006). The effects of the transition to parenthood and subsequent children on men's well-being and social participation. *Journal of Family Issues, 27*(11), 1532–1560.

Knopman, D. S. (2007). Cerebrovascular disease and dementia. *British Journal of Radiology, 80*(Special Issue 2), S121–S127. https://doi.org/10.1259/bjr/75681080

Kochanek, K. A., Murphy, S. L., Xu, J., & Tejeda-Vera, B. (2016). Deaths: Final data for 2017. *National Vital Statistics Report, 65.*

Kopp, C. B. (2011). Development in the early years: Socialization, motor development, and consciousness. *Annual Review of Psychology, 62*, 165–187. https://doi.org/10.1146/annurev.psych.121208.131625

Kosek, D. J., Kim, J.-S., Petrella, J. K., Cross, J. M., & Bamman, M. M. (2006). Efficacy of 3 days/wk resistance training on myofiber hypertrophy and myogenic mechanisms in young vs. older adults. *Journal of Applied Physiology, 101*(2), 531–544.

Kostka, T. (2005). Quadriceps maximal power and optimal shortening velocity in 335 men aged 23–88 years. *European Journal of Applied Physiology, 95*(2–3), 140–145.

Kraybill, J. H., & Bell, M. A. (2012). Infancy predictors of preschool and post-kindergarten executive function. *Developmental Psychobiology, 55*(5), 530–538. https://doi.org/10.1002/dev.21057

Kreider, R. M., & Ellis, R. (2011). Number, timing, and duration of marriages and divorces: 2009. *Current Population Reports P70-125.* U.S. Bureau of the Census.

Krouse, A., Craig, J., Watson, U., Matthews, Z., Kolski, G., & Isola, K. (2012). Bed-sharing influences, attitudes, and practices: Implications for promoting safe infant sleep. *Journal of Child Health Care, 16*(3), *274–283.* https://doi.org/10.1177/1367493511432300

Kryger, A. I., & Andersen, J. L. (2007). Resistance training in the oldest old: Consequences for muscle strength, fiber types, fiber size, and MHC isoforms. *Scandinavian Journal of Medicine and Science in Sports, 17*(4), 422–430. https://doi.org/10.1111/j.1600-0838.2006.00575.x

Kubzansky, L. D., Cole, S. R., Kawachi, I., Vokonas, P., & Sparrow, D. (2006). Shared and unique contributions of anger, anxiety, and depression to coronary heart disease: A prospective study in the Normative Aging Study. *Annals of Behavioral Medicine, 31*(1), 21–29.

Kuhl, P. K. (2010). Brain mechanisms in early language acquisition. *Neuron, 67*(5), 713–727. https://doi.org/10.1016/j.neuron.2010.08.038

Kujala, U. M. (2009). Evidence on the effects of exercise therapy in the treatment of chronic disease. *British Journal of Sports Medicine, 43*(8), 550–555. https://doi.org/10.1136/bjsm.2009.059808


## L


Labouvie-Vief, G., & Medler, M. (2002). Affect optimization and affect complexity: Modes and styles of regulation in adulthood. *Psychology and Aging, 17*(4), 571–588.

Lachman, M. E., Rosnick, C. B., Rocke, C., Bosworth, H. B., & Hertzog, C. (2009). The rise and fall of control beliefs and life satisfaction in adulthood: Trajectories of stability and change over ten years. In *Aging and cognition: Research methodologies and empirical advances* (pp. 143–160). American Psychological Association.

Lafreniere, D., & Mann, N. (2009). Anosmia: Loss of smell in the elderly. *Otolaryngology Clinics of North America, 42*(1), 123–131. https://doi.org/10.1016/j.otc.2008.09.001

Lagacé-Séguin, D. G., & Case, E. (2008). Extracurricular activity and parental involvement predict positive outcomes in elementary school children. *Early Child Development and Care, 180*(4), 453–462. https://doi.org/10.1080/03004430802040948

Lahelma, E., Aittomaki, A., Laaksonen, M., Lallukka, T., Martikainen, P., Piha, K., Rahkonen, O., & Saastamoinen, P. (2012). Cohort profile: The Helsinki health study. *International Journal of Epidemiology, 42*(3), 722–730. https://doi.org/10.1093/ije/dys039

Lancaster, S. M., Schick, U. M., Osman, M. M., & Enquobahrie, D. A. (2012). Risk factors associated with epidural use. *Journal of Clinical Medicine Research, 4*(2), 119–126. https://doi.org/10.4021/jocmr810w

Lancy, D., & Grove, M. A. (2011). Getting noticed. *Human Nature, 22*(3), 281–302. https://doi.org/10.1007/s12110-011-9117-5

Lang, F. R., & Carstensen, L. L. (1994). Close emotional relationships in late life: Further support for proactive aging in the social domain. *Psychology and Aging, 9*(2), 315–324.

Lang, F. R., & Carstensen, L. L. (2002). Time counts: Future time perspective, goals, and social relationships. *Psychology and Aging, 17*(1), 125–139.

Lang, T., Streeper, T., Cawthon, P., Baldwin, K., Taaffe, D. R., & Harris, T. B. (2009). Sarcopenia: Etiology, clinical consequences, intervention, and assessment. *Osteoporos International, 21,* 543–559. https://doi.org/10.1007/s00198-009-1059-y

Langberg, J., Dvorsky, M., & Evans, S. (2013). What specific facets of executive function are associated with academic functioning in youth with attention-deficit/hyperactivity disorder? *Journal of Abnormal Child Psychology, 41,* 1–15. https://doi.org/10.1007/s10802-013-9750-z

Lansford, J. E., Malone, P. S., Dodge, K. A., Pettit, G. S., & Bates, J. E. (2010). Developmental cascades of peer rejection, social information processing biases, and aggression during middle childhood. *Development and Psychopathology, 22*(3), 593–602. https://doi.org/10.1017/S0954579410000301

Lansford, J. E., Yu, T., Pettit, G. S., Bates, J. E., & Dodge, K. A. (2014). Pathways of peer relationships from childhood to young adulthood. *Journal of Applied Developmental Psychology, 35*(2), 111–117.

Lapalme, M.-È., Tremblay, M., & Simard, G. (2009). The relationship between career plateauing, employee commitment and psychological distress: The role of organizational and supervisor support. *International Journal of Human Resource Management, 20*(5), 1132–1145. https://doi.org/10.1080/09585190902850323

Larcom, M. J., & Isaacowitz, D. M. (2009). Rapid emotion regulation after mood induction: Age and individual differences. *Journals of Gerontology Series B: Psychological Sciences and Social Sciences, 64*(6), 733–741. https://doi.org/10.1093/geronb/gbp077

Lau, C. Q. (2012). The stability of same-sex cohabitation, different-sex cohabitation, and marriage. *Journal of Marriage and Family, 74*(5), 973–988.

Lauritsen, M. B. (2013). Autism spectrum disorder. *European Child & Adolescent Psychiatry, 22*(1), S37–S42. https://doi.org/10.1007/s00787-012-0359-5

Lease, S. H. (1998). Annual review, 1993–1997: Work attitudes and outcomes. *Journal of Vocational Behavior, 53*(2), 154–183.

Lecompte, V., Moss, E., Cyr, C., & Pascuzzo, K. (2014). Preschool attachment, self-esteem and the development of preadolescent anxiety and depressive symptoms. *Attachment & Human Development, 16*(3), 242–260. https://doi.org/10.1080/14616734.2013.873816

Lee, K., Bull, R., & Ho, R. M. H. (2013). Developmental changes in executive functioning. *Child Development, 84*(6), 1933–1953. https://doi.org/10.1111/cdev.12096

Lee, S. J., Ralson, H. J. P., Drey, E. A., Partridge, J. C., & Rosen, M. A. (2005). Fetal pain: A systematic multidisiplinary review of the evidence. *Journal of the American Medical Association, 294*(8), 947–954.

Lenhart, A. (2015). Teens, social media & technology overview 2015. *Pew Research Center, 9.*

Leonardelli, G. J., Hermann, A. D., Lynch, M. E., & Arkin, R. M. (2003). The shape of self-evaluation: Implicit theories of intelligence and judgments of intellectual ability. *Journal of Research in Personality, 37*(3), 141–168.

Leopold, T., & Skopek, J. (2015). Convergence or continuity? The gender gap in household labor after retirement. *Journal of Marriage and Family, 77*(4), 819–832. https://doi.org/10.1111/jomf.12199

Lerma, E. V. (2009). Anatomic and physiologic changes of the aging kidney. *Clinics in Geriatric Medicine, 25*(3), 325–329. https://doi.org/10.1016/j.cger.2009.06.007

Leung, R. K., Toumbourou, J. W., & Hemphill, S. A. (2014). The effect of peer influence and selection processes on adolescent alcohol use: A systematic review of longitudinal studies. *Health Psychology Review, 14*(8), 426–457.

Leve, L. D., DeGarmo, D. S., Bridgett, D. J., Neiderhiser, J. M., Shaw, D. S., Harold, G. T., Natsuaki, M. N., & Reiss, D. (2013). Using an adoption design to separate genetic, prenatal, and temperament influences on toddler executive function. *Developmental Psychology, 49*(6), 1045–1057.

Leveille, S. G. (2004). Musculoskeletal aging. *Current Opinions in Rheumatology, 16*(2), 114–118.

Levy, B. R., Slade, M. D., Kunkel, S. R., & Kasl, S. V. (2002). Longevity increased by positive self-perceptions of aging. *Journal of Personality and Social Psychology, 83*(2), 261–270.

Lewis, J. M., & Kreider, R. M. (2015). *Remarriage in the United States.* American Community Survey Reports, ACS-30, https://www.census.gov/content/dam/Census/library/publications/2015/acs/acs-30.pdf

Li, Y., Bebiroglu, N., Phelps, E., Lerner, R. M., & Lerner, J. V. (2016). Out-of-school time activity participation, school engagement and positive youth development: Findings from the 4-H Study of Positive Youth Development. *Journal of Youth Development, 3*(3).

Lillard, A. S., Lerner, M. D., Hopkins, E. J., Dore, R. A., Smith, E. D., & Palmquist, C. M. (2013). The impact of pretend play on children's development: A review of the evidence. *Psychological Bulletin, 139*(1), 1–34. https://doi.org/10.1037/a0029321

Lin, F., Friedman, E., Quinn, J., Chen, D.-G., & Mapstone, M. (2012). Effect of leisure activities on inflammation and cognitive function in an aging sample. *Archives of Gerontology and Geriatrics, 54*(3), e398–e404. https://doi.org/10.1016/j.archger.2012.02.002

Lindau, S. T., & Gavrilova, N. (2010). Sex, health, and years of sexually active life gained due to good health: Evidence from two US population based cross sectional surveys of ageing. *BMJ: British Medical Journal, 340.*

Lister, J. P., & Barnes, C. A. (2009). Neurobiological changes in the hippocampus during normative aging. *Archives of Neurology, 66*(7), 829–833. https://doi.org/10.1001/archneurol.2009.125

Livingstone, K. M., & Isaacowitz, D. M. (2015). Situation selection and modification for emotion regulation in younger and older adults. *Social Psychological and Personality Science, 6*(8), 904–910. https://doi.org/10.1177/1948550615593148

Lobjois, R., & Cavallo, V. (2009). The effects of aging on street-crossing behavior: From estimation to actual crossing. *Accident Analysis and Prevention, 41*(2), 259–267. https://doi.org/10.1016/j.aap.2008.12.001

Lodi-Smith, J., Jackson, J., Bogg, T., Walton, K., Wood, D., Harms, P., & Roberts, B. W. (2010). Mechanisms of health: Education and health-related behaviours partially mediate the relationship between conscientiousness and self-reported physical health. *Psychology & Health, 25*(3), 305–319. https://doi.org/10.1080/08870440902736964

Loehlin, J. C. (2012). The differential heritability of personality item clusters. *Behavioral Genetics, 42*(3), 500–507.

Lombardi, G., Tauchmanova, L., Di Somma, C., Musella, T., Rota, F., Savanelli, M. C., & Colao, A. (2005). Somatopause: Dismetabolic and bone effects. *Journal of Endocrinological Investigation, 28*(10), 36–42.

Lovas, G. S. (2011). Gender and patterns of language development in mother-toddler and father-toddler dyads. *First Language, 31*(1), 83–108. https://doi.org/10.1177/0142723709359241

Lovasi, G. S., Lemaitre, R. N., Siscovick, D. S., Dublin, S., Bis, J. C., Lumley, T., ... Psaty, B. M. (2007). Amount of leisure-time physical activity and risk of nonfatal myocardial infarction. *Annals of Epidemiology, 17*(6), 410–416. https://doi.org/10.1016/j.annepidem.2006.10.012

Low, K. S. D., Yoon, M., Roberts, B. W., & Rounds, J. (2005). The stability of vocational interests from early adolescence to middle adulthood: A quantitative review of longitudinal studies. *Psychological Bulletin, 131*(5), 713–737.

Lowe, N. K. (2002). The nature of labor pain. *American Journal of Obstetrics and Gynecology, 186*(5), S16–S24.

Lowry, L. W., & Beikirch, P. (1998). Effect of comprehensive care on pregnancy outcomes. *Applied Nursing Research, 11*(2), 55–61.

Lu, B., Qian, Z., Cunningham, A., & Li, C.-L. (2012). Estimating the effect of premarital cohabitation on timing of marital disruption: Using propensity score matching in event history analysis. *Sociological Methods & Research, 41*(3), 440–466. https://doi.org/10.1177/0049124112452395

Lucas, R. E., Clark, A. E., Georgellis, Y., & Diener, E. (2003). Reexamining adaptation and the set point model of happiness: Reactions to changes in marital status. *Journal of Personality and Social Psychology, 84*(3), 527–539.

Luna, B., & Sweeney, J. A. (2004). The emergence of collaborative brain function: FMRI studies of the development of response inhibition. *Annals of the New York Academy of Sciences, 1021*(1), 296–309.

Luo, Y., LaPierre, T. A., Hughes, M. E., & Waite, L. J. (2012). Grandparents providing care to grandchildren: A population-based study of continuity and change. *Journal of Family Issues, 33*(9), 1143–1167. https://doi.org/10.1177/0192513x12438685

Lupien, S. J., McEwen, B. S., Gunnar, M. R., & Heim, C. (2009). Effects of stress throughout the lifespan on the brain, behaviour and cognition. *Nature Reviews Neuroscience, 10*(6), 434–445. https://doi.org/10.1038/nrn2639

Luthar, S. S., & Latendresse, S. J. (2005). Children of the affluent: Challenges to well-being. *Current Directions in Psychological Science, 14*(1), 49–53.

Lyons, H. Z., & O'Brien, K. M. (2006). The role of person-environment fit in the job satisfaction and tenure intentions of African American employees. *Journal of Counseling Psychology, 53*(4), 387–396.

Lyssens-Danneboom, V., & Mortelmans, D. (2014). Living apart together and money: New partnerships, traditional gender roles. *Journal of Marriage and Family, 76*(5), 949–966. https://doi.org/10.1111/jomf.12136


## M


MacDorman, M., Declercq, E., & Menacker, F. (2011). Recent trends and patterns in cesarean and vaginal birth after cesarean (VBAC) deliveries in the United States. *Clinics in Perinatology, 38*(2), 179–192. https://doi.org/10.1016/j.clp.2011.03.007

MacDorman, M. F., & Mathews, T. J. (2010). Behind international rankings of infant mortality: How the United States compares with Europe. *International Journal of Health Services, 40*(4), 577–588.

Macias, M. M., & Twyman, K. A. (2011). Speech and language development and disorders. In *Developmental and behavioral pediatrics* (pp. 201–219). American Academy of Pediatrics.

MacKinnon, K., & McIntyre, M. (2006). From Braxton Hicks to preterm labour: The constitution of risk in pregnancy. *Canadian Journal of Nursing Research, 38*(2), 56–72.

Madden, D. J. (2001). Speed and timing of behavioural processes. In J. E. Birren & K. W. Schaie (Eds.), *Handbook of the psychology of aging* (5th ed.). Academic Press.

Magai, C. (2008). Attachment in middle and later life. In J. Cassidy, P. R. Shaver, J. Cassidy, & P. R. Shaver (Eds.), *Handbook of attachment: Theory, research, and clinical applications* (2nd ed.) (pp. 532–551). Guilford.

Magai, C., Consedine, N. S., Krivoshekova, Y. S., Kudadjie-Gyamfi, E., & McPherson, R. (2006). Emotion experience and expression across the adult lifespan: Insights from a multimodal assessment study. *Psychology and Aging, 21*(2), 303–317.

Magnuson, K., & Berger, L. M. (2009). Family structure states and transitions: Associations with children's well-being during middle childhood. *Journal of Marriage and Family, 71*(3), 575–591. https://doi.org/10.1111/j.1741-3737.2009.00620.x

Mah, V. K., & Ford-Jones, E. L. (2012). Spotlight on middle childhood: Rejuvenating the "forgotten years." *Paediatrics & Child Health, 17*(2), 81–83.

Mahlberg, R., Tilmann, A., Salewski, L., & Kunz, D. (2006). Normative data on the daily profile of urinary 6-sulfatoxymelatonin in healthy subjects between the ages of 20 and 84. *Psychoneuroendocrinology, 31*(5), 634–641.

Main, M. (1991). Metacognitive knowledge, metacognitive monitoring, and singular (coherent) vs. multiple (incoherent) models of attachment. In C. M. Parkes, J. Stevenson-Hinde, & P. Marris (Eds.), *Attachment across the life cycle* (p. 127–159). Tavistock/Routledge.

Majer, I. M., Nusselder, W. J., Mackenbach, J. P., & Kunst, A. E. (2011). Socioeconomic inequalities in life and health expectancies around official retirement age in 10 Western-European countries. *Journal of Epidemiology and Community Health, 65*(11), 972–979. https://doi.org/10.1136/jech.2010.111492

Malone, J. C., Cohen, S., Liu, S. R., Vaillant, G. E., & Waldinger, R. J. (2013). Adaptive midlife defense mechanisms and late-life health. *Personality and Individual Differences, 55*(2), 85–89.

Maltais, M. L., Desroches, J., & Dionne, I. J. (2009). Changes in muscle mass and strength after menopause. *Journal of Musculoskeletal and Neuronal Interactions, 9*(4), 186–197.

Mancini, A. D., & Bonanno, G. A. (2006). Marital closeness, functional disability, and adjustment in late life. *Psychology and Aging, 21*(3), 600–610.

Manini, T. M., Everhart, J. E., Anton, S. D., Schoeller, D. A., Cummings, S. R., Mackey, D. C., Delmonico, M. J., Bauer, D. C., Simonsick, E. M., Colbert, L. H., Visser, M., Tylavsky, F., Newman, L. B., & Harris, T. B. (2009). Activity energy expenditure and change in body composition in late life. *The American Journal of Clinical Nutrition, 90*(5), 1336–1342.

Manzoli, L., Villari, P., M Pirone, G., & Boccia, A. (2007). Marital status and mortality in the elderly: A systematic review and meta-analysis. *Social Science & Medicine, 64*(1), 77–94.

March of Dimes. (2003). Infant behavior, reflexes, and cues. *Perinatal nursing education: Understanding the behavior of term infants.*

Marcia, J. (1980). Identity in adolescence. In *Handbook of adolescent psychology* (pp. 159–187). Wiley.

Marcia, J. E., & Archer, S. L. (1993). Identity status in late adolescents: Scoring criteria. In *Ego Identity* (pp. 205–240). Springer.

Marcus, S. M. (2009). Depression during pregnancy: Rates, risks and consequences—Motherisk update 2008. *Canadian Journal of Clinical Pharmacology, 16*(1), e15–e22.

Markland, A. D., Richter, H. E., Burgio, K. L., Bragg, C., Hernandez, A. L., & Subak, L. L. (2009). Fecal incontinence in obese women with urinary incontinence: Prevalence and role of dietary fiber intake. *American Journal of Obstetrics and Gynecology, 200*(5), p566. e561–e566. https://doi.org/10.1016/j.ajog.2008.11.019

Marks, N. F. (1998). Does it hurt to care? Caregiving, work–family conflict, and midlife well-being. *Journal of Marriage and the Family, 60*(4), 951–966. https://doi.org/10.2307/353637

Markus, H., & Nurius, P. (1986). Possible selves. *American Psychologist, 41*(9), 954–969.

Markus, H. R., Ryff, C. D., Curhan, K. B., & Palmersheim, K. A. (2005). *In their own words: Well-being at midlife among high school-educated and college-educated adults. How healthy are we?* http://midus.wisc.edu/howhealthyarewe/

Marschall-Lévesque, S., Castellanos-Ryan, N., Vitaro, F., & Séguin, J. R. (2014). Moderators of the association between peer and target adolescent substance use. *Addictive Behaviors, 39*(1), 48–70.

Marsiglio, W., Amato, P., Day, R. D., & Lamb, M. E. (2002). Scholarship on fatherhood in the 1990s and beyond. *Journal of Marriage & the Family, 62*(4), 1173–1191.

Marson, S. M., & Powell, R. M. (2014). Goffman and the infantilization of elderly persons: A theory in development. *Journal of Sociology and Social Welfare, 41*(4), 143–158.

Martin, A. S., Palmer, B. W., Rock, D., Gelston, C. V., & Jeste, D. V. (2015). Associations of self-perceived successful aging in young-old versus old-old adults. *International Psychogeriatrics, 27*(4), 601–609. https://doi.org/10.1017/s104161021400221x

Martin, J. A., Hamilton, B. E., Osterman, M. J. K., Driscoll, A. K., & Mathews, T. J. (2017). Births: Final data for 2015. *National Vital Statistics Reports, 66*(1).

Martin, J. A., Hamilton, B. E., Ventura, S. J., Osterman, M., Kirmeyer, S., Mathews, T., & Wilson, E. C. (2011). Births: Final data for 2009. *National Vital Statistics Reports, 60*(1).

Marvin, R. S., Britner, P. A., Cassidy, J., & Shaver, P. (2008). Normative development: The ontogeny of attachment. In J. C. P. R. Shaver (Ed.), *Handbook of attachment.* Guilford.

Masataka, N. (1996). Perception of motherese in a signed language by 6-month-old deaf infants. *Developmental Psychology, 32*(5), 874–879.

Masayesva, B. G., Mambo, E., Taylor, R. J., Goloubeva, O. G., Zhou, S., Cohen, Y., Minhas, K., Koch, W., Sciubba, J., Alberg, J. A., Sidransky, D., & Califano, J. (2006). Mitochondrial DNA content increase in response to cigarette smoking. *Cancer Epidemiology Biomarkers and Prevention, 15*(1), 19–24.

Masuda, A. D., McNall, L. A., Allen, T. D., & Nicklin, J. M. (2012). Examining the constructs of work-to-family enrichment and positive spillover. *Journal of Vocational Behavior, 80*(1), 197–210. https://doi.org/10.1016/j.jvb.2011.06.002

Matricciani, L. A., Olds, T. S., Blunden, S., Rigney, G., & Williams, M. T. (2012). Never enough sleep: A brief history of sleep recommendations for children. *Pediatrics, 129*(3), 548–556.

Matthews, R. A., Bulger, C. A., & Barnes-Farrell, J. L. (2010). Work social supports, role stressors, and work-family conflict: The moderating effect of age. *Journal of Vocational Behavior, 76*(1), 78–90.

Matthews, S. H. (1986). *Friendships through the life course.* SAGE.

Maunder, R., & Hunter, J. (2009). Assessing pattern of adult attachment in medical patients. *General Hospital Psychiatry, 31*(2), 123–130.

Mayhew, P. M., Thomas, C. D., Clement, J. G., Loveridge, N., Beck, T. J., Bonfield, W., Burgoyne, C. J., & Reeve, J. (2005). Relation between age, femoral neck cortical stability, and hip fracture risk. *Lancet, 366*(9480), 129–135.

Maywald, M., & Rink, L. (2015). Zinc homeostasis and immunosenescence. *Journal of Trace Elements in Medicine and Biology, 29,* 24–30. https://doi.org/10.1016/j.jtemb.2014.06.003

McAdams, D. P. (2008). Generativity, the redemptive self, and the problem of a noisy ego in American life. In H. A. Wayment & J. J. Bauer (Eds.), *Transcending self-interest: Psychological explorations of the quiet ego* (pp. 235–242). American Psychological Association.

McAdams, D. P. (2011). Life narratives. In K. L. Fingerman, C. A. Berg, J. Smith, & T. C. Antonucci (Eds.), *Handbook of life-span development* (pp. 589–610). Springer.

McAdams, K. K., Lucas, R. E., & Donnellan, M. B. (2012). The role of domain satisfaction in explaining the paradoxical association between life satisfaction and age. *Social Indicators Research, 109*(2), 295–303. https://doi.org/10.1007/s11205-011-9903-9

McCandliss, B., Beck, I. L., Sandak, R., & Perfetti, C. (2003). Focusing attention on decoding for children with poor reading skills: Design and preliminary tests of the word building intervention. *Scientific Studies of Reading, 7*(1), 75–104. https://doi.org/10.1207/s1532799xssr0701_05

McCarthy, L. H., Bigal, M. E., Katz, M., Derby, C., & Lipton, R. B. (2009). Chronic pain and obesity in elderly people: Results from the Einstein aging study. *Journal of the American Geriatrics Society, 57*(1), 115–119. https://doi.org/10.1111/j.1532-5415.2008.02089.x

McCleane, G. (2007). Pharmacological pain management in the elderly patient. *Clinical Interventions in Aging, 2*(4), 637–643.

McDonald-Miszczak, L., Hertzog, C., & Hultsch, D. F. (1995). Stability and accuracy of metamemory in adulthood and aging: A longitudinal analysis. *Psychology and Aging, 10*(4), 553–564.

McEwen, B. S., & Getz, L. (2013). Lifetime experiences, the brain and personalized medicine: An integrative perspective. *Metabolism, 62*(1), S20–S26. https://doi.org/10.1016/j.metabol.2012.08.020

McEwen, B. S., & Stellar, E. (1993). Stress and the individual: Mechanisms leading to disease. *Archives of Internal Medicine, 153*(18), 2093–2101.

McHale, S. M., Updegraff, K. A., & Whiteman, S. D. (2012). Sibling relationships and influences in childhood and adolescence. *Journal of Marriage and Family, 74*(5), 913–930.

McKeith, I. G. (2006). Consensus guidelines for the clinical and pathologic diagnosis of dementia with Lewy bodies (DLB): Report of the Consortium on DLB International Workshop. *Journal of Alzheimer's Disease, 9*(3), 417–423.

McKenna, L. (2012, January 6). *Child labor is making a disturbing resurgence around the world.* http://www.businessinsider.com/countries-worst-child-labor-risks-2012-1?op=1#ixzz2VBRAHuND

McKhann, G., Drachman, D., Folstein, M., Katzman, R., Price, D., & Stadlan, E. M. (1984). Clinical diagnosis of Alzheimer's disease: Report of the NINCDS-ADRDA Work Group under the auspices of Department of Health and Human Services Task Force on Alzheimer's Disease. *Neurology, 34*(7), 939–944.

McLaughlin, S. J., Connell, C. M., Heeringa, S. G., Li, L. W., & Roberts, J. S. (2010). Successful aging in the United States: Prevalence estimates from a national sample of older adults. *Journals of Gerontology: Series B: Psychological Sciences and Social Sciences, 65B*(2), 216–226. https://doi.org/10.1093/geronb/gbp101

McLean, K. C. (2008). Stories of the young and the old: Personal continuity and narrative identity. *Developmental Psychology, 44*(1), 254–264. https://doi.org/10.1037/0012-1649.44.1.254

McMahon, C. A., Boivin, J., Gibson, F. L., Hammarberg, K., Wynter, K., Saunders, D., & Fisher, J. (2013). Pregnancy-specific anxiety, ART conception and infant temperament at 4 months post-partum. *Human Reproduction, 28*(4), 887–1005. https://doi.org/10.1093/humrep/det029

McNall, L. A., Masuda, A. D., & Nicklin, J. M. (2010). Flexible work arrangements, job satisfaction, and turnover intentions: The mediating role of work-to-family enrichment. *Journal of Psychology, 144*(1), 61–81.

McNamara, B., & Rosenwax, L. (2010). Which careers of family members at the end of life need more support from health services and why? *Social Science & Medicine, 70*(7), 1035–1041. https://doi.org/10.1016/j.socscimed.2009.11.029

McNeely, C. A., & Barber, B. K. (2010). How do parents make adolescents feel loved? Perspectives on supportive parenting from adolescents in 12 cultures. *Journal of Adolescent Research, 25*(4), 601–631.

MedlinePlus. (2020). *Fetal development.* http://www.nlm.nih.gov/medlineplus/ency/article/002398.htm

Mendle, J., & Ferrero, J. (2012). Detrimental psychological outcomes associated with pubertal timing in adolescent boys. *Developmental Review, 32*(1), 49–66.

Mendle, J., Turkheimer, E., & Emery, R. E. (2007). Detrimental psychological outcomes associated with early pubertal timing in adolescent girls. *Developmental Review, 27*(2), 151–171.

Mennella, J. A., Jagnow, C. P., & Beauchamp, G. K. (2001). Prenatal and postnatal flavor learning by human infants. *Pediatrics, 107*(6), E88.

Mennella, J. A., Johnson, A., & Beauchamp, G. K. (1995). Garlic ingestion by pregnant women alters the odor of amniotic fluid. *Chemical Senses, 20*(2), 207–209. https://doi.org/10.1093/chemse/20.2.207

Mercer, R. T., Ferketich, S., May, K., DeJoseph, J., & Sollid, D. (1988). Further exploration of maternal and paternal fetal attachment. *Research in Nursing and Health, 11*(2), 83–95.

Metsäpelto, R.-L., & Pulkkinen, L. (2011). Socioemotional behavior and school achievement in relation to extracurricular activity participation in middle childhood. *Scandinavian Journal of Educational Research, 56*(2), 167–182. https://doi.org/10.1080/00313831.2011.581681

Meunier, N., Beattie, J. H., Ciarapica, D., O'Connor, J. M., Andriollo-Sanchez, M., Taras, A., Coudray, C., & Polito, A. (2005). Basal metabolic rate and thyroid hormones of late-middle-aged and older human subjects: The ZENITH study. *European Journal of Clinical Nutrition, 59*(2), S53–S57. https://doi.org/10.1038/sj.ejcn.1602299

Mhaoláin, A. M. N., Gallagher, D., Connell, H. O., Chin, A. V., Bruce, I., Hamilton, F., Teehee, E., Coen, R., Coakley, D., Cunningham, C., Walsh, J. B., & Lawlor, B. A. (2012). Subjective well-being amongst community-dwelling elders: What determines satisfaction with life? Findings from the Dublin Healthy Aging Study. *International Psychogeriatrics, 24*(2), 316–323. https://doi.org/10.1017/s1041610211001360

Miche, M., Huxhold, O., & Stevens, N. L. (2013). A latent class analysis of friendship network types and their predictors in the second half of life. *Journals of Gerontology Series B: Psychological and Social Sciences, 68*(4), 644–652. https://doi.org/10.1093/geronb/gbt041

Miller, B. C. (2002). Family influences on adolescent sexual and contraceptive behavior. *Journal of Sex Research, 39*(1), 22–26.

Miller, P. J. E., Niehuis, S., & Huston, T. L. (2006). Positive illusions in marital relationships: A 13-year longitudinal study. *Personality and Social Psychology Bulletin, 32*(12), 1579–1594.

Mindell, J. (2020, September 25). *Sleep, infants and parents.* http://www.sleepfoundation.org/article/ask-the-expert/sleep-infants-and-parents

Mitchell, B. A., & Lovegreen, L. D. (2009). The empty nest syndrome in midlife families: A multimethod exploration of parental gender differences and cultural dynamics. *Journal of Family Issues, 30*(12), 1651–1670. https://doi.org/10.1177/0192513x09339020

Mitchell, S. L., Teno, J. M., Kiely, D. K., Shaffer, M. L., Jones, R. N., Prigerson, H. G., Volicer, L., Givens, J. L., & Hamel, M. B. (2009). The clinical course of advanced dementia. *New England Journal of Medicine, 361*, 1529–1538. https://doi.org/10.1056/NEJMoa0902234

Mitnick, D. M., Heyman, R. E., & Smith Slep, A. M. (2009). Changes in relationship satisfaction across the transition to parenthood: A meta-analysis. *Journal of Family Psychology, 23*(6), 848–852. https://doi.org/10.1037/a0017004

Mitty, E. (2009). Nursing care of the aging foot. *Geriatric Nursing, 30*(5), 350–354. https://doi.org/10.1016/j.gerinurse.2009.08.004

Miyake, A., Friedman, N. P., Emerson, M. J., Witzki, A. H., Howerter, A., & Wager, T. D. (2000). The unity and diversity of executive functions and their contributions to complex "frontal lobe" tasks: A latent variable analysis. *Cognitive Psychology, 41*(1), 49–100. https://doi.org/10.1006/cogp.1999.0734

Moen, P., Kim, J. E., & Hofmeister, H. (2001). Couples' work/retirement transitions, gender, and marital quality. *Social Psychology Quarterly, 64*(1), 55–71.

Moffitt, R. A., & Ribar, D. C. (2016). *Child age and gender differences in food security in a low-income inner-city population.* National Bureau of Economic Research.

Moilanen, K. L., Shaw, D. S., & Maxwell, K. L. (2010). Developmental cascades: Externalizing, internalizing, and academic competence from middle childhood to early adolescence. *Development and Psychopathology, 22*(3), 635–653.

Molinuevo, B., Bonillo, A., Pardo, Y., Doval, E., & Torrubia, R. (2010). Participation in extracurricular activities and emotional and behavioral adjustment in middle childhood in Spanish Boys and Girls. *Journal of Community Psychology, 38*(7), 842–857. https://doi.org/10.1002/jcop.20399

Moon, C., Lagercrantz, H., & Kuhl, P. K. (2013). Language experienced in utero affects vowel perception after birth: A two-country study. *Acta Paediatrica, 102*(2), 156–160. https://doi.org/10.1111/apa.12098

Moore, E. R., Anderson, G. C., & Bergman, N. (2007). Early skin-to-skin contact for mothers and their healthy newborn infants. *Cochrane Database of Systematic Reviews*, CD003519. https://doi.org/10.1002/14651858.CD003519.pub2

Moore, K. A., & Kahn, J. (2008). *Family and neighborhood risks: How they relate to involvement in out-of-school time activities.* https://www.childtrends.org/wp-content/uploads/2013/01/Family-NeighborhoodRisks.pdf

Moorman, S. M., Booth, A., & Fingerman, K. L. (2006). Women's romantic relationships after widowhood. *Journal of Family Issues, 27*(9), 1281–1304.

Morelli, G. A., & Tronick, E. Z. (1992). Efe fathers: One among many? A comparison of forager children's involvement with fathers and other males. *Social Development, 1*(1), 36–54.

Moro-Garcia, M. A., Fernandez-Garcia, B., Echeverria, A., Rodriguez-Alonso, M., Suarez-Garcia, F. M., Solano-Jaurrieta, J. J., López-Larrea, C., & Alonso-Arias, R. (2014). Frequent participation in high volume exercise throughout life is associated with a more differentiated adaptive immune response. *Brain Behavior and Immunity, 39*, 61–74. https://doi.org/10.1016/j.bbi.2013.12.014

Motta, M., Bennati, E., Ferlito, L., Malaguarnera, M., & Motta, L. (2005). Successful aging in centenarians: Myths and reality. *Archives of Gerontology and Geriatrics, 40*(3), 241–251.

Mozurkewich, E. L., Chilimigras, J. L., Berman, D. R., Perni, U. C., Romero, V. C., King, V. J., & Keeton, K. L. (2011). Methods of induction of labour: A systematic review. *BMC Pregnancy Childbirth, 11*(84). https://doi.org/10.1186/1471-2393-11-84

Mroczek, D. K., & Kolarz, C. M. (1998). The effect of age on positive and negative affect: A developmental perspective on happiness. *Journal of Personality and Social Psychology, 75*(5), 1333–1349.

Muchinsky, P. (1999). Application of Holland's theory in industrial and organizational settings. *Journal of Vocational Behavior, 55*(1), 127–125.

Mueller, M. M., Wilhelm, B., & Elder, G. H., Jr. (2002). Variations in grandparenting. *Research on Aging, 24*(3), 360–388.

Munakata, Y., Herd, S. A., Chatham, C. H., Depue, B. E., Banich, M. T., & O'Reilly, R. C. (2011). A unified framework for inhibitory control. *Trends in Cognitive Sciences, 15*(10), 453–459.

Mundy, P., & Neal, A. R. (2001). Neural plasticity, joint attention, and a transactional social-orienting model of autism. In L. M. Glidden (Ed.), *International review of research in mental retardation: Vol. 23. Autism* (pp. 139–168). Academic Press.

Muratore, A. M., & Earl, J. K. (2015). Improving retirement outcomes: The role of resources, pre-retirement planning and transition characteristics. *Ageing & Society, 35*(10), 2100–2140. https://doi.org/10.1017/s0144686x14000841

Murphy, D. R., Daneman, M., & Schneider, B. A. (2006). Why do older adults have difficulty following conversations? *Psychology and Aging, 21*(1), 49–61.

Murphy, N. A., & Isaacowitz, D. M. (2008). Preferences for emotional information in older and younger adults: A meta-analysis of memory and attention tasks. *Psychology and Aging, 23*(2), 263–286.

Murray, A. (2012). The relationship of parenting style to academic achievement in middle childhood. *Irish Journal of Psychology, 33*(4), 137–152. https://doi.org/10.1080/03033910.2012.724645

Murray, G. K., Jones, P. B., Kuh, D., & Richards, M. (2007). Infant developmental milestones and subsequent cognitive function. *Annals of Neurology, 62*(2), 128–136. https://doi.org/10.1002/ana.21120

Musil, C., Warner, C., Zauszniewski, J., Wykle, M., & Standing, T. (2009). Grandmother caregiving, family stress and strain, and depressive symptoms. *Western Journal of Nursing Research, 31*(3), 389–408.

Muuss, R. E. (1988). *Theories of adolescence*. Crown.

# N

National Alliance on Mental Illness. (2016). *Mental Health Facts: Children and teens*. https://www.nami.org/NAMI/media/NAMI-Media/Infographics/Children-MH-Facts-NAMI.pdf

National Association for Sport and Physical Education. (2002). *Active start: A statement of physical activity guidelines for children birth to five years*. NASPE Publications.

National Cancer Institute. (2020). *Cancer statistics*. https://www.cancer.gov/about-cancer/understanding/statistics

National Center for Health Statistics. (2010). *Marriage and cohabitation in the United States: A statistical portrait based on Cycle 6 (2002) of the National Survey of Family Growth* [Series 23, no. 28]. Vital and Health Statistics.

National Health Service. (2017). *Hormone replacement therapy (HRT)*. Author.

National Institute of Aging. (2009). *Caring for a person with Alzheimer's disease*. http://www.nia.nih.gov/NR/rdonlyres/6A0E9F3C-E429-4F03-818E-D1B60235D5F8/0/100711_LoRes2.pdf

National Institute of Dental and Craniofacial Research. (2019). *Older adults and oral health*. https://www.nidcr.nih.gov/OralHealth/OralHealthInformation/OlderAdults/

National Institute of Health. (2013). *Newborn hearing screening*. http://report.nih.gov/nihfactsheets/ViewFactSheet.aspx?csid=104

National Library of Medicine. (2010). *Melatonin*. http://www.nlm.nih.gov/medlineplus/druginfo/natural/patient-melatonin.html

Negash, S., Smith, G. E., Pankratz, S., Aakre, J., Geda, Y. E., Roberts, R. O., Knopman, D. S., Boeve, B. F., Ivnik, R. J., & Petersen, R. C. (2011). Successful aging: Definitions and prediction of longevity and conversion to mild cognitive impairment. *American Journal of Geriatric Psychiatry, 19*(6), 581–588. https://doi.org/10.1097/JGP.0b013e3181f17ec9

Neikrug, A. B., & Ancoli-Israel, S. (2009). Sleep disorders in the older adult: A mini-review. *Gerontology, 56*(2), 121–122. https://doi.org/10.1159/000236900

Neilson, J. P. (2008). Cochrane update: Effect of timing of umbilical cord clamping at birth of term infants on mother and baby outcomes. *Obstetrics & Gynecology, 112*(1), 177–178. https://doi.org/10.1097/AOG.0b013e31817f2169

Nelson, E. A., & Dannefer, D. (1992). Aged heterogeneity: Fact or fiction? The fate of diversity in gerontological research. *Gerontologist, 32*(1), 17–23.

Ness, A., Goldberg, J., & Berghella, V. (2005). Abnormalities of the first and second stages of labor. *Obstetrics and Gynecology Clinics of North America, 32*(2), 201–220. https://doi.org/10.1016/j.ogc.2005.01.007

Neugarten, B. L., & Weinstein, K. K. (1964). The changing American grandparent. *Journal of Marriage and the Family, 26*(2), 199–204.

Newborn Screening Authoring Committee. (2008). Newborn screening expands: Recommendations for pediatricians and medical homes—implications for the system. *Pediatrics, 121*(1), 192–217. https://doi.org/10.1542/peds.2007-3021

Ng, T. W. H., & Feldman, D. C. (2010). The relationships of age with job attitudes: A meta-analysis. *Personnel Psychology, 63*(3), 677–718. https://doi.org/10.1111/j.1744-6570.2010.01184.x

Ng, T. W. H., & Feldman, D. C. (2012). Evaluating six common stereotypes about older workers with meta-analytical data. *Personnel Psychology, 65*(4), 821–858. https://doi.org/10.1111/peps.12003

Nikitin, N. P., Loh, P. H., de Silva, R., Witte, K. K., Lukaschuk, E. I., Parker, A., Farnsworth, T. A., Alamgir, F. M., Clark, A. L., & Cleland, J. G. (2006). Left ventricular morphology, global and longitudinal function in normal older individuals: A cardiac magnetic resonance study. *International Journal of Cardiology, 108*(1), 76–83.

Niven, C., & Gijsbers, K. (1984). Obstetric and non-obstetric factors related to labour pain. *Journal of Reproductive and Infant Psychology, 2*(2), 61–78. https://doi.org/10.1080/02646838408403451

Noel, A., Stark, P., Redford, J., & Zukerberg, A. (2013). *Parent and family involvement in education, from the National Household Education Surveys Program of 2012.* National Center for Education Statistics.

Noll, J. G., Shenk, C. E., Barnes, J. E., & Putnam, F. W. (2009). Childhood abuse, avatar choices, and other risk factors associated with Internet-initiated victimization of adolescent girls. *Pediatrics, 123*(6), e1078–e1083.

Noone, J. H., Stephens, C., & Alpass, F. M. (2009). Preretirement planning and well-being in later life: A prospective study. *Research on Aging, 31*(1), 295–317.

Nordmann, A. J., Suter-Zimmermann, K., Bucher, H. C., Shai, I., Tuttle, K. R., Estruch, R., & Briel, M. (2011). Meta-Analysis comparing Mediterranean to low-fat diets for modification of cardiovascular risk factors. *American Journal of Medicine, 124*, 841–851.

Norsker, F. N., Espenhain, L., á Rogvi, S., Morgen, C. S., Andersen, P. K., & Andersen, A.-M. N. (2012). Socioeconomic position and the risk of spontaneous abortion: A study within the Danish National Birth Cohort. *BMJ Open, 2.* https://doi.org/10.1136/ bmjopen-2012-001077

Novin, S., Banerjee, R., Dadkhah, A., & Rieffe, C. (2009). Self-reported use of emotional display rules in the Netherlands and Iran: Evidence for sociocultural influence. *Social Development, 18*(2), 397–411. https://doi.org/10.1111/j.1467-9507.2008.00485.x

Novin, S., Rieffe, C., Banerjee, R., Miers, A. C., & Cheung, J. (2011). Anger response styles in Chinese and Dutch children: A socio-cultural perspective on anger regulation. *British Journal of Developmental Psychology, 29*(4), 806–822. https://doi.org/10.1348/2044-835x.002010

Nuru-Jeter, A. M., Sarsour, K., Jutte, D. P., & Thomas Boyce, W. (2010). Socioeconomic predictors of health and development in middle childhood: Variations by socioeconomic status measure and race. *Issues in Comprehensive Pediatric Nursing, 33*(2), 59–81. https://doi.org/10.3109/01460861003663953

# O


O'Connor, K. (2012). Auditory processing in autism spectrum disorder: A review. *Neuroscience & Biobehavioral Reviews, 36*(2), 836–854. https://doi.org/10.1016/j.neubiorev.2011.11.008

O'Donovan, D., Hausken, T., Lei, Y., Russo, A., Keogh, J., Horowitz, M., & Jones, K. L. (2005). Effect of aging on transpyloric flow, gastric emptying, and intragastric distribution in healthy humans—impact on glycemia. *Digestive Diseases and Sciences, 50*(4), 671–676.

O'Flaherty, M., Bandosz, P., Critchley, J., Capewell, S., Guzman-Castillo, M., Aspelund, T., Bennett, K., Kabir, K., Björk, L., Bruthans, J., Hotchkiss, J. W., Hughes, J., Laatikainen, T., Palmieri, L., Zdrojewski, T., & Zdrojewski, T. (2016). Exploring potential mortality reductions in 9 European countries by improving diet and lifestyle: A modelling approach. *International Journal of Cardiology, 207*, 286–291. https://doi.org/10.1016/j.ijcard.2016.01.147

O'Hara, M. W., & Segre, L. S. (2008). Psychological disorders of pregnancy and the postpartum. In D. N. Danforth & R. S. Gibbs (Eds.), *Danforth's obstetrics and gynecology.* Wolters Kluwer Health.

O'Keeffe, G. S., & Clarke-Pearson, K. (2011). The impact of social media on children, adolescents, and families. *Pediatrics, 127*(4), 800–804.

Odle-Dusseau, H. N., Britt, T. W., & Greene-Shortridge, T. M. (2012). Organizational work–family resources as predictors of job performance and attitudes: The process of work–family conflict and enrichment. *Journal of Occupational Health Psychology, 17*(1), 28–40. https://doi.org/10.1037/a0026428

Oken, B. S., Zajdel, D., Kishiyama, S., Flegal, K., Dehen, C., Haas, M., Kraemer, D. F., Lawrence, J., & Leyva, J. (2006). Randomized, controlled, six-month trial of yoga in healthy seniors: Effects on cognition and quality of life. *Alternative Therapies in Health and Medicine, 12*(1), 40–47.

Olsson, G., Hemstrom, O., & Fritzell, J. (2009). Identifying factors associated with good health and ill health: Not just opposite sides of the same coin. *International Journal of Behavioral Medicine, 16*(4), 323–330. https://doi.org/10.1007/s12529-009-9033-9

Ong, A. D., Bergeman, C. S., Bisconti, T. L., & Wallace, K. A. (2006). Psychological resilience, positive emotions, and successful adaptation to stress in later life. *Journal of Personality and Social Psychology, 91*(4), 730–749.

Orel, N. A., & Fruhauf, C. A. (2015). *The lives of LGBT older adults: Understanding challenges and resilience.* American Psychological Association.

Otsuki, T., Maeda, S., Kesen, Y., Yokoyama, N., Tanabe, T., Sugawara, J., Miyauchi, T., Kuno, S., Ajisaka, R., & Matsuda, M. (2006). Age-related reduction of systemic arterial compliance induces excessive myocardial oxygen consumption during sub-maximal exercise. *Hypertension Research, 29*, 65–73.

Ouwehand, C., de Ridder, D. T. D., & Bensing, J. M. (2007). A review of successful aging models: Proposing proactive coping as an important additional strategy. *Clinical Psychology Review, 27*(8), 873–884. https://doi.org/10.1016/j.cpr.2006.11.003

Owens, P. L., Thompson, J., Elixhauser, A., & Ryan, K. (2003). *Care of children and adolescents in U.S. hospitals.* Agency for Healthcare and Research Quality.

Owings, M., Uddin, S., & Williams, S. (2013). Trends in circumcision for male newborns in US hospitals. https://www.cdc.gov/nchs/data/hestat/circumcision_2013/circumcision_2013.pdf


# P


Pagani, L. S., Fitzpatrick, C., Barnett, T. A., & Dubow, E. (2010). Prospective associations between early childhood television exposure and academic, psychosocial, and physical well-being by middle childhood. *Archives of Pediatrics & Adolescent Medicine, 164*(5), 425–431. https://doi.org/10.1001/archpediatrics.2010.50

Pagani, L. S., Japel, C., Vaillancourt, T., & Tremblay, R. E. (2010). Links between middle-childhood trajectories of family dysfunction and indirect aggression. *Journal of Interpersonal Violence, 25*(12), 2175–2198. https://doi.org/10.1177/0886260509354886

Palmer, K. (2009, June 28). The new parenttrap: More boomers help adult kids out financially. *U.S. News & World Report.*

Panegyres, P., Berry, R., & Burchell, J. (2016). Early dementia screening. *Diagnostics, 6*(1), 6.

Parker, K., & Patten, E. (2013). *The sandwich generation rising financial burdens for middle-aged Americans.* http://www.pewsocialtrends.org/2013/01/30/the-sandwich-generation

Parker, L., & Anderson, G. C. (2002). Kangaroo care for adoptive parents and their critically ill preterm infant. *MCN American Journal of Maternal Child Nursing, 27*(3), 230–232.

Parslow, R. A., Lewis, V. J., & Nay, R. (2011). Successful aging: Development and testing of a multidimensional model using data from a large sample of older Australians. *Journal of the American Geriatrics Society, 59*(11), 2077–2083. https://doi.org/10.1111/j.1532-5415.2011.03665.x

Paterson, S. J., Heim, S., Thomas Friedman, J., Choudhury, N., & Benasich, A. A. (2006). Development of structure and function in the infant brain: Implications for cognition, language and social behaviour. *Neuroscience & Biobehavioral Reviews, 30*(8), 1087–1105. https://doi.org/10.1016/j.neubiorev.2006.05.001

Paul, K. I., & Moser, K. (2016). Unemployment impairs mental health: Meta-analyses. In G. J. Boyle, J. G. O'Gorman, & G. J. Fogarty (Eds.), *Work and organisational psychology: Research methodology; assessment and selection; organisational change and development; human resource and performance management; emerging trends: Innovation/globalisation/technology* (pp. 285–319). SAGE

Paulson, J. F., & Bazemore, S. D. (2010). Prenatal and postpartum depression in fathers and its association with maternal depression: A meta-analysis. *JAMA, 303*(19), 1961–1969. https://doi.org/10.1001/jama.2010.605

Pegula, S., Marsh, S. M., & Jackson, L. L. (2007). Fatal occupational injuries—United States, 2005. *Morbidity and Mortality Weekly Report, 56*(13), 297–301.

Pelaez, M. (2009). Joint attention and social referencing in infancy as precursors of derived relational responding. *Derived relational responding: Applications for learners with autism and other developmental disabilities*, 63–78.

Penedo, F. J., Brintz, C. E., Llabre, M. M., Arguelles, W., Isasi, C. R., Arredondo, E. M., Navas-Nacher, E. L., Perreira, K. M., Gonzáles, H. M., Rodriguez, C. J., Daviglus, M., Schneiderman, N., & Gallo, L. C. (2015). Family environment and the metabolic syndrome: Results from the Hispanic Community Health Study/Study of Latinos (HCHS/SOL) Sociocultural Ancillary Study (SCAS). *Annals of Behavioral Medicine, 49*(6), 793–801. https://doi.org/10.1007/s12160-015-9713-4

Peplau, L. A., & Fingerhut, A. W. (2007). The close relationships of lesbians and gay men. *Annual Review of Psychology, 58*, 405–424.

Pesonen, A. K., Raikkonen, K., Heinonen, K., Andersson, S., Hovi, P., Järvenpää, A. L., Eriksson, J. G., & Kajantie, E. (2008). Personality of young adults born prematurely: The Helsinki study of very low birth weight adults. *Journal of Child Psychology and Psychiatry, 49*(6), 609–617. https://doi.org/10.1111/j.1469-7610.2007.01874.x

Pesonen, A. K., Raikkonen, K., Kajantie, E., Heinonen, K., Strandberg, T. E., & Jarvenpaa, A. L. (2006). Fetal programming of temperamental negative affectivity among children born healthy at term. *Developmental Psychobiology, 48*(8), 633–643. https://doi.org/10.1002/dev.20153

Peterson, B. E. (2006). Generativity and successful parenting: An analysis of young adult outcomes. *Journal of Personality, 74*(3), 847–869. https://doi.org/10.1111/j.1467-6494.2006.00394.x

Peterson, C., & Whalen, N. (2001). Five years later: Children's memory for medical emergencies. *Applied Cognitive Psychology, 15*(7), S7–S24. https://doi.org/10.1002/acp.832

Petrofsky, J. S., McLellan, K., Bains, G. S., Prowse, M., Ethiraju, G., Lee, S., Guhman, S., Lohman, E., III, & Schwab, E. (2009). The influence of ageing on the ability of the skin to dissipate heat. *Medical Science Monitor, 15*(6), CR261–268.

Pettit, G. S., Laird, R. D., Dodge, K. A., Bates, J. E., & Criss, M. M. (2001). Antecedents and behavior-problem outcomes of parental monitoring and psychological control in early adolescence. *Child Development, 72*(2), 583–598.

Pew Research Center. (2009, June 29). *Growing old in America: Expectations vs. reality.* http://pewresearch.org/pubs/1269/aging-survey-expectations-versus-reality

Pfirrmann, C. W., Metzdorf, A., Elfering, A., Hodler, J., & Boos, N. (2006). Effect of aging and degeneration on disc volume and shape: A quantitative study in asymptomatic volunteers. *Journal of Orthopedics Research, 24*(5), 1086–1094.

Piaget, J. (1962). *Play, dreams and imitation*, Vol. 24 Norton.

Picchioni, M. M., & Murray, R. M. (2007). Schizophrenia. *BMJ: British Medical Journal, 14*, 91–95.

Pienta, A. M. (2003). Partners in marriage: An analysis of husbands' and wives' retirement behavior. *Journal of Applied Gerontology, 22*(3), 340–358. https://doi.org/10.1177/0733464803253587

Pierce, K., Bolt, D., & Vandell, D. (2010). Specific features of after-school program quality: Associations with children's functioning in middle childhood. *American Journal of Community Psychology, 45*, 381–393. https://doi.org/10.1007/s10464-010-9304-2

Pierret, C. R. (2006). Sandwich generation: Women caring for parents and children. *Monthly Laboratory Review, 129.*

Pietschmann, P., Rauner, M., Sipos, W., & Kerschan-Schindl, K. (2009). Osteoporosis: An age-related and gender-specific disease—A mini-review. *Gerontology, 55*(1), 3–12. https://doi.org/10.1159/000166209

Pinker, S. (1994). *The language instinct: The new science of language and mind*, Vol. 7529 Penguin.

Plantin, L., Olukoya, A. A., & Ny, P. (2011). Positive health outcomes of father involvement in pregnancy and childbirth paternal support: A scope study literature review. *Fathering, 9*(1), 87–102.

Plaut, V. C., Markus, H. R., & Lachman, M. E. (2003). Place matters: Consensual features and regional variation in American well-being and self. *Journal of Personality & Social Psychology, 83*(1), 160–184.

Pluess, M., & Belsky, J. (2010). Differential susceptibility to parenting and quality child care. *Developmental Psychology, 46*(2), 379–390. https://doi.org/10.1037/a0015203

Podulka, J., Stranges, E., & Steiner, C. (2011). *Hospitalizations related to childbirth, 2008* [Statistical brief no. 110]. Agency for Healthcare and Research Quality.

Pollet, T. V., Nelissen, M., & Nettle, D. (2009). Lineage based differences in grandparental investment: Evidence from a large British cohort study. *Journal of Biosocial Science, 41*(3), 355–379.

Pongchaiyakul, C., Nguyen, T. V., Kosulwat, V., Rojroongwasinkul, N., Charoenkiatkul, S., & Rajatanavin, R. (2005). Effect of urbanization on bone mineral density: A Thai epidemiological study. *BMC Musculoskeletal Disorders, 6*(1), 5.

Porrett, L., Barkla, S., Knights, J., de Costa, C., & Harmen, S. (2013). An exploration of the perceptions of male partners involved in the birthing experience at a regional Australian hospital. *Journal of Midwifery and Women's Health, 58*(1), 92–97. https://doi.org/10.1111/j.1542-2011.2012.00238.x

Porter, J. S., Stern, M., Mazzeo, S. E., Evans, R. K., & Laver, J. (2013). Relations among teasing, body satisfaction, self-esteem, and depression in treatment-seeking obese African American adolescents. *Journal of Black Psychology, 39*(4), 375–395. https://doi.org/10.1177/0095798412454680

Prediger, D. J., & Vansickle, T. R. (1992). Locating occupations on Holland's hexagon: Beyond RIASEC. *Journal of Vocational Behavior, 40*(2), 111–128. https://doi.org/10.1016/0001-8791(92)90060-d

Previti, D., & Amato, P. R. (2004). Is infidelity a cause or a consequence of poor marital quality? *Journal of Social and Personal Relationships, 21*(2), 217–230.

Priem, J. S., Solomon, D. H., & Steuber, K. R. (2009). Accuracy and bias in perceptions of emotionally supportive communication in marriage. *Personal Relationships, 16*(4), 531–551.

Pruchno, R. A., & McKenney, D. (2002). Psychological well-being of Black and White grandmothers raising grandchildren: Examination of a two-factor model. *Journals of Gerontology Series B: Psychological Sciences and Social Sciences, 57*(5), P444–P452.

Pulkki-Raback, L., Elovainio, M., Kivimaki, M., Raitakari, O. T., & Keltikangas-Jarvinen, L. (2005). Temperament in childhood predicts body mass in adulthood: The Cardiovascular Risk in Young Finns Study. *Health Psychology, 24*(3), 307–315.

# Q

Querleu, D., Renard, X., Versyp, F., Paris-Delrue, L., & Crèpin, G. (1988). Fetal hearing. *European Journal of Obstetrics & Gynecology and Reproductive Biology, 28*, 191–212. https://doi.org/10.1016/0028-2243(88)90030-5

# R

Rachon, D. (2015). Endocrine disrupting chemicals (EDCs) and female cancer: Informing the patients. *Reviews in Endocrine and Metabolic Disorders, 16*, 359–364. https://doi.org/10.1007/s11154-016-9332-9

Raj, I. S., Bird, S. R., & Shield, A. J. (2010). Aging and the force-velocity relationship of muscles. *Experimental Gerontology, 45*(2), 81–90. https://doi.org/10.1016/j.exger.2009.10.013

Rawson, N. E. (2006). Olfactory loss in aging. *Science of Aging Knowledge Environment, 2006*(5), pe6.

Reeves, N. D., Narici, M. V., & Maganaris, C. N. (2006). Myotendinous plasticity to ageing and resistance exercise in humans. *Experimental Physiology, 91*(3), 483–498.

Reichstadt, J., Depp, C. A., Palinkas, L. A., Folsom, D. P., & Jeste, D. V. (2007). Building blocks of successful aging: A focus group study of older adults' perceived contributors to successful aging. *American Journal of Geriatric Psychiatry, 15*(3), 194–201.

Reitzes, D. C., & Mutran, E. J. (2004). Grandparent identity, intergenerational family identity, and well-being. *Journals of Gerontology Series B: Psychological Sciences and Social Sciences, 59B*(4), S213–S219.

Resnick, B., Shaughnessy, M., Galik, E., Scheve, A., Fitten, R., Morrison, T., Michael, K., & Agness, C. (2009). Pilot testing of the PRAISEDD intervention among African American and low-income older adults. *Journal of Cardiovascular Nursing, 24*(5), 352–361. https://doi.org/10.1097/JCN.0b013e3181ac0301

Rhoades, G. K., Stanley, S. M., & Markman, H. J. (2009). The pre-engagement cohabitation effect: A replication and extension of previous findings. *Journal of Family Psychology, 23*(1), 107–111.

Rick, S. I., Small, D. A., & Finkel, E. J. (2011). Fatal (fiscal) attraction: Spendthrifts and tightwads in marriage. *Journal of Marketing Research, 48*(2), 228–237. https://doi.org/10.1509/jmkr.48.2.228

Ridgway, C. L., Ong, K. K., Tammelin, T., Sharp, S. J., Ekelund, U., & Jarvelin, M. R. (2009). Birth size, infant weight gain, and motor development influence adult physical performance. *Medicine and Science in Sports and Exercise, 41*(6), 1212–1221. https://doi.org/10.1249/MSS.0b013e31819794ab

Riordan, C. M., Griffith, R. W., & Weatherly, E. W. (2003). Age and work-related outcomes: The moderating effects of status characteristics. *Journal of Applied Social Psychology, 33*, 37–57.

Ritchie, R. A., Meca, A., Madrazo, V. L., Schwartz, S. J., Hardy, S. A., Zamboanga, B. L., Weisskurch, R. C., Kim, S. Y., Whitbourne, S. K., Ham, L. S., & Lee, R. M. (2013). Identity dimensions and related processes in emerging adulthood: Helpful or harmful? *Journal of Clinical Psychology, 69*(4), 415–432.

Roberson, E. D., & Mucke, L. (2006). 100 years and counting: Prospects for defeating Alzheimer's disease. *Science, 314*(5800), 781–784.

Roberts, B. W., & DelVecchio, W. F. (2000). The rank-order consistency of personality traits from childhood to old age: A quantitative review of longitudinal studies. *Psychological Bulletin, 126*(1), 3–25.

Roberts, B. W., Donnellan, M. B., & Hill, P. L. (2013). Personality trait development in adulthood. In H. Tennen, J. Suls, & I. B. Weiner (Eds.), *Handbook of Psychology: Vol. 5. Personality and social psychology* (2nd ed.) (pp. 183–196). Wiley.

Robins, R. W., Trzesniewski, K. H., Tracy, J. L., Gosling, S. D., & Potter, J. (2002). Global self-esteem across the lifespan. *Psychology and Aging, 17*(3), 423–434.

Rodella, L. F., Bonazza, V., Labanca, M., Lonati, C., & Rezzani, R. (2014). A review of the effects of dietary silicon intake on bone homeostasis and regeneration. *Journal of Nutrition Health and Aging, 18*(9), 820–826. https://doi.org/10.1007/s12603-014-0484-6

Roig, M., Macintyre, D. L., Eng, J. J., Narici, M. V., Maganaris, C. N., & Reid, W. D. (2010). Preservation of eccentric strength in older adults: Evidence, mechanisms and implications for training and rehabilitation. *Experimental Gerontology, 45*(6), 400–409. https://doi.org/10.1016/j.exger.2010.03.008

Romeo, R. D. (2003). Puberty: A period of both organizational and activational effects of steroid hormones on neurobehavioural development. *Journal of Neuroendocrinology, 15*(12), 1185–1192.

Rottinghaus, P. J., Coon, K. L., Gaffey, A. R., & Zytowski, D. G. (2007). Thirty-year stability and predictive validity of vocational interests. *Journal of Career Assessment, 15*(1), 5–22.

Rovee-Collier, C., & Cuevas, K. (2009). Multiple memory systems are unnecessary to account for infant memory development: An ecological model. *Developmental Psychology, 45*(1), 160–174. https://doi.org/10.1037/a0014538

Rowe, J. W., & Kahn, R. L. (1998). *Successful aging: The MacArthur foundation study*. Pantheon.

Rubin, D. C., Rahhal, T. A., & Poon, L. W. (1998). Things learned in early adulthood are remembered best. *Memory and Cognition, 26*(1), 3–19.

Ruitenberg, M. F., Abrahamse, E. L., & Verwey, W. B. (2013). Sequential motor skill in preadolescent children: The development of automaticity. *Journal of Experimental Child Psychology, 115*(4), 607–623.

Rupp, D. E., Vodanovich, S. J., & Crede, M. (2006). Age bias in the workplace: The impact of ageism and causal attributions. *Journal of Applied Social Psychology, 36*, 1337–1364.

Rusnáková, Š., & Rektor, I. (2012). The neurocognitive networks of the executive functions. *Advances in Clinical Neurophysiology*, 161.

Ryder, K. M., Shorr, R. I., Bush, A. J., Kritchevsky, S. B., Harris, T., Stone, K., Caluey, J., & Tylavsky, F. A. (2005). Magnesium intake from food and supplements is associated with bone mineral density in healthy older white subjects. *Journal of the American Geriatrics Society, 53*(11), 1875–1180.

# S


Saarento, S., Kärnä, A., Hodges, E. V., & Salmivalli, C. (2013). Student-, classroom-, and school-level risk factors for victimization. *Journal of School Psychology, 51*(3), 421–434.

Sadeh, A., Tikotzky, L., & Scher, A. (2010). Parenting and infant sleep. *Sleep Medicine Reviews, 14*(2), 89–96. https://doi.org/10.1016/j.smrv.2009.05.003

Safdar, S., Friedlmeier, W., Matsumoto, D., Yoo, S. H., Kwantes, C. T., Kakai, H., & Shigemasu, E. (2009). Variations of emotional display rules within and across cultures: A comparison between Canada, USA, and Japan. *Canadian Journal of Behavioural Science, 41*(1), 1–10.

Sahni, S., Hannan, M. T., Blumberg, J., Cupples, L. A., Kiel, D. P., & Tucker, K. L. (2009). Inverse association of carotenoid intakes with 4-y change in bone mineral density in elderly men and women: The Framingham Osteoporosis Study. *American Journal of Clinical Nutrition, 89*(1), 416–424. https://doi.org/10.3945/ajcn.2008.26388

Saito, M., & Marumo, K. (2009). Collagen cross-links as a determinant of bone quality: A possible explanation for bone fragility in aging, osteoporosis, and diabetes mellitus. *Osteoporos International, 21,* 195–214. https://doi.org/10.1007/s00198-009-1066-z

Salari, S. M., & Rich, M. (2001). Social and environmental infantilization of aged persons: Observations in two adult day care centers. *International Journal of Aging and Human Development, 52*(2), 115–134.

Sales, J. M., Fivush, R., & Peterson, C. (2003). Parental reminiscing about positive and negative events. *Journal of Cognition and Development, 4*(2), 185–209.

Salloway, S. (2008). Taking the next steps in the treatment of Alzheimer's disease: Disease-modifying agents. *CNS Spectrum, 13*(3), 11–14.

Salthouse, T. (2012). Consequences of age-related cognitive declines. *Annual Review of Psychology, 63*(1), 201–226. https://doi.org/10.1146/annurev-psych-120710-100328

Saltzman, W., & Ziegler, T. E. (2014). Functional significance of hormonal changes in mammalian fathers. *Journal of Neuroendocrinology, 26*(10), 685–696. https://doi.org/10.1111/jne.12176

Samanez-Larkin, G. R., Robertson, E. R., Mikels, J. A., Carstensen, L. L., & Gotlib, I. H. (2009). Selective attention to emotion in the aging brain. *Psychology and Aging, 24*(3), 519–529. https://doi.org/10.1037/a0016952

Sameroff, A. J., & MacKenzie, M. J. (2003). Research strategies for capturing transactional models of development: The limits of the possible. *Development and Psychopathology, 15*(3), 613–640.

Sanchis-Gomar, F., Pareja-Galeano, H., Mayero, S., Perez-Quilis, C., & Lucia, A. (2014). New molecular targets and lifestyle interventions to delay aging sarcopenia. *Frontiers in Aging and Neuroscience, 6,* 156. https://doi.org/10.3389/fnagi.2014.00156

Santrock, J. (2015). *A topical approach to lifespan development.* McGraw-Hill.

Satizabal, C. L., Beiser, A. S., Chouraki, V., Chêne, G., Dufouil, C., & Seshadri, S. (2016). Incidence of dementia over three decades in the Framingham heart study. *New England Journal of Medicine, 374*(6), 523–532. https://doi.org/10.1056/NEJMoa1504327

Sbarra, D. A., & Emery, R. E. (2008). Deeper into divorce: Using actor-partner analyses to explore systemic differences in coparenting conflict following custody dispute resolution. *Journal of Family Psychology, 22*(1), 144–152. https://doi.org/10.1037/0893-3200.22.1.144

Scharte, M., & Bolte, G. (2013). Increased health risks of children with single mothers: The impact of socio-economic and environmental factors. *European Journal of Public Health, 23*(3), 469–475.

Schiffman, S. S. (2009). Effects of aging on the human taste system. *Annals of the New York Academy of Science, 1170*(1), 725–729. https://doi.org/10.1111/j.1749-6632.2009.03924.x

Schmid, B., Blomeyer, D., Buchmann, A. F., Trautmann-Villalba, P., Zimmermann, U. S., Schmidt, M. H., Esser, G., Banaschewski, T., & Laucht, M. (2011). Quality of early mother-child interaction associated with depressive psychopathology in the offspring: A prospective study from infancy to adulthood. *Journal of Psychiatric Research, 4(10)5,* 1387–1394. https://doi.org/10.1016/j.jpsychires.2011.05.010

Schoenborn, C. A., & Heyman, K. M. (2009). Health characteristics of adults aged 55 years and over: United States 2004–2007. *National Health Statistics Reports,* no. 16. National Center for Health Statistics.

Schoenfeld, E. A., Bredow, C. A., & Huston, T. L. (2012). Do men and women show love differently in marriage? *Personality and Social Psychology Bulletin, 38*(11), 1396–1409. https://doi.org/10.1177/0146167212450739

Schoenhofen, E. A., Wyszynski, D. F., Andersen, S., Pennington, J., Young, R., Terry, D. F., & Perls, T. T. (2006). Characteristics of 32 supercentenarians. *Journal of the American Geriatrics Society, 54*(8), 1237–1240.

Schonert-Reichl, K. A. (1994). Gender differences in depressive symptomatology and egocentrism in adolescence. *Journal of Early Adolescence, 14*(1), 49–65.

Schwartz, C., Chabanet, C., Laval, C., Issanchou, S., & Nicklaus, S. (2013). Breast-feeding duration: Influence on taste acceptance over the first year of life. *British Journal of Nutrition, 109*(6), 1154–1161. https://doi.org/10.1017/S0007114512002668

Schwartz, D., Lansford, J. E., Dodge, K. A., Pettit, G. S., & Bates, J. E. (2014). Peer victimization during middle childhood as a lead indicator of internalizing problems and diagnostic outcomes in late adolescence. *Journal of Clinical Child & Adolescent Psychology, 44*(3), 393–404.

Scollon, C. N., & Diener, E. (2006). Love, work, and changes in extraversion and neuroticism over time. *Journal of Personality and Social Psychology, 91*(6), 1152–1165.

Section on Breastfeeding. (2012). Breastfeeding and the use of human milk. *Pediatrics, 129*(3), e827–841. https://doi.org/10.1542/peds.2011-3552

Seeman, T. E., Singer, B. H., Rowe, J. W., Horwitz, R. I., & McEwen, B. S. (1997). Price of adaptation: Allostatic load and its health consequences: MacArthur studies of successful aging. *Archives of Internal Medicine, 157*(19), 2259–2268.

Segal, D. L., Needham, T. N., & Coolidge, F. L. (2009). Age differences in attachment orientations among younger and older adults: Evidence from two self-report measures of attachment. *International Journal of Aging and Human Development, 69*(2), 119–132.

Selvarajan, T. T., Cloninger, P. A., & Singh, B. (2013). Social support and work–family conflict: A test of an indirect effects model. *Journal of Vocational Behavior, 83*(3), 486–499. https://doi.org/10.1016/j.jvb.2013.07.004

Serste, T., & Bourgeois, N. (2006). Ageing and the liver. *Acta Gastro-enterologica Belgium, 69*, 296–298.

Shackelford, T. K., Schmitt, D. P., & Buss, D. M. (2005). Mate preferences of married persons in the newlywed year and three years later. *Cognition and Emotion, 19*(8), 1262–1270. https://doi.org/10.1080/02699930500215249

Sharma, K. K., & Santhoshkumar, P. (2009). Lens aging: Effects of crystallins. *Biochimica et Biophysica Acta, 1790*(1), 1095–1108. https://doi.org/10.1016/j.bbagen.2009.05.008

Sharma, M., Naik, V., & Deogaonkar, M. (2016). Emerging applications of deep brain stimulation. *Journal of Neurosurgical Science, 60*(2), 242–255.

Sheu, Y., Cauley, J. A., Wheeler, V. W., Patrick, A. L., Bunker, C. H., Kammerer, C. M., & Zmuda, J. M. (2009). Natural history and correlates of hip BMD loss with aging in men of African ancestry: The Tobago Bone Health Study. *Journal of Bone Mineral Research, 24*(7), 1290–1298. https://doi.org/10.1359/jbmr.090221

Shiah, Y.-J., Huang, Y., Chang, F., Chang, C.-F., & Yeh, L.-C. (2012). School-based extracurricular activities, personality, self-concept, and college career development skills in Chinese society. *Educational Psychology, 33*(2), 135–154. https://doi.org/10.1080/01443410.2012.747240

Shim, Y. S., Roe, C. M., Buckles, V. D., & Morris, J. C. (2013). Clinicopathologic study of Alzheimer's disease: Alzheimer mimics. *Journal of Alzheimer's Disease, 35*(4), 799–811. https://doi.org/10.3233/jad-121594

Shu, C. H., Hummel, T., Lee, P. L., Chiu, C. H., Lin, S. H., & Yuan, B. C. (2009). The proportion of self-rated olfactory dysfunction does not change across the lifespan. *American Journal of Rhinology and Allergy, 23*(4), 413–416. https://doi.org/10.2500/ajra.2009.23.3343

Shumway-Cook, A., Guralnik, J. M., Phillips, C. L., Coppin, A. K., Ciol, M. A., Bandinelli, S., & Ferrucci, L. (2007). Age-associated declines in complex walking task performance: The Walking InCHIANTI toolkit. *Journal of the American Geriatrics Society, 55*(1), 58–65.

Siebert, D. C., Mutran, E. J., & Reitzes, D. C. (2002). Friendship and social support: The importance of role identity to aging adults. *Social Work, 44*(6), 522–533.

Siegler, I. C., Costa, P. T., Brummett, B. H., Helms, M. J., Barefoot, J. C., Williams, R. B., Dahlstrom, G. W., Kaplan, H. B., Vitaliano, P. P., Nichaman, M. Z., Day, S. R., & Rimer, B. K. (2003). Patterns of change in hostility from college to midlife in the UNC Alumni Heart Study predict high-risk status. *Psychosomatic Medicine, 65*(5), 738–745.

Sigurdsson, G., Aspelund, T., Chang, M., Jonsdottir, B., Sigurdsson, S., Eiriksdottir, G., Gudmundsson, A., Harris, T. B., Gudnason, V., & Lang, T. F. (2006). Increasing sex difference in bone strength in old age: The Age, Gene/Environment Susceptibility-Reykjavik Study (AGES-REYKJAVIK). *Bone, 39*(3), 644–651.

Silverman, B. L., Rizzo, T. A., Cho, N. H., & Metzger, B. E. (1998). Long-term effects of the intrauterine environment. The Northwestern University Diabetes in Pregnancy Center. *Diabetes Care, 21*(2), B142–B149.

Silverman, J. M., Schmeidler, J., Beeri, M. S., Rosendorff, C., Sano, M., Grossman, H. T., Carrión-Baralt, J. R., Bespalova, I. N., West, R., & Haroutunian, V. (2012). C-reactive protein and familial risk for dementia: A phenotype for successful cognitive aging. *Neurology, 79*(11), 1116–1123. https://doi.org/10.1212/WNL.0b013e3182698c89

Silverstein, M., & Parker, M. G. (2002). Leisure activities and quality of life among the oldest old in Sweden. *Research on Aging, 24*(5), 528–547.

Sindi, S., Fiocco, A. J., Juster, R. P., Lord, C., Pruessner, J., & Lupien, S. J. (2014). Now you see it, now you don't: Testing environments modulate the association between hippocampal volume and cortisol levels in young and older adults. *Hippocampus, 24*(12), 1623–1632. https://doi.org/10.1002/hipo.22341

Siu, O.-l., Lu, J.-f., Brough, P., Lu, C.-q., Bakker, A. B., Kalliath, T., O'Driscoll, M., Phillips, D. R., Chen, W.-q., Lo, D., Sit, C., & Shi, K. (2010). Role resources and work–family enrichment: The role of work engagement. *Journal of Vocational Behavior, 77*(3), 470–480. https://doi.org/10.1016/j.jvb.2010.06.007

Skultety, K. M., & Whitbourne, S. K. (2004). Gender differences in identity processes and self-esteem in middle and later adulthood. *Journal of Women and Aging, 16*(1–2), 175–188.

Slining, M., Adair, L. S., Goldman, B. D., Borja, J. B., & Bentley, M. (2010). Infant overweight is associated with delayed motor development. *Journal of Pediatrics, 157*(1), 20–25. e21. https://doi.org/10.1016/j.jpeds.2009.12.054

Sluiter, J. K. (2006). High-demand jobs: Age-related diversity in work ability? *Applied Ergonomics, 37*(4), 429–440.

Smith, A. R., Chein, J., & Steinberg, L. (2014). Peers increase adolescent risk taking even when the probabilities of negative outcomes are known. *Developmental Psychology, 50*(5), 1564–1568.

Smith, D. B., Hanges, P. J., & Dickson, M. W. (2001). Personnel selection and the five-factor model: Reexamining the effects of applicant's frame of reference. *Journal of Applied Physiology, 86*, 304–315.

Smith, J., & Freund, A. M. (2002). The dynamics of possible selves in old age. *Journals of Gerontology Series B: Psychological Sciences and Social Sciences, 57*(6), P492–P500.

Smith-Ruig, T. (2009). Exploring career plateau as a multi-faceted phenomenon: Understanding the types of career plateaux experienced by accounting professionals. *British Journal of Management, 20*(4), 610–622. https://doi.org/10.1111/j.1467-8551.2008.00608.x

Sneed, J. R., & Whitbourne, S. K. (2003). Identity processing and self-consciousness in middle and later adulthood. *Journals of Gerontology Series B: Psychological Sciences and Social Sciences, 58*(6), P313–P319.

Soldz, S., & Vaillant, G. E. (1998). A 50-year longitudinal study of defense use among inner city men: A validation of the DSM-IV defense axis. *Journal of Nervous and Mental Disease, 186*(2), 104–111.

Solomon, J., & George, C. (1996). Defining the caregiving system: Toward a theory of caregiving. *Infant Mental Health Journal, 17*(3), 183–197.

Speece, D. L., Ritchey, K. D., Silverman, R., Schatschneider, C., Walker, C. Y., & Andrusik, K. N. (2010). Identifying children in middle childhood who are at risk for reading problems. *School Psychology Review, 39*(2), 258–276.

Spira, A. P., Stone, K., Beaudreau, S. A., Ancoli-Israel, S., & Yaffe, K. (2009). Anxiety symptoms and objectively measured sleep quality in older women. *American Journal of Geriatric Psychiatry, 17*(2), 136–143. https://doi.org/10.1097/JGP.0b013e3181871345

Spooner, A. L., Evans, M. A., & Santos, R. (2005). Hidden shyness in children: Discrepancies between self-perceptions and the perceptions of parents and teachers. *Merrill-Palmer Quarterly, 51* (4), 437–466.

Sroufe, L. A., & Fleeson, J. (1988). The coherence of family relationships. *Relationships within families: Mutual influences*, 27–47.

Stack, D. M., & Jean, A. D. (2011). Communicating through touch: Touching during parent–infant interactions. In *The handbook of touch: Neuroscience, behavioral, and health perspectives* (pp. 273–298). Springer.

Stanley, S. M., Amato, P. R., Johnson, C. A., & Markman, H. J. (2006). Premarital education, marital quality, and marital stability: Findings from a large, random household survey. *Journal of Family Psychology, 20*(1), 117–126.

Stansfeld, S. A., Bosma, H., Hemingway, H., & Marmot, M. G. (1998). Psychosocial work characteristics and social support as predictors of SF-36 health functioning: The Whitehall II study. *Psychosomatic Medicine, 60*(3), 247–255. https://doi.org/10.1097/00006842-199805000-00004

Stansfeld, S. A., Shipley, M. J., Head, J., Fuhrer, R., & Kivimaki, M. (2013). Work characteristics and personal social support as determinants of subjective well-being. *PloS One, 8*(11), e81115. https://doi.org/10.1371/journal.pone.0081115

Starr, J. M., Deary, I. J., Fox, H. C., & Whalley, L. J. (2007). Smoking and cognitive change from age 11 to 66 years: A confirmatory investigation. *Addictive Behaviors, 32*(1), 63–68.

Staudinger, U. M., & Kunzmann, U. (2005). Positive adult personality development: Adjustment and/or growth? *European Psychologist, 10*(4), 320–329.

Steinberg, L. (2007). Risk taking in adolescence: New perspectives from brain and behavioral science. *Current Directions in Psychological Science, 16*(2), 55–59.

Steinberg, L. (2008). A social neuroscience perspective on adolescent risk-taking. *Developmental Review, 28*(1), 78–106.

Stella, F., Radanovic, M., Canineu, P. R., de Paula, V. J., & Forlenza, O. V. (2015). Anti-dementia medications: Current prescriptions in clinical practice and new agents in progress. *Therapeutic Advances in Drug Safety, 6*(4), 151–165. https://doi.org/10.1177/2042098615592116

Stenberg, G. (2009). Selectivity in infant social referencing. *Infancy, 14*(4), 457–473. https://doi.org/10.1080/15250000902994115

Stengel, B., Couchoud, C., Cenee, S., & Hemon, D. (2000). Age, blood pressure and smoking effects on chronic renal failure in primary glomerular nephropathies. *Kidney International, 57*(6), 2519–2526.

Stephansson, O., Kieler, H., Haglund, B., Artama, M., Engeland, A., Furu, K., Gissler, M., Nörgaard, M., Nielsen, R. B., Zoega, H., & Valdimarsdottir, U. (2013). Selective serotonin reuptake inhibitors during pregnancy and risk of stillbirth and infant mortality. *JAMA, 309*(1), 48–54. https://doi.org/10.1001/jama.2012.153812

Stephenson, R., Baschieri, A., Clements, S., Hennink, M., & Madise, N. (2006). Contextual influences on the use of health facilities for childbirth in Africa. *American Journal of Public Health, 96*, 84–93. https://doi.org/10.2105/AJPH.2004.057422

Sternberg, R. J. (2004). Culture and Intelligence. *American Psychologist, 59*(5), 325–338.

Sternberg, R. J. (2011). The theory of successful intelligence. In R. J. Sternberg & S. B. Kaufman (Eds.), *The Cambridge handbook of intelligence* (pp. 504–527). Cambridge University Press.

Sterns, H. L., & Gray, J. H. (1999). Work, leisure, and retirement. In J. C. Cavanaugh & S. K. Whitbourne (Eds.), *Gerontology: Interdisciplinary perspectives* (pp. 355–390). Oxford University Press.

Stevens, E., Plumert, J. M., Cremer, J. F., & Kearney, J. K. (2013). Preadolescent temperament and risky behavior: Bicycling across traffic-filled intersections in a virtual environment. *Journal of pediatric psychology, 38*(3), 285–295.

Stevens, E. E., Patrick, T. E., & Pickler, R. (2009). A history of infant feeding. *Journal of Perinatal Education, 18*(2), 32–39. https://doi.org/10.1624/105812409X426314

Stewart, L., Holman, C., Hart, R., Bulsara, M., Preen, D., & Finn, J. (2012). In vitro fertilization and breast cancer: Is there cause for concern? *Fertility and Sterility, 98*(2), 334–349.

Storch, E. A., & Ledley, D. R. (2005). Peer victimization and psychosocial adjustment in children: Current knowledge and future directions. *Clinical Pediatrics, 44*(1), 29–38.

Story, M., & Stang, J. (2005). *Nutrition needs of adolescents.* Center for. Leadership, Education and Training in Maternal and Child Nutrition.

Story, T. N., Berg, C. A., Smith, T. W., Beveridge, R., Henry, N. J., & Pearce, G. (2007). Age, marital satisfaction, and optimism as predictors of positive sentiment override in middle-aged and older married couples. *Psychology and Aging, 22*(4), 719–727. https://doi.org/10.1037/0882-7974.22.4.719

Straif, K., Benbrahim-Tallaa, L., Baan, R., Grosse, Y., Secretan, B., El Ghissassi, F., Bouvard, V., Guha, N., Freeman, C., Galichet, L., & Cogliano, V. (2009). A review of human carcinogens—Part C: Metals, arsenic, dusts, and fibres. *Lancet Oncology, 10*(5), 453–454.

Strange, D., & Hayne, H. (2013). The devil is in the detail: Children's recollection of details about their prior experiences. *Memory, 21*(4), 431–443.

Strauss, R. S. (2000). Childhood obesity and self-esteem. *Pediatrics, 105*(1), e15.

Stricker, P. (2009, November 2). *Mental capacity for sports in the pre-teen years.* http://www.healthychildren.org/English/ages-stages/gradeschool/fitness/Pages/Mental-Capacity-for-Sports-in-the-Pre-Teen-Years.aspx

Stroebe, M., Schut, H., & Stroebe, W. (2007). Health outcomes of bereavement. *Lancet, 370*(9603), 1960–1973.

Stuenkel, C. A., Davis, S. R., Gompel, A., Lumsden, M. A., Murad, M. H., Pinkerton, J. V., & Santen, R. J. (2015). Treatment of symptoms of the menopause: An endocrine society clinical practice guideline. *Journal of Clinical Endocrinology and Metabolism, 100*(11), 3975–4011. https://doi.org/10.1210/jc.2015-2236

Suarez, E. C., Williams, R. B., Kuhn, C. M., & Zimmerman, E. A. (1991). Biobehavioral basis of coronary-prone behavior in middle-aged men: II. Serum cholesterol, the type A behavior pattern, and hostility as interactive modulators of physiological reactivity. *Psychosomatic Medicine, 53*(5), 528–537.

Sullivan, S. E., Martin, D. F., Carden, W. A., & Mainiero, L. A. (2003). The road less traveled: How to manage the recycling career stage. *Journal of Leadership & Organizational Studies, 10*(2), 34–42. https://doi.org/10.1177/107179190301000204

Super, D. E. (1957). *The psychology of careers.* Harper.

Super, D. E. (1990). A lifespan, life-space approach to career development. In D. Brown & L. Brooks (Eds.), *Career choice and development* (2nd ed.). Jossey-Bass.

Susskind, J. M., Lee, D. H., Cusi, A., Feiman, R., Grabski, W., & Anderson, A. K. (2008). Expressing fear enhances sensory acquisition. *Nature Neuroscience, 11*(7), 843–850.

Sutin, A. R., Terracciano, A., Deiana, B., Naitza, S., Ferrucci, L., Uda, M., Schlessinger, D., & Costa, P. T. (2009). High neuroticism and low conscientiousness are associated with interleukin-6. *Psychological Medicine, 40*(9) 1–9. https://doi.org/10.1017/S0033291709992029

Sutin, A. R., Terracciano, A., Deiana, B., Uda, M., Schlessinger, D., Lakatta, E. G., & Costa, P. T., Jr. (2010). Cholesterol, triglycerides, and the five-factor model of personality. *Biological Psychology, 184*(2), 186–191. https://doi.org/10.1016/j.biopsycho.2010.01.012

Sweeney, M. M., & Cancian, M. (2004). The changing importance of white women's economic prospects for assortative mating. *Journal of Marriage and Family, 66*(4), 1015–1028.

Sweeper, S., & Halford, K. (2006). Assessing adult adjustment to relationship separation: The Psychological Adjustment to Separation Test (PAST). *Journal of Family Psychology, 20*(4), 632–640.

Swift, D., Lavie, C., Johannsen, N., Arena, R., Earnest, C., O'Keefe, J., Milani, R. V., Blair, S. N., & Church, T. (2013). Physical activity, cardiorespiratory fitness, and exercise training in primary and secondary coronary prevention. *Circulation, 77*(2), 281–292.

Sword, W., Landy, C. K., Thabane, L., Watt, S., Krueger, P., Farine, D., & Foster, G. (2011). Is mode of delivery associated with postpartum depression at 6 weeks: A prospective cohort study. *BJOG, 118*(8), 966–977. https://doi.org/10.1111/j.1471-0528.2011.02950.x


# T


Tabor, A., Vestergaard, C. H. F., & Lidegaard, Ø. (2009). Fetal loss rate after chorionic villus sampling and amniocentesis: An 11-year national registry study. *Ultrasound in Obstetrics and Gynecology, 34*(1), 19–24. https://doi.org/10.1002/uog.6377

Takahashi, K., Takahashi, H. E., Nakadaira, H., & Yamamoto, M. (2006). Different changes of quantity due to aging in the psoas major and quadriceps femoris muscles in women. *Journal of Musculoskeletal and Neuronal Interactions, 6*(2), 201–205.

Tallal, P. (2004). Improving language and literacy is a matter of time. *Nature Reviews Neuroscience, 5*(9), 721–728. https://doi.org/10.1038/nrn1499

Tanaka, C., Matsui, M., Uematsu, A., Noguchi, K., & Miyawaki, T. (2012). Developmental trajectories of the fronto-temporal lobes from infancy to early adulthood in healthy individuals. *Developmental Neuroscience, 34*(6), 477–487.

Tang, H. Y., Harms, V., Speck, S. M., Vezeau, T., & Jesurum, J. T. (2009). Effects of audio relaxation programs for blood pressure reduction in older adults. *European Journal of Cardiovascular Nursing, 8*(5), 329–336. https://doi.org/10.1016/j.ejcnurse.2009.06.001

Taras, H. (2005). Nutrition and student performance at school. *Journal of School Health, 75*(6), 199–213.

Tasker, S. L., Nowakowski, M. E., & Schmidt, L. A. (2010). Joint attention and social competence in deaf children with cochlear implants. *Journal of Developmental and Physical Disabilities, 22*(5), 509–532. https://doi.org/10.1007/s10882-010-9189-x

Task Force on Sudden Infant Death Syndrome. (2005). The changing concept of sudden infant death syndrome: Diagnostic coding shifts, controversies regarding the sleeping environment, and new variables to consider in reducing risk. *Pediatrics, 116*(5), 1245–1255. https://doi.org/10.1542/peds.2005-1499

Taylor, J. S., Risica, P. M., & Cabral, H. J. (2003). Why primiparous mothers do not breastfeed in the United States: A national survey. *Acta Paediatr, 92*(11), 1308–1313.

Taylor, R. J., Forsythe-Brown, I., Lincoln, K. D., & Chatters, L. M. (2017). Extended family support networks of Caribbean Black adults in the United States. *Journal of Family Issues, 38*(4), 522–546. https://doi.org/10.1177/0192513x15573868

Teichtahl, A. J., Wluka, A. E., Wang, Y., Hanna, F., English, D. R., Giles, G. G., & Cicuttini, F. M. (2009). Obesity and adiposity are associated with the rate of patella cartilage volume loss over 2 years in adults without knee osteoarthritis. *Annals of the Rheumatic Diseases, 68*(6), 909–913. https://doi.org/10.1136/ard.2008.093310

Tement, S. (2014). The role of personal and key resources in the family-to-work enrichment process. *Scandinavian Journal of Psychology, 55*(5), 489–496. https://doi.org/10.1111/sjop.12146

Terracciano, A., & Costa, P. T. J. (2004). Smoking and the five-factor model of personality. *Addiction, 99*(4), 472–481.

Terracciano, A., Lockenhoff, C. E., Crum, R. M., Bienvenu, O. J., & Costa, P. T., Jr. (2008). Five-factor model personality profiles of drug users. *BMC Psychiatry, 8.*

Thomaes, S., Reijntjes, A., Orobio de Castro, B., Bushman, B. J., Poorthuis, A., & Telch, M. J. (2010). I like me if you like me: On the interpersonal modulation and regulation of preadolescents' state self-esteem. *Child Development, 81*(3), 811–825.

Thomas, A., Chess, S., & Birch, H. G. (1970). The origin of personality. *Scientific American, 223*(2), 102–109.

Thomas, R., & Zimmer-Gembeck, M. J. (2011). Accumulating evidence for parent–child interaction therapy in the prevention of child maltreatment. *Child Development, 82*(1), 177–192. https://doi.org/10.1111/j.1467-8624.2010.01548.x

Thomas, T. L., Strickland, O., Diclemente, R., & Higgins, M. (2013). An opportunity for cancer prevention during preadolescence and adolescence: Stopping human papillomavirus (HPV)-related cancer through HPV vaccination. *Journal of Adolescent Health, 52*(5), S60–S68.

Thompson, A. L., Adair, L. S., & Bentley, M. E. (2013). Maternal characteristics and perception of temperament associated with infant TV exposure. *Pediatrics, 131*(2), e390–e397. https://doi.org/10.1542/peds.2012-1224

Thompson, J., & Nelson, A. (2011). Middle childhood and modern human origins. *Human Nature, 22*, 249–280. https://doi.org/10.1007/s12110-011-9119-3

Thorsell, M., Lyrenas, S., Andolf, E., & Kaijser, M. (2011). Induction of labor and the risk for emergency cesarean section in nulliparous and multiparous women. *Acta Obstetricia et Gynecologica Scandinavica, 90*(10), 1094–1099. https://doi.org/10.1111/j.1600-0412.2011.01213.x

Tinetti, M. E., & Kumar, C. (2010). The patient who falls: "It's always a trade-off." *Journal of the American Medical Association, 303*(3), 258–266. https://doi.org/10.1001/jama.2009.2024

Tobin, J., Hsueh, Y., & Karasawa, M. (2009). *Preschool in three cultures revisited: China, Japan, and the United States.* University of Chicago Press.

Tolomio, S., Ermolao, A., Travain, G., & Zaccaria, M. (2008). Short-term adapted physical activity program improves bone quality in osteopenic/osteoporotic postmenopausal women. *Journal of Physical Activity and Health, 5*(6), 844–853.

Tomás, J., Sancho, P., Galiana, L., & Oliver, A. (2016). A double test on the importance of spirituality, the "forgotten factor," in successful aging. *Social Indicators Research, 127*, 1377–1389. https://doi.org/10.1007/s11205-015-1014-6

Tomasello, M. (2009). *Constructing a language: A usage-based theory of language acquisition.* Harvard University Press.

Toossi, M. (2009). Labor force projections to 2018: Older workers stay active despite their age. *Monthly Labor Review*, 30–51. http://www.bls.gov/opub/mlr/2009/11/art3full.pdf

Travison, T. G., Araujo, A. B., Beck, T. J., Williams, R. E., Clark, R. V., Leder, B. Z., & McKinlay, J. B. (2009). Relation between serum testosterone, serum estradiol, sex hormone–binding globulin, and geometrical measures of adult male proximal femur strength. *Journal of Clinical Endocrinology and Metabolism, 94*(3), 853–860. https://doi.org/10.1210/jc.2008-0668

Tremblay, S., & Pierce, T. (2011). Perceptions of fatherhood: Longitudinal reciprocal associations within the couple. *Canadian Journal of Behavioural Science, 43*(2), 99–110. https://doi.org/10.1037/a0022635

Tronick, E. Z., Morelli, G. K., & Ivey, P. K. (1992). The Efe forager infant and toddler's pattern of social relationships: Multiple and simultaneous. *Developmental Psychology, 28*(4), 568–577.

Trouillet, R. l., Gana, K., Lourel, M., & Fort, I. (2009). Predictive value of age for coping: The role of self-efficacy, social support satisfaction and perceived stress. *Aging and Mental Health, 13*(3), 357–366.

Tucker, K. L. (2009). Osteoporosis prevention and nutrition. *Current Osteoporosis Reports, 7*(4), 111–117.

Tucker-Samaras, S., Zedayko, T., Cole, C., Miller, D., Wallo, W., & Leyden, J. J. (2009). A stabilized 0.1% retinol facial moisturizer improves the appearance of photodamaged skin in an eight-week, double-blind, vehicle-controlled study. *Journal of Drugs and Dermatology, 8*(10), 932–936.

Turcotte, M. (2006, March). Parents with adult children living at home. *Canadian Social Trends,* 11–14.

Turiano, N. A., Mroczek, D. K., Moynihan, J., & Chapman, B. P. (2013). Big 5 personality traits and interleukin-6: Evidence for 'healthy neuroticism' in a US population sample. *Brain, Behavior, and Immunity, 28,* 83–89. https://doi.org/10.1016/j.bbi.2012.10.020

# U

Uchino, B. N., Berg, C. A., Smith, T. W., Pearce, G., & Skinner, M. (2006). Age-related differences in ambulatory blood pressure during daily stress: Evidence for greater blood pressure reactivity with age. *Psychology and Aging, 21*(2), 231–239.

Uematsu, A., Matsui, M., Tanaka, C., Takahashi, T., Noguchi, K., Suzuki, M., & Nishijo, H. (2012). Developmental trajectories of amygdala and hippocampus from infancy to early adulthood in healthy individuals. *PloS One, 7*(10), e46970.

Urien, B., & Kilbourne, W. (2011). Generativity and self-enhancement values in eco-friendly behavioral intentions and environmentally responsible consumption behavior. *Psychology & Marketing, 28*(1), 69–90. https://doi.org/10.1002/mar.20381

U.S. Bureau of the Census. (2019). *Historical living arrangements of children.* https://www.census.gov/data/tables/time-series/demo/families/children.html

U.S. Bureau of the Census. (2018). *America's families and living arrangements: 2016.* https://www.census.gov/data/tables/2016/demo/families/cps-2016.html

U.S. Bureau of the Census. (2017b). *American fact finder.* https://factfinder.census.gov/faces/tableservices/jsf/pages/productview.xhtml?pid=ACS_15_1YR_B11009&prodType=table

U.S. Bureau of the Census. (2017c). *Characteristics of same-sex couple households: 2005 to present.* https://www.census.gov/data/tables/time-series/demo/same-sex-couples/ssc-house-characteristics.html

U.S. Bureau of the Census. (2017d). *Stats for stories: Singles awareness day.* https://www.census.gov/newsroom/stories/2017/february/singles_awarenss_day.html

U.S. Department of Energy Genome Programs. (2019). *The Human Genome Project.* http://genomics.energy.gov

U.S. Department of Labor. (2017). *Gender wage gap.* Author.

U.S. Bureau of Labor Statistics. (n.d.). *Injuries, illnesses, and fatalities.* http://www.bls.gov/iif/#News

U.S. Bureau of Labor Statistics. (2014). *Women in the labor force: A databook.* https://www.bls.gov/opub/reports/womens-databook/archive/women-in-the-labor-force-a-databook-2014.pdf

U.S. Bureau of Labor Statistics. (2016, September). *Labor force characteristics by race and ethnicity, 2015.* https://www.bls.gov/opub/reports/race-and-ethnicity/2015/home.htm

U.S. Bureau of Labor Statistics. (2019). *Employment projections.* https://www.bls.gov/emp/ep_chart_001.htm

U.S. Bureau of Labor Statistics. (2020a). *The employment situation—July 2017.* https://www.bls.gov/news.release/pdf/empsit.pdf

U.S. Bureau of Labor Statistics. (2020b). *Employment situation of veterans summary.* https://www.bls.gov/news.release/vet.nr0.htm

U.S. Bureau of Labor Statistics. (2020c). *Labor force statistics from the Current Population Survey.* https://www.bls.gov/cps/cpsaat07.htm

U.S. Bureau of Labor Statistics. (2017). *Women's median earnings 82 percent of men's in 2016.* https://www.bls.gov/opub/ted/2017/womens-median-earnings-82-percent-of-mens-in-2016.htm

U.S. Bureau of Labor Statistics. (2017e). Median *weekly earnings by educational attainment in 2014.* https://www.bls.gov/opub/ted/2015/median-weekly-earnings-by-education-gender-race-and-ethnicity-in-2014.htm

Uvnäs-Moberg, K. (2012). Short-term and long-term effects of oxytocin released by suckling and of skin-to-skin contact in mothers and infants. In D. Narváez, J. Panksepp, A. N. Schore, & T. R. Gleason (Eds.), *Evolution, early experience and human development: From research to practice and policy.* Oxford University Press.

# V

Vahia, I. V., Thompson, W. K., Depp, C. A., Allison, M., & Jeste, D. V. (2012). Developing a dimensional model for successful cognitive and emotional aging. *International Psychogeriatrics, 24(4),* 515–523. https://doi.org/10.1017/s1041610211002055

Vaillant, G. E. (2000). Adaptive mental mechanisms: Their role in a positive psychology. *American Psychologist, 55*(1), 89–98.

Valiathan, R., Ashman, M., & Asthana, D. (2016). Effects of ageing on the immune system: Infants to elderly. *Scandinavian Journal of Immunology, 83*(4), 255–266. https://doi.org/10.1111/sji.12413

Valkenburg, P. M., Sumter, S. R., & Peter, J. (2011). Gender differences in online and offline self-disclosure in pre-adolescence and adolescence. *British Journal of Developmental Psychology, 29*(2), 253–269.

van de Bongardt, D., Yu, R., Deković, M., & Meeus, W. H. (2015). *Romantic relationships and sexuality in adolescence and young adulthood: The role of parents, peers, and partners.* Taylor & Francis.

van der Kooy, J., Poeran, J., de Graaf, J. P., Birnie, E., Denktass, S., Steegers, E. A., & Bonsel, G. J. (2011). Planned home compared with planned hospital births in the Netherlands: Intrapartum and early neonatal death in low-risk pregnancies. *Obstetrics and Gynecology, 118*(5), 1037–1046. https://doi.org/10.1097/AOG.0b013e3182319737

van Hooff, M. L., Geurts, S. A., Taris, T. W., Kompier, M. A., Dikkers, J. S., Houtman, I. L., & van den Heuvel, F. M. (2005). Disentangling the causal relationships between work-home interference and employee health. *Scandinavian Journal of Work and Environmental Health, 31*(1), 15–29.

Van Ness, P. H., & Larson, D. B. (2002). Religion, senescence, and mental health: The end of life is not the end of hope. *American Journal of Geriatric Psychiatry, 10*(4), 386–397.

Vannorsdall, T. D., Waldstein, S. R., Kraut, M., Pearlson, G. D., & Schretlen, D. J. (2009). White matter abnormalities and cognition in a community sample. *Archives of Clinical Neuropsychology, 24*(3), 209–217. https://doi.org/10.1093/arclin/acp037

Varendi, H., Christensson, K., Porter, R. H., & Winberg, J. (1998). Soothing effect of amniotic fluid smell in newborn infants. *Early Human Development, 51*(1), 47–55.

Velkoff, V. A., & Lawson, V. A. (1998). *Gender and aging: Caregiving.* Washington, DC: U.S. Department of Commerce.

Verghese, J., Wang, C., Katz, M. J., Sanders, A., & Lipton, R. B. (2009). Leisure activities and risk of vascular cognitive impairment in older adults. *Journal of Geriatric Psychiatry and Neurology, 22*(2), 110–118.

Véronneau, M.-H., Vitaro, F., Brendgen, M., Dishion, T. J., & Tremblay, R. E. (2010). Transactional analysis of the reciprocal links between peer experiences and academic achievement from middle childhood to early adolescence. *Developmental psychology, 46*(4), 773–790.

Verweij, L. M., van Schoor, N. M., Deeg, D. J., Dekker, J., & Visser, M. (2009). Physical activity and incident clinical knee osteoarthritis in older adults. *Arthritis Rheumatology, 61*(2), 152–157. https://doi.org/10.1002/art.24233

Vespa, J. (2009). Gender ideology construction: A life course and intersectional approach. *Gender & Society, 23*(3), 363–387. https://doi.org/10.1177/0891243209337507

Vespa, J., Lewis, J. M., & Kreider, R. M. (2013). America's families and living arrangements: 2012. *Current Population Reports.* U.S. Census.

Villa, J. C., Gianakos, A., & Lane, J. M. (2016). Bisphosphonate treatment in osteoporosis: Optimal duration of therapy and the incorporation of a drug holiday. *Musculoskeletal Journal of Hospital for Special Surgery, 12*(1), 66–73. https://doi.org/10.1007/s11420-015-9469-1

Vogelzangs, N., Comijs, H. C., Oude Voshaar, R. C., Stek, M. L., & Penninx, B. W. (2014). Late-life depression symptom profiles are differentially associated with immunometabolic functioning. *Brain Behavior and Immunology, 41*, 109–115. https://doi.org/10.1016/j.bbi.2014.05.004

Volpe, F. M. (2011). Correlation of cesarean rates to maternal and infant mortality rates: An ecologic study of official international data. *Revista Panamericana Salud Publica, 29*(5), 303–308.

von Arnim, C. A. F., Herbolsheimer, F., Nikolaus, T., Peter, R., Biesalski, H. K., Ludolph, A. C., Riepe, M., & Nagel, G. (2012). Dietary antioxidants and dementia in a population-based case-control study among older people in South Germany. *Journal of Alzheimer's Disease, 31*(4), 717–724.

von Muhlen, D., Laughlin, G. A., Kritz-Silverstein, D., & Barrett-Connor, E. (2007). The Dehydroepiandrosterone and WellNess (DAWN) Study: Research design and methods. *Contemporary Clinical Trials, 28*(2), 153–168.

Vural, E. M., van Munster, B. C., & de Rooij, S. E. (2014). Optimal dosages for melatonin supplementation therapy in older adults: A systematic review of current literature. *Drugs & Aging, 31*(6), 441–451. https://doi.org/10.1007/s40266-014-0178-0

Vygotsky, L. S. (1967). Play and its role in the mental development of the child. *Journal of Russian and East European Psychology, 5*(3), 6–18.


## W


Wagner, K., & Dobkins, K. R. (2011). Synaesthetic associations decrease during infancy. *Psychological Science, 22*(8), 1067–1072. https://doi.org/10.1177/0956797611416250

Waite, L. J., Laumann, E. O., Das, A., & Schumm, L. P. (2009). Sexuality: Measures of partnerships, practices, attitudes, and problems in National Social Life, Health, and Aging Study. *Journals of Gerontology: Series B: Psychological Sciences and Social Sciences, 64B*(1), I56–I66.

Walker, L. O., Cooney, A. T., & Riggs, M. W. (1999). Psychosocial and demographic factors related to health behaviors in the 1st trimester. *Journal of Obstetric, Gynecologic, & Neonatal Nursing, 28*(6), 606–614.

Walker, V. (2012). *Transition to preschool.* http://www.handsandvoices.org/articles/early_intervention/V8-4_transition.htm

Walster, E., Walster, G. W., & Berscheid, E. (1978). *Equity: Theory and research.* Allyn & Bacon.

Wang, J., Iannotti, R. J., & Nansel, T. R. (2009). School bullying among adolescents in the United States: Physical, verbal, relational, and cyber. *Journal of Adolescent Health, 45*(4), 368–375.

Wang, M. (2007). Profiling retirees in the retirement transition and adjustment process: Examining the longitudinal change patterns of retirees' psychological well-being. *Journal of Applied Psychology, 92*(2), 455–474.

Wang, M., Henkens, K., & van Solinge, H. (2011). Retirement adjustment: A review of theoretical and empirical advancements. *American Psychologist, 66*(3), 204–213. https://doi.org/10.1037/a0022414

Wang, M.-T., & Eccles, J. S. (2013). School context, achievement motivation, and academic engagement: A longitudinal study of school engagement using a multidimensional perspective. *Learning and Instruction, 28*, 12–23.

Wang, M. T., & Fredricks, J. A. (2014). The reciprocal links between school engagement, youth problem behaviors, and school dropout during adolescence. *Child Development, 85*(2), 722–737.

Wang, S. Q., & Dusza, S. W. (2009). Assessment of sunscreen knowledge: A pilot survey. *British Journal of Dermatology, 161*(3), 28–32. https://doi.org/10.1111/j.1365-2133.2009.09446.x

Ward, R. A., Spitze, G., & Deane, G. (2009). The more the merrier? Multiple parent-adult child relations. *Journal of Marriage and Family, 71*(1), 161–173.

Warr, P. (1994). Age and employment. In H. C. Triandis, M. D. Dunnette, & L. M. Hough (Eds.), *Handbook of industrial and organizational psychology* (pp. 485–550). Consulting Psychologists Press.

Warren, J. B., & Phillipi, C. A. (2012). Care of the well newborn. *Pediatrics in Review, 33*(1), 4–18.

Watamura, S. E., Phillips, D. A., Morrissey, T. W., McCartney, K., & Bub, K. (2011). Double jeopardy: Poorer social-emotional outcomes for children in the NICHD SECCYD experiencing home and child-care environments that confer risk. *Child Development, 82*(1), 48–65. https://doi.org/10.1111/j.1467-8624.2010.01540.x

Wax, J. R., Pinette, M. G., Cartin, A., & Blackstone, J. (2010). Maternal and newborn morbidity by birth facility among selected United States 2006 low-risk births. *American Journal of Obstetrics and Gynecology, 202*(2), 152.e151–152.e155.

Wayne, J. H., Randel, A. E., & Stevens, J. (2006). The role of identity and work-family support in work-family enrichment and its work-related consequences. *Journal of Vocational Behavior, 69*(3), 445–461.

Weinberger, M. I., Hofstein, Y., & Whitbourne, S. K. (2008). Intimacy in young adulthood as a predictor of divorce in midlife. *Personal Relationships, 15*(4), 551–557. https://doi.org/10.1111/j.1475-6811.2008.00215.x

Weinberger, M. I., & Whitbourne, S. K. (2010). Depressive symptoms, self-reported physical functioning, and identity in community-dwelling older adults. *Ageing International, 35*, 276–285. https://doi.org/10.1007/s12126-010-9053-4

Weiss, A., & Costa, P. T., Jr. (2005). Domain and facet personality predictors of all-cause mortality among Medicare patients aged 65 to 100. *Psychosomatic Medicine, 67*(5), 724–733. https://doi.org/10.1097/01.psy.0000181272.58103.18

Weiss, M., Ryan, P., Lokken, L., & Nelson, M. (2004). Length of stay after vaginal birth: Sociodemographic and readiness-for-discharge factors. *Birth, 31*(2), 93–101. https://doi.org/10.1111/j.0730-7659.2004.00286.x

Welge-Lussen, A. (2009). Ageing, neurodegeneration, and olfactory and gustatory loss. *B-ENT, 5*(13), 129–132.

Weltman, A., Weltman, J. Y., Roy, C. P., Wideman, L., Patrie, J., Evans, W. S., & Veldhuis, J. D. (2006). Growth hormone response to graded exercise intensities is attenuated and the gender difference abolished in older adults. *Journal of Applied Physiology, 100*(5), 1623–1629.

Wentzel, K. R., & Asher, S. R. (1995). The academic lives of neglected, rejected, popular, and controversial children. *Child Development, 66*(3), 754–763.

Werner, P., Buchbinder, E., Lowenstein, A., & Livni, T. (2005). Mediation across generations: A tri-generational perspective. *Journal of Aging Studies, 19*(4), 489–502.

West, R. L., Thorn, R. M., & Bagwell, D. K. (2003). Memory performance and beliefs as a function of goal setting and aging. *Psychological Aging, 18*(1), 111–125.

Whisman, M. A., Johnson, D. P., Li, A., & Robustelli, B. L. (2014). Intimate relationship involvement, intimate relationship quality, and psychiatric disorders in adolescents. *Journal of Family Psychology, 28*(6), 908–914.

Whitbourne, S. K. (1985). The life-span construct as a model of adaptation in adulthood. In J. E. Birren & K. W. Schaie (Eds.), *Handbook of the psychology of aging* (2nd ed.) (pp. 594–618). Van Nostrand Reinhold.

Whitbourne, S. K. (1986). *The me I know: A study of adult identity*. Springer-Verlag.

Whitbourne, S. K. (1996). *The aging individual: Physical and psychological perspectives*. Springer.

Whitbourne, S. K. (2001). *Adult development and aging: Biopsychosocial perspectives*. Wiley.

Whitbourne, S. K. (2010). *The search for fulfillment*. Ballantine.

Whitbourne, S. K. (2015). Differential aging. In J. D. Wright (Ed.), *International encyclopedia of the social & behavioral sciences (Second Edition)*, 378-383. Elsevier. https://doi.org/10.1016/B978-0-08-097086-8.31039-X

Whitbourne, S. K., & Bookwala, J. (2015). Gender and aging: Perspectives from geropsychology. In P. A. Lichtenberg & Mast, B. T. (Eds.), *APA Handbook of Clinical Geropsychology* (pp. 443–458). American Psychological Association.

Whitbourne, S. K., & Collins, K. C. (1998). Identity and physical changes in later adulthood: Theoretical and clinical implications. *Psychotherapy, 35*(4), 519–530.

Whitbourne, S. K., Culgin, S., & Cassidy, E. (1995). Evaluation of infantilizing intonation and content of speech directed at the aged. *International Journal of Aging and Human Development, 41*(2), 107–114.

Whitbourne, S. K., Sneed, J. R., & Skultety, K. M. (2002). Identity processes in adulthood: Theoretical and methodological challenges. *Identity, 2*(1), 29–45.

Whitbourne, S. K., & Wills, K.-J. (1993). Psychological issues in institutional care of the aged. In S. B. Goldsmith (Ed.), *Long-term care administration handbook* (pp. 19–32). Aspen.

Whitbourne, S. K., & Whitbourne, S. B. (2012). Demography of aging: Behavioral and social implications. In S. K. Whitbourne & M. J. Sliwinksi (Eds.), *The Wiley-Blackwell Handbook of Adulthood and Aging* (pp. 25–48). Wiley.

Whiting, W. L., Madden, D. J., Pierce, T. W., & Allen, P. A. (2005). Searching from the top down: Ageing and attentional guidance during singleton detection. *Quarterly Journal of Experimental Psychology: Section A, 58*(1), 72–97. https://doi.org/10.1080/02724980443000205

Whitlock, G., Lewington, S., Sherliker, P., Clarke, R., Emberson, J., Halsey, J., ... Peto, R. (2009). Body-mass index and cause-specific mortality in 900 000 adults: Collaborative analyses of 57 prospective studies. *Lancet, 373*(9669), 1083–1096. https://doi.org/10.1016/S0140-6736(09)60318-4

Whitton, S. W., Rhoades, G. K., Stanley, S. M., & Markman, H. J. (2008). Effects of parental divorce on marital commitment and confidence. *Journal of Family Psychology, 22*(5), 789–793. https://doi.org/10.1037/a0012800

Wickremaratchi, M. M., & Llewelyn, J. G. (2006). Effects of ageing on touch. *Postgraduate Medical Journal, 82*(967), 301–304.

Wieser, M. J., Muhlberger, A., Kenntner-Mabiala, R., & Pauli, P. (2006). Is emotion processing affected by advancing age? An event-related brain potential study. *Brain Research, 1096*(1), 138–147.

Wiik, K. L., Loman, M. M., Van Ryzin, M. J., Armstrong, J. M., Essex, M. J., Pollak, S. D., & Gunnar, M. R. (2011). Behavioral and emotional symptoms of post-institutionalized children in middle childhood. *Journal of Child Psychology and Psychiatry, 52*(1), 56–63. https://doi.org/10.1111/j.1469-7610.2010.02294.x

Wilcox, A. J., Weinberg, C. R., O'Connor, J. F., Baird, D. D., Schlatterer, J. P., Canfield, R. E., Armstrong, E. G., & Nisula, B. C. (1988). Incidence of early loss of pregnancy. *New England Journal of Medicine, 319*, 189–194.

Wilcox, S., Evenson, K. R., Aragaki, A., Wassertheil-Smoller, S., Mouton, C. P., & Loevinger, B. L. (2003). The effects of widowhood on physical and mental health, health behaviors, and health outcomes: The Women's Health Initiative. *Health Psychology, 22*(5), 513–522.

Wilks, T., Gerber, R. J., & Erdie-Lalena, C. (2010). Developmental milestones: Cognitive development. *Pediatrics in Review, 31*(9), 364–367. https://doi.org/10.1542/pir.31-9-364

Wille, B., & De Fruyt, F. (2014). Vocations as a source of identity: Reciprocal relations between big five personality traits and RIASEC characteristics over 15 years. *Journal of Applied Psychology, 99*(2), 262–281. https://doi.org/10.1037/a0034917

Williams, B. R., Zhang, Y., Sawyer, P., Mujib, M., Jones, L. G., Feller, M. A., Ekundayo, J., Iban, I. B., Love, T. E., Lott, A., & Ahmed, A. (2011). Intrinsic association of widowhood with mortality in community-dwelling older women and men: Findings from a prospective propensity-matched population study. *Journals of Gerontology: Series A: Biological Sciences and Medical Sciences, 66A*(12), 1360–1368. https://doi.org/10.1093/gerona/glr144

Williams, K., & Dunne-Bryant, A. (2006). Divorce and adult psychological well-being: Clarifying the role of gender and child age. *Journal of Marriage and Family, 68*(5), 1178–1196.

Williams, K. N., & Warren, C. A. (2009). Communication in assisted living. *Journal of Aging Studies, 23*(1), 24–36. https://doi.org/10.1016/j.jaging.2007.09.003

Williams, P. G., Rau, H. K., Cribbet, M. R., & Gunn, H. E. (2009). Openness to experience and stress regulation. *Journal of Research in Personality, 43*(5), 777–784.

Wilsgaard, T., Emaus, N., Ahmed, L. A., Grimnes, G., Joakimsen, R. M., Omsland, T. K., & Berntsen, G. R. (2009). Lifestyle impact on lifetime bone loss in women and men: The Tromso Study. *American Journal of Epidemiology, 169*(7), 877–886. https://doi.org/10.1093/aje/kwn407

Wilson, M. N. (1986). The Black extended family: An analytical consideration. *Developmental Psychology, 22*(2), 246–258.

Wilson, R. S., Arnold, S. E., Tang, Y., & Bennett, D. A. (2006). Odor identification and decline in different cognitive domains in old age. *Neuroepidemiology, 26*(2), 61–67.

Wilson, R. S., Schneider, J. A., Arnold, S. E., Bienias, J. L., & Bennett, D. A. (2007). Conscientiousness and the incidence of Alzheimer's disease and mild cognitive impairment. *Archives of General Psychiatry, 64*(10), 1204–1212. https://doi.org/10.1001/archpsyc.64.10.1204

Winch, R. F. (1958). *Mate selection: A study of complementary needs.* Harper & Row.

Wolak, J., Evans, L., Nguyen, S., & Hines, D. A. (2013). Online predators: Myth versus reality. *New England Journal of Public Policy, 25*(1), 6. https://scholarworks.umb.edu/nejpp/vol25/iss1/6

Wolak, J., Finkelhor, D., Mitchell, K. J., & Ybarra, M. L. (2008). Online "predators" and their victims: Myths, realities, and implications for prevention and treatment. *American Psychologist, 63*(2), 111–128.

Wood, R. G., Goesling, B., & Avellar, S. (2007). *The effects of marriage on health.* ASPE Research Brief.

World Health Organization. (1948). *Preamble to the Constitution of the World Health Organization as adopted by the International Health Conference.* Author.

World Health Organization. (2002a). *Active ageing: A policy framework.* Author.

World Health Organization. (2002b). *Infant and young child nutrition: Global strategy on infant and young child feeding.* Author.

World Health Organization. (2009). *WHO guidelines for the management of postpartum haemorrhage and retained placenta.* Author.

World Health Organization. (2010). *Maternal mortality.* http://www.who.int/mediacentre/factsheets/fs348/en/index.html

World Health Organization. (2013a). *Genes and human disease.* http://www.who.int/genomics/public/geneticdiseases/en/index2.html

World Health Organization. (n.d.). *Male circumcision for HIV prevention.* http://www.who.int/hiv/topics/malecircumcision/en/

World Health Organization. (2017c). *Chronic obstructive pulmonary disease (COPD).* http://www.who.int/respiratory/copd/en/

World Health Organization. (2018). *Cancer.* http://www.who.int/mediacentre/factsheets/fs297/en/

World Health Organization. (n.d.). *Cardiovascular diseases (CVD).* http://www.who.int/mediacentre/factsheets/fs317/en/

World Health Organization. (2018). *Noncommunicable diseases.* http://www.who.int/mediacentre/factsheets/fs355/en/

World Health Organization. (2020, September 1). *Dementia.* http://www.who.int/mediacentre/factsheets/fs362/en/

World Health Organization. (n.d.). *Diabetes.* http://www.who.int/diabetes/en/

World Health Organization. (2020, April 1). *Obesity and overweight.* http://www.who.int/mediacentre/factsheets/fs311/en/

World Health Organization. (2020). *Tobacco.* http://www.who.int/mediacentre/factsheets/fs339/en/

Wright, D. M., Rosato, M., & O'Reilly, D. (2015). Urban/rural variation in the influence of widowhood on mortality risk: A cohort study of almost 300,000 couples. *Health Place, 34,* 67–73. https://doi.org/10.1016/j.healthplace.2015.04.003

# X

Xu, Y. (2008). Children's social play sequence: Parten's classic theory revisited. *Early Child Development and Care, 180*(4), 489–498. https://doi.org/10.1080/03004430802090430

# Y

Yabiku, S. T., & Gager, C. T. (2009). Sexual frequency and the stability of marital and cohabiting unions. *Journal of Marriage & the Family, 71*(4), 983–1000.

Yamamoto, Y., Uede, K., Yonei, N., Kishioka, A., Ohtani, T., & Furukawa, F. (2006). Effects of alpha-hydroxy acids on the human skin of Japanese subjects: The rationale for chemical peeling. *Journal of Dermatology, 33*(1), 16–22.

Yarcheski, A., Mahon, N. E., Yarcheski, T. J., Hanks, M. M., & Cannella, B. L. (2009). A meta-analytic study of predictors of maternal-fetal attachment. *International Journal of Nursing Studies, 46*(5), 708–715. https://doi.org/10.1016/j.ijnurstu.2008.10.013

Yin, H., Lin, S.-J., Kong, S. X., Benzeroual, K., Crawford, S. Y., Hedeker, D., Lambert, B. L. L., & Muramatsu, N. (2011). The association between physical functioning and self-rated general health in later life: The implications of social comparison. *Applied Research in Quality of Life, 6,* 1–19. https://doi.org/10.1007/s11482-010-9109-3

Yohannes, A. M., & Tampubolon, G. (2014). Changes in lung function in older people from the English Longitudinal Study of Ageing. *Expert Review of Respiratory Medicine, 8*(4), 515–521. https://doi.org/10.1586/17476348.2014.919226

Yong, H. H. (2006). Can attitudes of stoicism and cautiousness explain observed age-related variation in levels of self-rated pain, mood disturbance and functional interference in chronic pain patients? *European Journal of Pain, 10*(5), 399–407.

Yu, R., Branje, S., Keijsers, L., & Meeus, W. H. (2014). Personality effects on romantic relationship quality through friendship quality: A ten-year longitudinal study in youths. *PloS One, 9*(9), e102078.

Yung, L. M., Laher, I., Yao, X., Chen, Z. Y., Huang, Y., & Leung, F. P. (2009). Exercise, vascular wall and cardiovascular diseases: An update (Part 2). *Sports Medicine, 39*(1), 45–63.

# Z

Zachrisson, H. D., Dearing, E., Lekhal, R., & Toppelberg, C. O. (2013). Little evidence that time in child care causes externalizing problems during early childhood in Norway. *Child Development, 84*(4), 1152–1170. https://doi.org/10.1111/cdev.12040

Zalewski, M., Lengua, L. J., Wilson, A. C., Trancik, A., & Bazinet, A. (2011). Associations of coping and appraisal styles with emotion regulation during preadolescence. *Journal of Experimental Child Psychology, 110*(2), 141–158. https://doi.org/10.1016/j.jecp.2011.03.001

Zamboni, M., Mazzali, G., Fantin, F., Rossi, A., & Di Francesco, V. (2008). Sarcopenic obesity: A new category of obesity in the elderly. *Nutrition, Metabolism, and Cardiovascular Diseases, 18*(5), 388–395. https://doi.org/10.1016/j.numecd.2007.10.002

Zeleznik, J. (2003). Normative aging of the respiratory system. *Clinics in Geriatric Medicine, 19*(1), 1–18.

Zhang, C., Wu, B., Beglopoulos, V., Wines-Samuelson, M., Zhang, D., Dragatsis, I., Sudhöf, T. C., & Shen, J. (2009). Presenilins are essential for regulating neurotransmitter release. *Nature, 460*, 632–636. https://doi.org/10.1038/nature08177

Zhang, F., & Labouvie-Vief, G. (2004). Stability and fluctuation in adult attachment style over a 6-year period. *Attachment and Human Development, 6*(4), 419–437.

Zhang, Y., Qiu, C., Lindberg, O., Bronge, L., Aspelin, P., Backman, L., Fratiglioni, L., & Wahlund, L. O. (2010). Acceleration of hippocampal atrophy in a non-demented elderly population: The SNAC-K study. *International Psychogeriatrics, 22*(1), 14–25. https://doi.org/10.1017/S1041610209991396

CPSIA information can be obtained
at www.ICGtesting.com
Printed in the USA
LVHW011254310822
727219LV00002B/18

9 781793 534996